DRUGS AND PEPTIC ULCER
Volume I
Therapeutic Agents for Peptic Ulcer Disease
Volume II
Pathogenesis of Ulcer Induction Revealed by Studies in Humans and Animals

CANCER OF THE ESOPHAGUS

ANIMAL MODELS FOR INTESTINAL DISEASE

Animal Models for Intestinal Disease

Editor

Carl J. Pfeiffer, Ph.D.

Professor
Division of Veterinary Biology and Clinical Studies
Virginia-Maryland Regional College of Veterinary Medicine
Virginia Polytechnic Institute and State University
Blacksburg, Virginia

CRC Series on Gastrointestinal Disease

Editor-in-Chief

Carl J. Pfeiffer

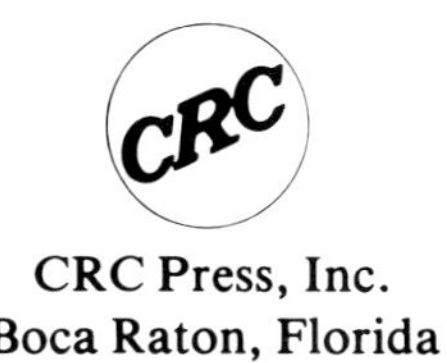

CRC Press, Inc.
Boca Raton, Florida

Library of Congress Cataloging in Publication Data
Main entry under title:

Animal models for intestinal disease.

  (CRC series on gastrointestinal disease)
  Includes bibliography and index.
  1. Intestines—Diseases—Animal models.
2. Veterinary gastroenterology. I. Pfeiffer, Carl J.
II. Series. [DNLM: 1. Intestinal Diseases. 2. Disease Models, Animal. WI 400 A598]
RC860.A55 1985   616.3'4027   84-7696
ISBN 0-8493-6215-6

Direct all inquiries to CRC Press, Inc., 2000 Corporate Blvd., N.W., Boca Raton, Florida, 33431.

© 1985 by CRC Press, Inc.

International Standard Book Number 0-8493-6215-6

Library of Congress Card Number 84-7696
Printed in the United States

PREFACE

The biomedical scientist, the clinician in both human and veterinary medicine, and the public health worker are often confronted with maladies of the alimentary tract. Indeed, diseases of the gut account for the majority of human patient complaints, of reasons for hospitalization, and of problems for the practicing veterinarian. They play a predominant role in contributing to high infant mortality in lesser developed countries, and contribute to huge economic losses to most nations at any level of development and are therefore of major public health concern. To study such diseases, animals of many species have served mankind for many years. In some diseases where the etiology remains obscure, such as some types of colitis in humans or lower animals, of cancers, or in other cases where the causative agent has been identified such as in transmissible gastroenteritis of neonatal pigs caused by *Clostridium prefringens* or human cholera caused by *Vibrio cholerae,* animal models have been invaluable in elucidating the pathogenesis. In the future it can be expected that animal models will continue to be of great value in the study of human diseases (despite growing movements to replace partially animal experiments with theoretical or nonanimal investigations), not because of tradition but because of scientific necessity. Likewise, research on the human, which has been the most thoroughly investigated animal, has provided insight into disease mechanisms and has provided the incentive for drug development and other therapeutic measures which have been adopted by the veterinarian for improving animal health. It is because of this reciprocal and essential cooperation between the medical scientist for human disease and the veterinarian, with the animal as the vital intermediary link, that the present volume was designed. The editor, who has worked with many species and in both human medical and veterinary academic institutions, is eager to encourage such cooperations. While the scope of intestinal disease is too large for one volume to be all-comprehensive, the present chapters provide a multidisciplinary and up-to-date review of significant findings and concepts on selected animal models for various intestinal diseases. The important role of many different species used in the study of intestinal maladies is clearly indicated in these chapters. These data and current reviews on animal models for intestinal disease will, it is hoped, encourage the clinician, research worker, or student of either human or animal disease to elucidate further the pathophysiology of such intestinal diseases.

Carl J. Pfeiffer

THE EDITOR

Carl J. Pfeiffer, Ph.D., is Professor, Division of Veterinary Biology and Clinical Studies, Virginia-Maryland Regional College of Veterinary Medicine, Virginia Tech., Blacksburg, Virginia. Formerly, he has held posts as Professor of Gastrointestinal Physiology and Director, Laboratory of Investigative Gastroenterology at the Faculty of Medicine, Memorial University of Newfoundland, St. John's, Newfoundland, Canada, and Director of Research, Institute of Gastroenterology, Presbyterian-University of Pennsylvania School of Medicine, Philadelphia. He was recently Visiting Professor, Kyoto University, School of Medicine, First Department of Surgery, Kyoto, Japan.

Professor Pfeiffer received a B.A. from Duke University, an M.A. and Ph.D. in Physiology-Pharmacology from Southern Illinois University, and his M.Sc. from Harvard University School of Public Health. He has trained numerous postdoctoral and other trainees from several countries, and has been active in cancer research for many years and in the development of diverse animal models for peptic ulcer, colitis, and esophageal cancer. In 1977-78 he was awarded the American Cancer Society-Eleanor Roosevelt-International Cancer Fellowship.

He is the editor or author of *Peptic Ulcer, Gastric Cancer, Drugs and Peptic Ulcer, Gastrointestinal Ultrastructure, Cancer of the Esophagus,* and other books, as well as author or co-author of more than 100 scientific papers and chapters. Professor Pfeiffer is a member of the Comparative Gastroenterological Society, the American Physiological Society, the Society of Toxicology, the International Society for Diseases of the Esophagus, among others. One of his chief interests is promoting international cooperation in medical and veterinary research and education.

CONTRIBUTORS

Robert A. Argenzio, Ph.D.
Professor of Physiology
Department of Anatomy, Physiological
  Sciences, and Radiology
School of Veterinary Medicine
North Carolina State University
Raleigh, North Carolina

Edgar C. Boedeker, M.D.
Chief
Department of Gastroenterology
Department of the Army
Walter Reed Army Institute of
  Research
Washington, D.C.

Edward A. Carter, Ph.D.
Director
Pediatric/Adult Breath-Analysis
  Laboratory
Massachusetts General Hospital
Shriner Burns Hospital
Children's Hospital Medical Center
Boston, Massachusetts

Phillip B. Carter, Ph.D.
Professor
Department of Microbiology,
  Pathology, and Parasitology
School of Veterinary Medicine
North Carolina State University
Raleigh, North Carolina

Laura V. Chalifoux, B.A.
Associate in Comparative Pathology
Harvard Medical School
New England Regional Primate
  Research Center
Southborough, Massachusetts

Christopher P. Cheney, Ph.D.
12910 Sutters Lane
Bowie, Maryland

Ronnie E. Cimprich, V.M.D.
Box 786
Elmer, New Jersey

Helen J. Cooke, Ph.D.
Associate Professor
Department of Physiology
University of Nevada School of
  Medicine
Reno, Nevada

Charles H. Domermuth, Ph.D.
Professor
Division of Agricultural and Urban
  Practice
Virginia-Maryland Regional College of
  Veterinary Medicine
Virginia Polytechnic Institute and State
  University
Blacksburg, Virginia

F. Robert Fekety, Jr., M.D.
Professor and Chief
Division of Infectious Diseases
Department of Medicine
University of Michigan Medical Center
Ann Arbor, Michigan

Walter B. Gross, D.V.M., Ph.D.
Professor
Division of Agricultural and Urban
  Practice
Virginia-Maryland Regional College of
  Veterinary Medicine
Virginia Polytechnic Institute and State
  University
Blacksburg, Virginia

Rudolph Hesterberg, M.D.
Department of Operative Medicine
University of Marburg
Marburg, West Germany

Syun Hosoda, M.D.
Chief
Laboratory of Pathology
Aichi Cancer Center Research Institute
Nagoya, Japan

Ronald D. Hunt, D.V.M.
Professor of Comparative Pathology
  and Director
New England Regional Primate
  Research Center
Southborough, Massachusetts

Bernhard Huskamp, Dr. med. vet.
Tierklinik Hochmoor
Gescher-Hochmoor, West Germany

James C. Keith, Jr., D.V.M., Ph.D.
Assistant Professor
Division of Veterinary Biology and
  Clinical Studies
Virginia-Maryland Regional College of
  Veterinary Medicine
Virginia Polytechnic Institute and State
  University
Blacksburg, Virginia

Charles E. King, M.D.
Associate Professor
Division of Gastroenterology,
  Hepatology, and Nutrition
University of Florida College of
  Medicine
Gainesville, Florida

Norval W. King, Jr., D.V.M.
Associate Professor of Comparative
  Pathology and Chairman
Division of Comparative Pathology
New England Regional Primate
  Research Center
Southborough, Massachusetts

Isamu Kino, M.D.
Professor
First Department of Pathology
School of Medicine
University of Hamamatsu
Hamamatsu, Japan

Jürgen Kusche, M.D.
Second Department of Surgery
Biochemistry and Experimental
  Division
University of Cologne
Cologne, West Germany

Wilfried Lorenz, M.D.
Professor
Department of Theoretical Surgery
Center of Operative Medicine I
University of Marburg
Marburg, West Germany

Akihiko Maekawa, M.D.
Section Chief
Division of Pathology
Biological Safety Research Center
National Institute of Hygienic Sciences
Tokyo, Japan

J. G. W. Matthews, M.Ch.,
  F.R.C.S.(Eng.)
Consultant Surgeon
Coleraine Hospital
Coleraine, Northern Ireland

Shinichi Nakamura, M.D.
First Department of Pathology
School of Medicine
University of Hamamatsu
Hamamatsu, Japan

Tomio Narisawa, M.D.
Associate Professor
Department of Surgery
Akita University School of Medicine
Akita, Japan

Toshiaki Ogiu, M.D.
Section Head
Laboratory of Ultrastructure Research
Aichi Cancer Center Research Institute
Nagoya, Japan

Brian D. Perry, D.V.M.
Assistant Professor
Virginia-Maryland Regional College of
  Veterinary Medicine
Virginia Polytechnic Institute and State
  University
Blacksburg, Virginia

Carl J. Pfeiffer, Ph.D.
Professor
Division of Veterinary Biology and
  Clinical Studies
Virginia-Maryland Regional College of
  Veterinary Medicine
Virginia Polytechnic Institute and State
  University
Blacksburg, Virginia

Gary D. Rifkin, M.D.
Associate Professor of Clinical
  Medicine
University of Illinois College of
  Medicine
Rockford, Illinois

Toshiko Saito
Research Assistant
Laboratory of Pathology
Aichi Cancer Center Research Institute
Nagoya, Japan

Motokazu Suyama, M.D.
Second Department of Surgery
Aichi Cancer Center Hospital
Nagoya, Japan

Phillip P. Toskes, M.D.
Professor and Director
Division of Gastroenterology,
  Hepatology, and Nutrition
University of Florida College of
  Medicine
Gainesville, Florida

A. David Weaver, Ph.D., F.R.C.V.S.
Senior Lecturer
Glasgow University Veterinary Hospital
Glasgow, Scotland
Department of Veterinary Medicine and
  Surgery
College of Veterinary Medicine
University of Missouri
Columbia, Missouri

J. D. Wood, Ph.D.
Professor and Chairman
Department of Physiology
University of Nevada School of
  Medicine
Reno, Nevada

Seiji Yamada, V.M.D.
Laboratory of Pathology
Aichi Cancer Center Research Institute
Nagoya, Japan

DEDICATION

This monograph is dedicated to the living memory of the late Marion duPont Scott who, after a lifetime of dedication to the breeding, training, and racing of fine horses, was the generous benefactor of the Marion duPont Scott Equine Medical Center at Morven Park near Leesburg, Virginia. This new medical center is a component of the Virginia-Maryland Regional College of Veterinary Medicine, and is located on land donated by the Westmoreland Davis Memorial Foundation.

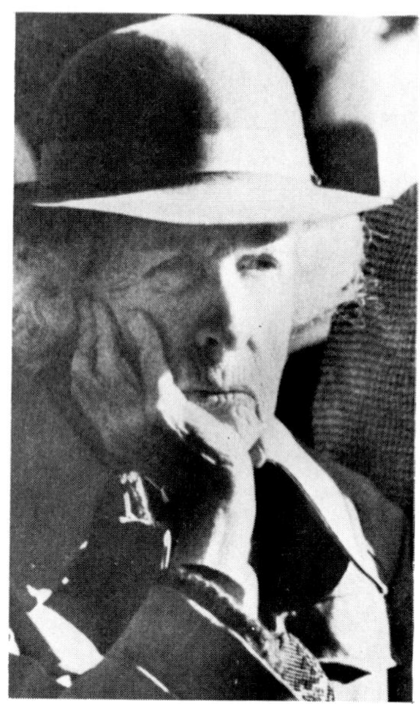

Marion duPont Scott

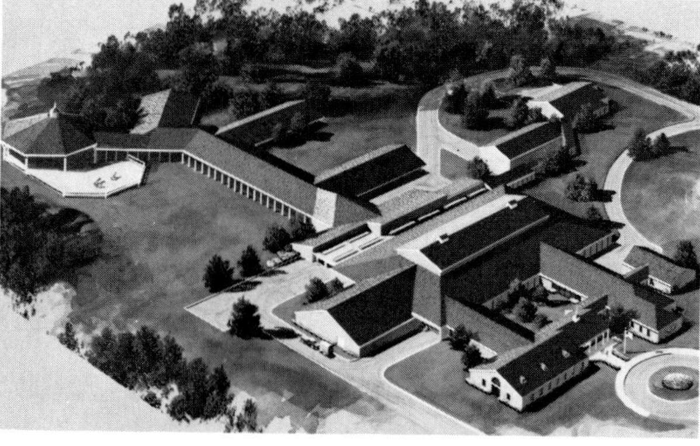

Marion duPont Scott Equine Medical Center

TABLE OF CONTENTS

PART I: SPONTANEOUS AND EXPERIMENTAL INFECTIOUS DISEASES OF THE ANIMAL INTESTINE

PART II: SPONTANEOUS OR INDUCED CANCERS OR CHRONIC INFLAMMATORY CONDITIONS OF THE INTESTINAL TRACT

Part I
Spontaneous and Experimental Infectious
Diseases of the Animal Intestine

Chapter 1

PATHOPHYSIOLOGY OF SWINE DYSENTERY

Robert A. Argenzio

TABLE OF CONTENTS

I. INTRODUCTION

Swine dysentery is an inflammatory, bacterial, diarrheal disease which is confined to the large intestine. As will be discussed below, the pathophysiology of this disease is unlike other common bacterial diarrheas such as salmonellosis or colibacillosis. In fact, although the etiology and pathologic lesions of swine dysentery are quite different from inflammatory bowel disease (IBD) in humans (ulcerative colitis and Crohn's disease), the pathophysiological changes in colonic ion transport are similar. Therefore, while the precise nature of the mechanisms producing the diarrhea in these conditions is at present unknown, further study may reveal pathogenetic mechanisms common to both.

II. ETIOLOGY, CLINICAL SIGNS, AND PATHOLOGY OF SWINE DYSENTERY

Swine dysentery is an infectious, bacterial disease most commonly seen in weanling-age swine, and characterized by a mucohemorrhagic diarrhea.[1] The organism producing the disease is a spirochete, the presence of which has been clearly demonstrated within and between colonic epithelial cells of dysentery-affected swine.[2] The agent was initially isolated and grown in pure culture by Taylor and Alexander[3] and by Harris et al.[4] and when inoculated into pigs would reproduce the disease. The agent was named *Treponema hyodysenteriae.*[4]

The classic clinical signs are a bloody diarrhea with mucus and fibrin in the feces. The animals are listless, anorectic, and emaciated, and may become prostrate and comatose prior to death.[5] The disease can be characterized by four separate syndromes: peracute, acute, subacute, and chronic.[6] In the peracute cases, the animals are found dead in the absence of prior clinical signs. Acute cases exhibit the classical signs of diarrhea with blood and mucus in the feces. Subacute cases are those characterized by weight loss associated with mild or intermittent diarrhea. In chronic cases, a watery diarrhea develops and the animals undergo progressive emaciation showing no signs of recovery, and eventually die. The mortality rates range from 40 to 60% in weanling animals to 10 to 20% in older stock, with the average about 25%.[5,7] Loss of fluid and electrolytes is the cause of death in swine dysentery.[2,8]

The gross lesions are confined to the cecum and colon. The serosa of the colon appears edematous and hyperemic. The mucosal lesions may be characterized by a catarrhal, hemorrhagic, mucohemorrhagic, or fibrinonecrotic enteritis. In more advanced cases, diptheritic pseudomembranes may be formed from the fibrinonecrotic exudate. In acute cases, it is common to see areas of mucosal ulceration, erosion, and edema of the colonic wall.[2,3,6]

Microscopically, the lesions involve primarily the upper one third of the mucosa. In the early stages of the disease, the goblet cells undergo hyperplasia and secrete large amounts of mucus. Later, these cells become exhausted and collapse.[2,5] Most of the damage is on the epithelial surface of the mucosa. The cells lose their attachment to the underlying structures and are sloughed into the lumen. Pseudomembranes may be formed from combinations of sloughed epithelial cells, fibrin, leukocytes, bacteria, and cellular debris (Figure 1). Focal areas of necrosis and erosions into deeper layers can be seen in more severe cases.[9,10]

III. NORMAL LARGE INTESTINAL FUNCTION

Because the disease is limited to the cecum and colon, much of the clinical course of the disease can be predicted by considering the consequences of interrupting normal

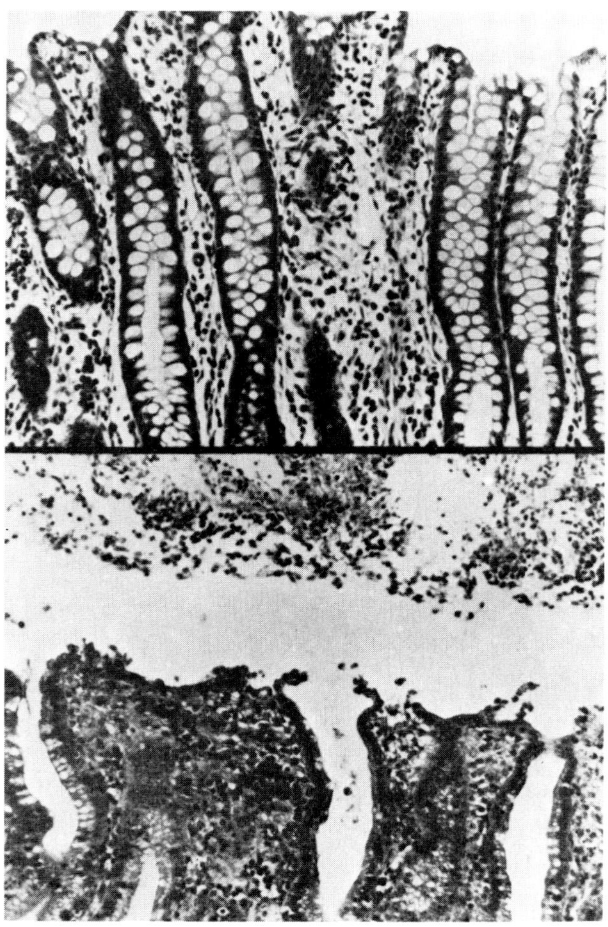

FIGURE 1. Photomicrographs showing histology of colonic mucosa from a normal pig and from a pig with swine dysentery. (Top) Mucosa from colonic loop of normal pig exposed to saline. (Bottom) Mucosa from colonic loop of infected pig exposed to saline, showing epithelial erosion, crypt dilatation, and hypercellularity of lamina propria. A fibrinonecrotic pseudomembrane is artifactually separated from the luminal surface. (From Argenzio, R. A., Whipp, S. C., and Glock, R. D., *J. Infect. Dis.*, 142, 676, 1980. With permission.)

function. Therefore, this section will briefly review the major quantitative functions of the porcine large intestine.

The large intestine of the pig, as well as numerous other omnivorous and herbivorous species, performs two major functions. The first of these is *microbial digestion* and the second is *reabsorption of electrolytes and water.* Table 1 shows the total quantity of volatile fatty acids produced in the large intestine of normal, 50-kg pigs per day. These values were obtained by the in vitro, zero time-fermentation rate method described by Hungate et al.,[11] but are good estimations of production rates in vivo. These organic acids arise from microbial fermentation of carbohydrate and consist chiefly of acetic, propionic, and butyric acids. The acids provide a source of energy to the host animal, and the percentage of the animal's maintenance energy requirement they supply is also shown in Table 1. Thus, the production and absorption of these organic acids provide an important source of energy to the growing animal.

Table 1
VOLATILE FATTY ACID PRODUCTION
RATES IN PIGS FED A HIGH FIBER (1) OR
HIGH GRAIN (2) DIET[49]

	Cecum (m M/day)	Proximal colon[a] (m M/day)	Distal colon (m M/day)	ME[b] (%)
Ration 1	193 ± 3	664 ± 130	521 ± 195	19 ± 5
Ration 2	485 ± 114	984 ± 105	606 ± 98	25 ± 3

[a]   Colon was divided at central flexure of spiral.
[b]   Maintenance energy.

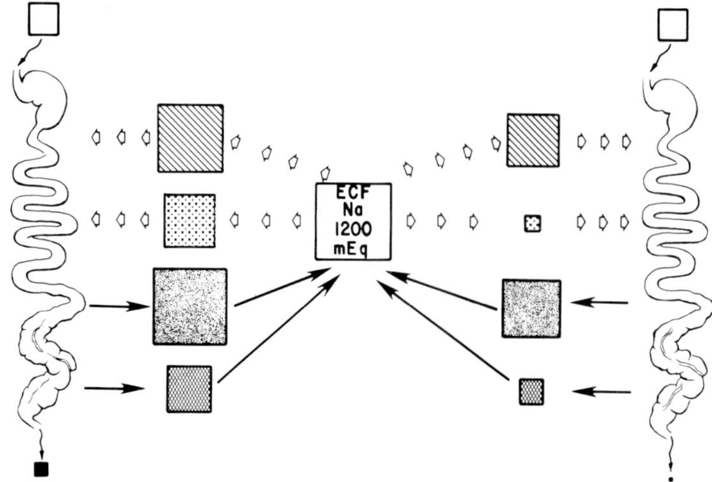

FIGURE 2.   Dietary and endogenous Na recycled into and out of digestive tract during a 24-hr period in 40-kg pigs fed a high fiber (left) or low fiber (right) diet. Animals were prepared with duodenal, mid-jejunal, and terminal ileal reentrant cannulas. Flow of digesta Na per 24 hr was measured at each of these three sites along with dietary intake and fecal excretion. Data were recalculated to estimate net Na secretion anterior to duodenum and between duodenum and mid-jejunum, as well as net absorption of Na between mid-jejunum and terminal ileum, and between terminal ileum and feces. The relative quantities of Na moving into or out of the segments is indicated by the shaded blocks, which are drawn in proportional size to the block indicating the quantity of extracellular fluid Na. (Calculated from data of Reference 12.)

The second major function of the large bowel (electrolyte and H_2O reabsorption) is more critical to the animal's immediate survival. This function is much more important in weaned and older animals than in the neonate. For example, in 3 day to 3-week-old pigs, some 90% of the endogenous and exogenous fluid load is reabsorbed by the small intestine.[48] However, in weaned pigs, a significant fraction of the animal's extracellular fluid volume (ECFV) is presented to the large bowel for absorption. The quantity of fluid is largely dependent on the type of diet and reflects primarily *endogenous* secretions. The approximate fraction of the ECV Na (and H_2O) entering and being reabsorbed daily from the bowel of normal 40-kg pigs is shown in Figure 2.[12] The secretory fluids largely represent salivary, gastric, pancreatic, and biliary secretions, but it is noteworthy that the upper small intestine is also in a state of net secretion or close to

Table 2
NET SOLUTE AND WATER
TRANSPORT FROM COLONS OF
CONTROL PIGS AND PIGS
INFECTED WITH *TREPONEMA
HYODYSENTERIAE*[13]

Net transport (per 2 hr)	Control (n = 20)	Infected (n = 18)
H_2O (mℓ/g)	10.7 ± 1.3	−0.3 ± 0.5
Solute (mosmol/g)	4.23 ± 0.3	0.2 ± 0.2

Note: Results expressed as mean ± SE per gram of dry mucosa. Positive values designate net absorption, negative value net secretion.

zero net movement of fluid. Thus, the lower small bowel and large intestine reabsorb the majority of these endogenous secretions. In the case of the large intestine, a volume equivalent to some 40% of the ECFV must be reabsorbed in animals fed the fiber diet.

Two important points are apparent from these data considering the age of dysentery-affected pigs. First, the contribution of the large bowel to energy balance in weaned pigs is substantial, and a failure of this process could easily explain the deterioration noted in chronically affected pigs. Second, while the contribution of the large bowel to fluid balance in neonatal pigs is insignificant, a critical fraction of the ECFV is absorbed daily by the colon of weaned pigs. It cannot be emphasized too strongly that the majority of these fluids *originate* from the ECFV and therefore *must* be reabsorbed to preserve the ECFV and arterial pressure. Thus, these figures would indicate that total colonic absorptive failure alone could rapidly result in serious dehydration; net secretion of fluid by the large bowel is unnecessary to produce a fatal diarrhea.

IV. INTESTINAL FUNCTION IN SWINE DYSENTERY

Because death in swine dysentery is a result of fluid and electrolyte loss, studies were conducted to examine the nature of colonic fluid and electrolyte transport in infected pigs — particularly to determine if colonic secretion was an important component.[13] Weaned pigs weighing 20 to 30 kg were infected with the organism and 1 to 2 days after diarrhea developed the colons of the anesthetized pigs were prepared with isolated loops into which experimental solutions were placed. Net transport of solute and water was determined with a nonabsorbable marker.

Table 2 compares rates of net transport of solute and water between control and infected pigs. Clearly, net water and ion absorption from the colons of the infected pigs was completely abolished. In addition, a *net* secretory response was not observed.

Although these results suggest an interruption of normal absorptive function, the net movement of ions and water across the mucosa is the result of bidirectional transmural fluxes. Thus, an increase in blood-to-lumen fluxes or a decrease in lumen-to-blood fluxes could equally well result in zero net movement and therefore a secretory component in this disease cannot be ruled out. Further studies were therefore carried out to determine bidirectional movements of Na and Cl, employing radioisotopes.[13] The results of these studies, shown in Table 3, demonstrate that the zero net movement of these ions, previously observed, can be entirely attributed to a decrease in the unidirectional movement of Na and Cl from lumen to blood; a significant increase in the oppositely directed fluxes was not observed. The results of these two studies indicate

Table 3

UNIDIRECTIONAL NA AND CL TRANSPORT
FROM COLONS OF CONTROL PIGS AND PIGS
WITH *TREPONEMA HYODYSENTERIAE*[13]

Transport (per 2 hr)	Control (n = 15)		Infected (n = 8)	
	Na	Cl	Na	Cl
Influx (meq/g)	2.3 ± 0.2	1.8 ± 0.1	1.1 ± 0.1	0.9 ± 0.1
Efflux (meq/g)	0.7 ± 0.1	0.5 ± 0.1	0.8 ± 0.2	0.8 ± 0.2
Net flux (meq/g)	1.6 ± 0.1	1.3 ± 0.1	0.3 ± 0.2	0.2 ± 0.1

Note: Results expressed as mean ± SE per gram dry mucosa.

that the fluid losses in these pigs may be a consequence of colonic absorptive failure alone. Neither an active nor a passive secretory process appears to be associated with this disease.

As pointed out in Section III, colonic absorptive failure alone theoretically could be sufficient to result in dehydration and death in pigs of this age. It was questioned, however, as to whether or not the small bowel might be involved. For example, previous studies of salmonellosis had shown that marked net secretion occurred in the jejunum of infected monkeys, even though minimal morphologic damage and little bacterial invasion was observed.[14] Thus, an enterotoxin or a colonic factor released from the inflamed colon could possibly alter small-bowel function.

Further studies were therefore conducted to examine the small-bowel function in pigs affected with swine dysentery.[15] These pigs were surgically prepared with a small cannula placed in the proximal jejunum and a second cannula near the terminal ileum. One to two days following the onset of diarrhea, the small intestines of the conscious pigs were perfused with either a glucose-Ringer solution or a mannitol-Ringer solution, and changes in net solute and water transport were determined. As shown in Figure 3, the net rates of solute and water absorption from the glucose solution between control and infected pigs were identical. Furthermore, the net rate of appearance of endogenous secretions into the mannitol solution was also identical. Thus, these results indicate that small-bowel function is normal, and the dehydration observed must be entirely the consequence of the failure of the colon to reabsorb the animal's own endogenous secretions. These factors illustrate the importance of normal colonic absorptive function in animals of this age.

V. PATHOPHYSIOLOGIC MECHANISMS OF DIARRHEA

Results of the functional studies discussed above indicate that colonic absorptive failure can explain the fluid losses; however, they give no indication of the mechanism of this absorptive failure. Several alternative mechanisms documented in other diarrheal diseases are possible and it is necessary to consider each of these.

The pathophysiology of most diarrheal illnesses can be grouped into at least four mechanistic classifications:

1. Osmotic diarrhea caused by tbe presence of nonabsorbable solutes in the gut lumen
2. Filtration secretion or malabsorption caused by an increase in mucosal permeability and tissue hydrostatic pressure
3. Cyclic nucleotide-mediated secretory diarrhea caused by bacterial enterotoxins and various other compounds such as prostaglandins or neuroendocrine agents

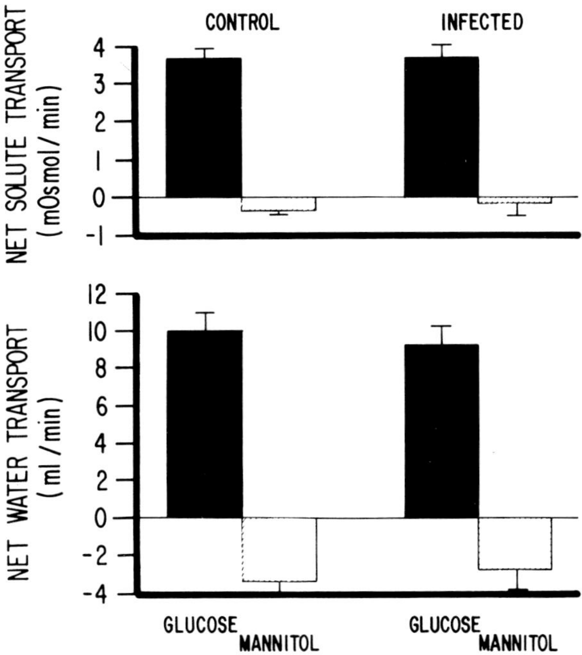

FIGURE 3. Net solute and net water transport in small intestine of control and infected pigs with 80-m M glucose or mannitol solutions. Entire small intestine was perfused in conscious pigs. Mean ± SE (n = 9).[15]

4. Deletion or inhibition of a normal absorptive mechanism such as occurs in villous atrophy and possibly other mucosal diseases

The first of these classifications can probably be ruled out as a major underlying mechanism operating in dysentery because the above studies demonstrating a defect in mucosal transport function can entirely account for the diarrhea.

In the second classification, an increase in mucosal permeability can lead to the abolition of net ion and fluid transport and has been cited as at least one of the causes of the diarrhea associated with bile acid malabsorption.[16] An experimental model demonstrating that increased mucosal permeability associated with elevated tissue hydrostatic pressure can lead to net intestinal secretion has been documented by Yablonski and Lifson.[17] Histologically, the lesions of swine dysentery suggest the possibility for such a mechanism. The epithelial erosions, submucosal edema, and appearance of blood in the lumen strongly suggest that an increased tissue permeability and possibly increased tissue hydrostatic pressure could explain the absorptive failure.

Cyclic nucleotide-mediated intestinal and colonic secretion has been well documented in noninvasive bacterial diarrheas associated with enterotoxin production such as cholera toxin and heat-labile enterotoxin of *Escherichia coli,* both of which activate the adenyl cyclase-cyclic AMP system.[18] Recent studies have shown that the heat-stable enterotoxin of *E. coli* activates the guanyl cyclase-cyclic GMP system, which also causes active electrolyte secretion by both small- and large-bowel mucosa.[19,20] Even in invasive bacterial diarrheas, such as salmonellosis, the cAMP system has been implicated. Although the histologic appearance of the lesions in salmonellosis suggested an increase in mucosal permeability as a factor in the fluid loss, two separate studies failed to reveal an increase in mucosal permeability.[21,22] Additional studies showed elevation of cAMP concentrations in the ileal loops of rabbits infected with a *Salmonella* strain producing severe inflammation and secretion.[23] Blocking the inflammatory response with nitrogen mustard or pretreatment of the loops with indomethacin abolished the secretory response. Thus, the possibility of a prostaglandin-mediated activation of adenyl cyclase was postulated.[24,25] Prostaglandins of the E series have been shown to induce electrolyte secretion in isolated rat colon and have been implicated in the pathogenesis of bile acid diarrhea as well as IBD.[26,27] Elevated PG levels have been demonstrated in both of these conditions. Thus, the involvement of the cAMP system must be considered in any situation that results in mucosal damage, inflammation, and PG release. Although numerous assays have failed to demonstrate an enterotoxigenic component in swine dysentery,[28] the possibility of a PG-cAMP component is a likely possibility.

The fourth category has been documented in viral-induced malabsorption in pigs infected with the transmissible gastroenteritis corona virus.[29,30] Impairment of the coupled Na-glucose absorptive mechanism in the small bowel was demonstrated in vitro. It would seem intuitively reasonable that any disease resulting in destruction of the mucosa could similarly result in malabsorption, but this premise is poorly documented.

Several investigations have demonstrated increased PG levels and adenyl cyclase in mucosa obtained from patients with active ulcerative colitis which was not further increased upon addition of PGE_2.[31] However, good evidence of net secretory response mediated by cAMP is lacking. Rather, a number of studies suggest a decrease in net absorption. Impaired Na transport and a fall in rectal transmural potential difference (PD) have been shown to occur in ulcerative colitis and Crohn's disease.[32,33] In addition, these mucosae were unresponsive to mineralocorticoid treatment in generating an increase in PD and net Na transport, suggesting an overall impairment in transport mechanisms.[33,34] One study of in vitro-isolated colonic mucosa taken from IBD patients demonstrated a decrease in the mucosal-to-serosal flux of Na, while flux in the opposite direction was unaffected.[35] No secretory response was observed, but since all but one patient had been treated with sulfasalazine (a prostaglandin inhibitor), a secretory response may have been masked. Nevertheless, specific inhibitors of the cyclooxygenase enzyme (which leads to PG production), such as indomethacin and flurbiprofen, have not only failed to improve the colonic appearance and Na transport, but have actually led to deterioration.[36,37] Thus, the hypothesis of PG-activation of adenyl cyclase and active electrolyte secretion in IBD is inconclusive.

Therefore, although the underlying mechanism causing the impaired absorption in IBD mucosa is unknown, the similarity to the net effects observed in dysentery suggests that a similar pathophysiologic mechanism is not an unlikely possibility.

VI. EXPERIMENTAL APPROACH TO PATHOPHYSIOLOGY OF SWINE DYSENTERY

As outlined above, several pathophysiologic mechanisms could be operating in dysentery and a systematic examination of each is necessary. An experimental approach to the consequences of increased mucosal permeability and cAMP-mediated diarrhea on fluid and electrolyte transport has been examined in the pig colon.[38] Ethylenediamine tetraacetic acid (EDTA) and deoxycholic acid (DCA) are agents that cause erosions of the colonic epithelium and result in a mucosal appearance not unlike that observed in dysentery. The effects of these two agents and an agent that elevates intracellular levels of cAMP (theophylline) were examined in isolated colonic loops of the normal pig. Net fluid transport was assessed, together with mucosal permeability, by utilizing an intravenous injection of ^{14}C-mannitol and measuring the appearance of ^{14}C in the loop.

Figure 4 shows the results of net water movement and ^{14}C-mannitol clearance into loops containing saline, 25 m*M* EDTA, 6 m*M* DCA, or EDTA + DCA. EDTA or

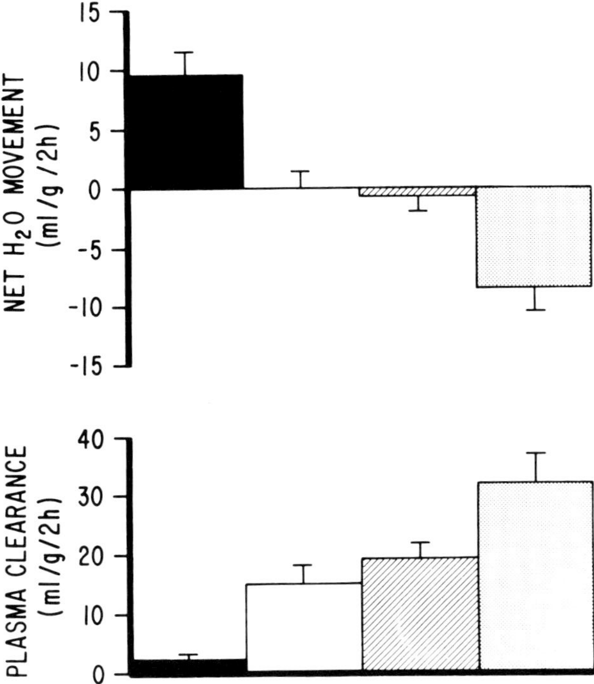

FIGURE 4. Effect of control, ■; 25 m*M* EDTA, □; 6 m*M* DCA, ◪; or EDTA + DCA ◩ solutions on net water transport and plasma clearance of ^{14}C-mannitol into colonic loops. Values expressed as mean ± SE per gram dry weight mucosa (n = 8). (From Argenzio, R. A. and Whipp, S. C., *Am. J. Vet. Res.*, 44, 1480, 1983. With permission.)

DCA completely abolished all net ion and water movement and the presence of both elicited net water and electrolyte secretion. Mannitol clearance into DCA- or EDTA-treated loops was increased tenfold from that observed in control loops and the presence of both EDTA and DCA resulted in a greater mannitol clearance than when either one was present alone. Thus, the changes in mannitol clearance appeared to reflect the changes in net water transport.

The effects of theophylline, 6 m*M* DCA, or theophylline plus DCA on net water transport and mannitol clearance are shown in Figure 5. Both theophylline and DCA abolished net water transport, but the two together had no further effect than either one alone. The clearance of mannitol was increased in loops exposed to DCA, as before, however, theophylline had no significant effect upon mannitol clearance, alone or in combination with DCA.

Thus, net absorptive failure in the pig, resembling that seen in swine dysentery, can be brought about by agents that increase mucosal permeability or result in an elevation in intracellular cAMP. The model was employed in an attempt to determine if one of these mechanisms was operating in dysentery.

A. Role of Mucosal Permeability in Swine Dysentery

Mucosal permeability was assessed in swine dysentery-affected pigs by the methods described above.[13] Figure 6 (upper) compares mucosal permeability to mannitol in control and infected pigs in which colonic loops contained normal saline or saline plus EDTA. No significant difference in permeability in saline loops between control and infected pigs was present and, in loops treated with EDTA, the increased mucosal

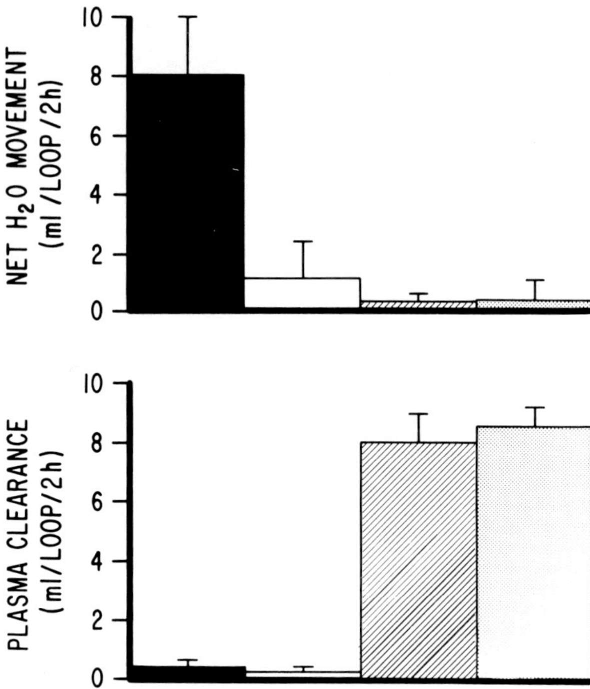

FIGURE 5.   Effect of control, ■; 20 m*M* theophylline, □; 6 m*M*
DCA, ▨; or theophylline + DCA, ▨ solutions on net water transport and plasma clearance of ^{14}C-mannitol into colonic loops. Values are mean ± SE (n = 8). (From Argenzio, R. A. and Whipp, S.
C., *Am. J. Vet. Res.*, 44, 1480, 1983. With permission.)

permeability was even reduced in infected pigs. Mucosal permeability in the direction
of lumen to blood was also assessed with polyethylene glycol 400, a compound with
eight different molecular weights ranging from 200 to 600 daltons, each of which can
be quantified by gas-liquid chromatography.[39] As shown in the lower portion of Figure
6, essentially identical results were obtained as with ^{14}C-mannitol. No differences between control and infected pigs were seen in loops exposed to saline, whereas with
EDTA the response in infected pigs was blunted.

Results of net fluid and ion transport recorded from these studies with EDTA are
shown in Table 4. As before, EDTA abolished ion and water transport in control pigs;
however, in dysentery-affected pigs significant net secretion of ions and water was
observed.

It was suggested that mucosal permeability was unaltered in dysentery; however, in
the presence of EDTA a tissue hydrostatic pressure may have been uncovered which
was otherwise ineffective. Possibly the mucofibrinous layer seen on the mucosa of
infected pigs provides a diffusion barrier similar to the normal mucosa. This would be
a fortunate occurrence, indeed, to prevent further fluid losses arising from pressure-
induced filtration secretion. However, it is clear that the absorptive failure in infected
pigs cannot simply be ascribed to an increase in mucosal permeability.

B. Role of Cyclic Nucleotides in Swine Dysentery

As shown above, theophylline results in an abolition of net fluid transport and the
mechanism of theophylline action in the pig colon was further investigated and defined.[20] These in vivo studies showed that theophylline results in the abolition of the

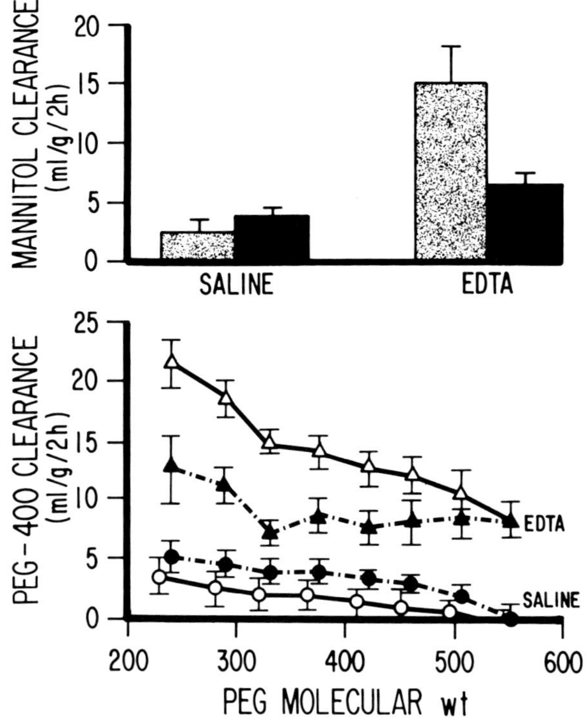

FIGURE 6. (Top) Mannitol clearance from plasma to loop in control pigs (▣), n = 10) and in pigs infected with *Treponema hyodysenteriae* (■, n = 8) after exposure to saline or EDTA. (Bottom) Polyethylene glycol (PEG-400) clearance from loop to plasma in control (O, △, n = 6) and infected (●, ▲, n = 6) pigs exposed to saline or EDTA. (From Argenzio, R. A., Whipp, S. C., and Glock, R. D., *J. Infect. Dis.*, 142, 676, 1980. With permission.)

Table 4
NET SOLUTE AND WATER TRANSPORT FROM COLONS OF CONTROL PIGS AND PIGS INFECTED WITH *TREPONEMA HYODYSENTERIAE* AFTER EXPOSURE TO EDTA SOLUTIONS[13]

Net transport (per 2 hr)	Control (n = 10)	Infected (n = 8)
H_2O (mℓ/g)	0.1 ± 1.6	-4.3 ± 1.5
Solute (mosmol/g)	0.7 ± 0.5	-1.5 ± 0.5

Note: Results expressed as mean ± SE per gram of dry mucosa. Positive values designate net absorption, negative values net secretion.

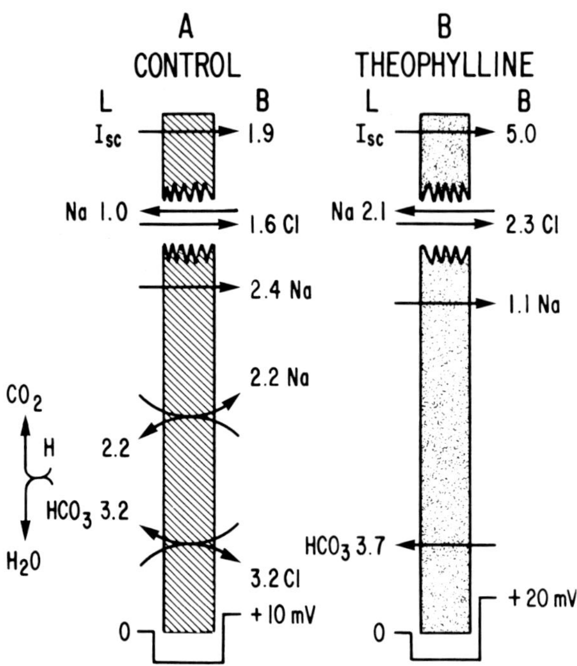

FIGURE 7.   Possible mechanisms to account for in vivo results obtained with Ringer or theophylline-Ringer solutions in pig colon. For simplicity, the models assume a single barrier to transport from lumen (L) to blood (B). In all likelihood, the H and HCO_3 ions which are exchanged for Na and Cl are produced by intracellular hydration of CO_2. All values are expressed in $\mu eq/cm^2 \times hr$. Values for short circuit current (Isc) obtained from parallel in vitro experiments are included and are in reasonably good agreement with current flows calculated from in vivo experiments. Arrows between barriers represent net passive ion flows traversing the tissue in response to transepithelial potential difference shown at bottom. (From Argenzio, R. A. and Whipp, S. C., *J. Physiol. (London)*, 320, 469, 1981. With permission.)

operation of electrically neutral Na and Cl absorptive mechanisms and elicits electrogenic HCO_3 secretion that results in an increase in the transmural PD (Figure 7). Net Cl absorption appears unaffected because the increased PD drives Cl passively across the mucosa from lumen to blood. Theophylline also caused a two- to threefold increase in cAMP and cGMP, the time course of which paralleled the electrical response.

Experiments were conducted by Schmall et al.[40] to examine the similarities or differences in colonic ion transport observed in the presence of theophylline or dysentery. Control or infected pigs were prepared with colonic loops into which a control Ringer solution or Ringer Plus 40 m*M* theophylline was placed. As shown in Table 5, in control pigs theophylline abolished net Na absorption and resulted in net HCO_3 secretion, whereas net Cl absorption was unaffected. In infected pigs, however, it may be seen that in loops exposed to normal Ringer, although net Na absorption is abolished similar to that noted in control pigs with theophylline, net Cl and HCO_3 movements are also abolished. Thus, dysentery and theophylline do not produce similar net transport results. As shown in the right-hand column of Table 5, addition of theophylline to loops of infected pigs resulted in no further effect, suggesting that the cAMP-mediated mechanisms in causing HCO_3 secretion were totally inoperative.

Table 5

NET WATER AND SOLUTE TRANSPORT FROM COLONS
OF CONTROL PIGS AND PIGS INFECTED WITH
TREPONEMA HYODYSENTERIAE AFTER EXPOSURE TO
SALINE OR 40 m*M* THEOPHYLLINE-SALINE SOLUTIONS[40]

	Control		Infected	
Net transport/hr	Saline (n = 6)	Theophylline (n = 6)	Saline (n = 12)	Theophylline (n = 14)
H_2O (mℓ/g)	3.0 ± 0.7	0.1 ± 0.4	-1.2 ± 0.4	-1.1 ± 0.3
Solute (mosmol/g)	1.5 ± 0.2	0.4 ± 0.2	-0.2 ± 0.2	-0.2 ± 0.1
Na (meq/g)	0.7 ± 0.1	0.1 ± 0.1	0.1 ± 0.1	0.0 ± 0.1
Cl (meq/g)	0.7 ± 0.1	0.5 ± 0.1	0.0 ± 0.2	0.0 ± 0.1
HCO_3 (meq/g)	-0.1 ± 0.1	-0.4 ± 0.1	0.1 ± 0.0	-0.1 ± 0.0

Note: Results expressed as mean $\pm$ SE per gram of dry mucosa. Positive values
designate net absorption, negative values net secretion.

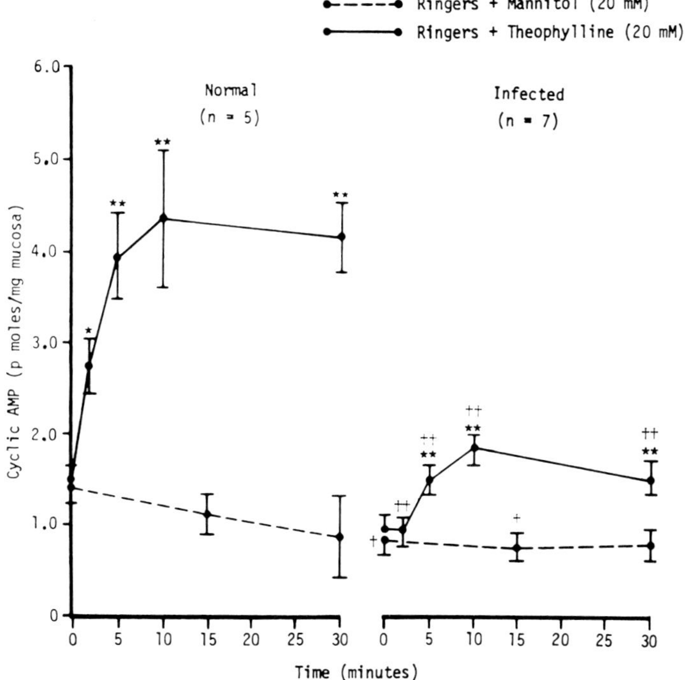

FIGURE 8. Cyclic AMP concentrations in colonic mucosa of normal and
infected pigs exposed to Ringer solution + 20 m*M* mannitol or Ringer solution + 20 m*M* theophylline in vitro. Values are mean $\pm$ SE. *$p < 0.05$, **$p <$
0.01; differences from time 0 in either normal or infected mucosa. †$p < 0.05$,
††$p < 0.01$: differences between corresponding solutions in normal and infected mucosa. (From Schmall, L. M., Argenzio, R. A., and Whipp, S. C.,
Am. J. Vet. Res., 44, 1480, 1983. With permission.)

Schmall et al.[40] also directly measured cyclic nucleotide levels in colonic mucosa of
control and infected pigs in the presence or absence of theophylline. Colonic tissue,
stripped of its underlying muscle, was incubated in oxygenated Ringer solution in vitro

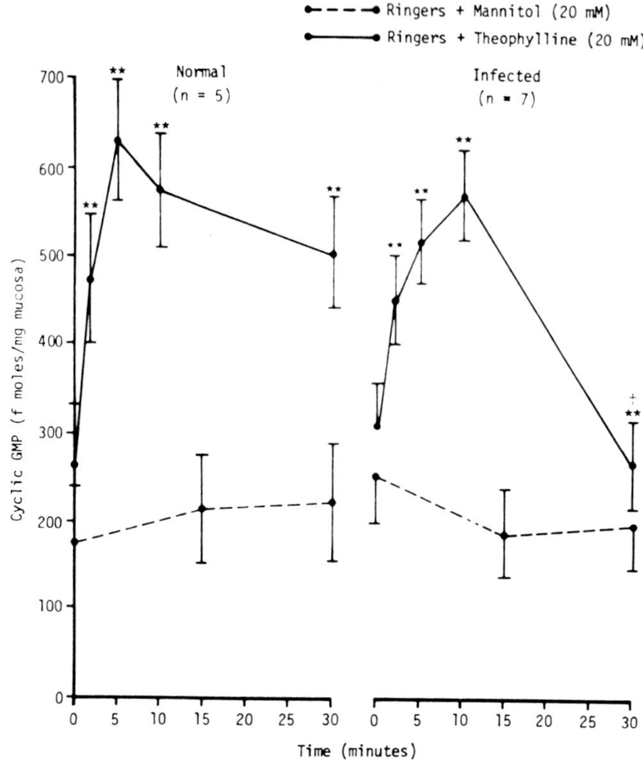

FIGURE 9.   Cyclic GMP concentrations in colonic mucosa of normal and infected pigs exposed to Ringer solution + 20 mM mannitol or Ringer solution + 20 mM theophylline in vitro. Values are mean ± SE. *$p < 0.05$, **$p < 0.01$; differences from time 0 in either normal or infected mucosa. †$p < 0.05$, ††$p < 0.01$: differences between corresponding solutions in normal and infected mucosa. (From Schmall, L. M., Argenzio, R. A., and Whipp, S. C., *Am. J. Vet. Res.*, 44, 1480, 1983. With permission.)

and samples were removed for 30 min following theophylline exposure. Results of these studies are shown in Figures 8 and 9. Basal levels of cyclic nucleotides in control and infected pigs are similar, suggesting firstly that these nucleotides are not mediating the absorptive failure and confirming the transport studies discussed above. Secondly, although the responses of both cAMP and cGMP to theophylline were reduced in infected pigs, the mucosa was still capable of a response. Thus, these results also suggest that mediators of the cAMP or cGMP mechanisms are not involved in the pathogenesis of swine dysentery.

VII. CONCLUSIONS

To date, the studies in the pig have uniformly failed to elucidate the underlying mechanism(s) causing the absorptive failure in swine dysentery. The failure to demonstrate increased levels of intracellular cAMP in an inflamed mucosa still capable of responding to theophylline is difficult to explain. However, it should be noted that the effects of isolated prostaglandins on the colonic mucosa of the pig have not been investigated, nor have the effects of mucosal damage upon tissue prostaglandin levels been examined. Knoop[41] has placed a pathogenic strain of *Treponema hyodysenteriae* in rabbit ileal loops which resulted in epithelial erosion and net fluid *secretion* similar to that observed with cholera toxin. More recent studies by Saheb et al.[42] have shown that a hemolysin obtained from culture filtrates of *T. hyodysenteriae* caused fluid accumulation and mucosal damage in ileal loops of the rat. These results are entirely consistent with PG-mediated intestinal secretion operating through the cAMP system. Thus, the role of PGs in the pig colon needs to be investigated.

On the other hand, studies with human colon affected with shigellosis have also demonstrated that basal levels of adenyl cyclase were unaffected, but still capable of partially responding to PGE_2.[31] These results are very similar to those described in the pig by Schmall et al.[40] and would suggest the alternative hypothesis: that PGs may not be involved in these two diseases.

Recent evidence has now implicated the lipoxygenase pathway of the arachidonic acid cascade in colonic secretion. Addition of either 5-hydroperoxyeicosatetraenoic acid (5-HPETE) or 5-hydroxyeicosatetraenoic acid (5-HETE) to isolated rabbit colonic mucosa resulted in active Cl secretion by a *non* cAMP-, cGMP-, or Ca-mediated mechanism.[43] These same agents were ineffective in rabbit ileum. Thus, the possibility arises that some products of the inflammatory response are operating through colonic secretory mechanisms which are at present unknown.

These recent findings have important therapeutic implications in diseases involving inflammation of the colon. As mentioned above, at least two antagonists of cyclooxygenase have failed to bring about remission in IBD. Currently, the therapy of choice in IBD is sulfasalazine, which is claimed to be effective because its metabolite, 5-aminosulfasalazine, released by colonic bacteria, inhibits PG synthesis.[44] However, there is also evidence that the drug acts by inhibiting PG 15-OH-dehydrogenase and thus potentiates the *cytoprotective* actions of endogenous PGs.[45] PG-cytoprotection is a well-known phenomenon in the stomach and upper small bowel,[46] and administration of 16,16-dimethyl PGE_2 to hamsters protected the colon from clindamycin-associated colitis.[47]

Thus, the role of these arachidonic acid metabolites and interactions among metabolites arising from the cyclooxygenase and lipoxygenase pathways must be explored in colonic function, and their participation in inflammatory processes of the colon quantified. Such studies may provide clues as to the underlying mechanisms operating in inflammatory conditions of the colon, as well as to superior therapeutic agents to be used in their control.

REFERENCES

1. Whiting, R. A., Swine dysentery, *J. Am. Vet. Med. Assoc.*, 17, 600, 1924.
2. Glock, R. D., Studies on the Etiology, Hematology, and Pathology of Swine Dysentery, Ph.D. thesis, Iowa State University, Ames, 1971.
3. Taylor, D. J. and Alexander, T. J. L., The production of dysentery in swine by feeding cultures containing a spirochete, *Br. Vet. J.*, 127, 58, 1971.
4. Harris, D. L., Glock, R. D., Christensen, C. R., and Kinyon, J. M., Swine dysentery. I. Inoculation of pigs with *Treponema hyodysenteriae* (New Species) and reproduction of the disease, *Vet. Med. Small Anim. Clin.*, 67, 61, 1972.
5. Whiting, R. A., Doyle, L. P., and Spray, R. S., Swine dysentery, *Purdue Univ. Agric. Exp. Stn. Bull.*, 257, 1, 1921.
6. Lussier, G., Vibrionic dysentery of swine in Ontario. I. Clinical aspects and pathology, *Can. Vet. J.*, 3, 228, 1962.
7. Doyle, L. P., Enteritis in swine, *Cornell Vet.*, 35, 103, 1955.

8. Ruth, R., Experimental Vibrionic Colitis in Swine, Master's thesis, Michigan State University, East Lansing, 1967.
9. Taylor, D. J. and Blakemore, W. F., Spirochaetal invasion of the colonic epithelium in swine dysentery, *Res. Vet. Sci.,* 12, 177, 1971.
10. Glock, R. D. and Harris, D. L., Swine dysentery. II. Characterization of lesions in pigs inoculated with *Treponema hyodysenteriae* in pure and mixed cultures, *Vet. Med. Small Anim. Clin.,* 67, 65, 1972.
11. Hungate, R. E., Mah, R. A., and Simesen, M., Rates of production of individual volatile fatty acids in the rumen of lactating cows, *Appl. Microbiol.,* 9, 554, 1961.
12. Partridge, I. G., Studies on digestion and absorption in the intestines of growing pigs. IV. Effects of dietary cellulose and sodium levels on mineral absorption, *Br. J. Nutr.,* 39, 539, 1978.
13. Argenzio, R. A., Whipp, S. C., and Glock, R. D., Pathophysiology of swine dysentery: colonic transport and permeability studies, *J. Infect. Dis.,* 142, 676, 1980.
14. Rout, W. R., Formal, S. B., Dammin, G. J., and Giannella, R. A., Pathophysiology of Salmonella diarrhea in the Rhesus monkey: intestinal transport, morphological, and bacteriological studies, *Gastroenterology,* 67, 59, 1974.
15. Argenzio, R. A., Glucose-stimulated fluid absorption by the pig small intestine during the early stage of swine dysentery, *Am. J. Vet. Res.,* 41, 2000, 1980.
16. Rummel, W., Nell, G., and Wanitschke, R., Action mechanisms of antiabsorptive and hydragogue drugs, in *Intestinal Absorption and Malabsorption,* Csaky, T. Z., Ed., Raven Press, New York, 1975, 209.
17. Yablonski, M. E. and Lifson, N., Mechanism of production of intestinal secretion by elevated venous pressure, *J. Clin. Invest.,* 57, 904, 1976.
18. Field, M., Regulation of small intestinal ion transport by cyclic nucleotides and calcium, in *Secretory Diarrhea,* Field, M., Fordtran, J. S., and Schultz, S. G., Eds., American Physiological Society, Bethesda, Md., 1980, 21.
19. Field, M., Graf, L. H., Laird, W. J., and Smith, P. L., Heat stable enterotoxin of *Escherichia coli: in vitro* effects of guanylate cyclase activity, cyclic GMP concentration, and ion transport in small intestine, *Proc. Natl. Acad. Sci. U.S.A.,* 75, 2800, 1978.
20. Argenzio, R. A. and Whipp, S. C., Effect of *Escherichia coli* heat-stable enterotoxin, choleratoxin and theophylline on ion transport in porcine colon, *J. Physiol. (London),* 320, 469, 1981.
21. Kinsey, M. D., Dammin, G. J., Formal, S. B., and Giannella, R. A., The role of altered intestinal permeability in the pathogenesis of *Salmonella* diarrhea in the Rhesus monkey, *Gastoenterology,* 71, 429, 1976.
22. Giannella, R. A., Rout, W. R., Formal, S. B., and Collins, H., Role of plasma filtration in the intestinal fluid secretion mediated by infections with *Salmonella typhimurium, Infect. Immunol.,* 13, 470, 1976.
23. Giannella, R. A., Gots, R. E., Charney, A. N., Greenough, W. B., III, and Formal, S. B., Pathogenesis of *Salmonella* mediated intestinal fluid secretion. Activation of adenylate cyclase and inhibition by indomethacin, *Gastroenterology,* 69, 1238, 1975.
24. Giannella, R. A., Rout, W. R., and Formal, S. B., Effect of indomethacin on intestinal water transport on *Salmonella* infected Rhesus monkeys, *Infect. Immunol.,* 17, 136, 1977.
25. Giannella, R. A., Importance of the intestinal inflammatory response in *Salmonella* mediated intestinal secretion, *Infect. Immunol.,* 23, 140, 1979.
26. Beubler, E. and Juan, H., PGE-mediated laxative effect of diphenolic laxatives, *Naunyn-Schmiedegag's Arch. Pharmacol.,* 305, 91, 1978.
27. Kimberg, D. V., The ubiquitous prostaglandins and their role in ulcerative colitis, *Gastroenterology,* 75, 748, 1978.
28. Whipp, S. C., Harris, D. L., Kinyon, J. M., Songer, J. G., and Glock, R. D., Enteropathogenicity testing of *Treponema hyodysenteriae* in ligated colonic loops of swine, *Am. J. Vet. Res.,* 39, 1293, 1978.
29. Kerzner, B., Kelly, M. H., Gall, D. G., Butler, D. G., and Hamilton, J. R., Transmissible gastroenteritis: sodium transport and the intestinal epithelium during the course of viral enteritis, *Gastroenterology,* 72, 457, 1977.
30. Shepherd, R. W., Gall, D. G., Butler, D. G., and Hamilton, J. R., Determinants of diarrhea in viral enteritis. The role of ion transport and epithelial changes in the ileum in transmissible gastroenteritis in piglets, *Gastroenterology,* 76, 20, 1979.
31. Rachmilewitz, D., Karmeli, F., and Selinger, Z., Increased colonic adenylate cyclase activity in active ulcerative colitis, *Gastroenterology,* 85, 12, 1983.
32. Edmonds, C. J. and Pilcher, D., Electrical potential difference and sodium and potassium fluxes across rectal mucosa in ulcerative colitis, *Gut,* 14, 784, 1973.
33. Ruddell, W. S., Blendis, L. M., and Lovell, D., Rectal potential difference and histology in Crohn's disease, *Gut,* 18, 284, 1977.

34. Edmonds, C. J., Electical potential of the sigmoid colon and rectum in irritable bowel syndrome and ulcerative colitis, *Gut,* 11, 867, 1970.
35. Hawker, P. C., McKay, J. S., and Turnberg, L. A., Electrolyte transport across colonic mucosa from patients with inflammatory bowel disease, *Gastroenterology,* 81, 508, 1980.
36. Gould, S. R., Brash, A. R., Conolly, M. C., and Lennard-Jones, J. E., Studies of prostaglandins and sulphasalazine in ulcerative colitis, *Prostaglandins Med.* 6, 165, 1981.
37. Rampton, D. S. and Sladen, G. E. , Prostaglandin synthesis inhibitors in ulcerative colitis: flurbiprofen compared with conventional treatment, *Prostaglandins,* 21(3), 417, 1981.
38. Argenzio, R. A. and Whipp, S. C., Comparison of the effects of disodium ethylenediaminetetraacetate, theophylline, and deoxycholate on colonic ion transport and permeability, *Am. J. Vet. Res.,* 44, 1480, 1983.
39. Chadwick, V. S., Phillips, S. F., and Hofmann, A. F., Measurements of intestinal permeability using low molecular weight polyethylene glycols (PEG-400). I. Chemical analysis and biological properties of PEG-400, *Gastroenterology,* 73, 241, 1977.
40. Schmall, L. M., Argenzio, R. A., and Whipp, S. C., Pathophysiologic features of swine dysentery: cyclic nucleotide-independent production of diarrhea, *Am. J. Vet. Res.,* 44, 1309, 1983.
41. Knoop, F. C., Experimental infection of rabbit ligated loops with *Treponema hyodysenteriae, Infect. Immunol.,* 26, 1196, 1979.
42. Saheb, S. A., Lallier, R., Massicotte, L., Lafleur, L., and Lemieux, S., Biological activity of Treponema hyodysenteriae hemolysin, *Curr. Microbiol.,* 5, 91, 1981.
43. Musch, M. W., Miller, R. J., Field, M., and Siegel, M. I., Stimulation of colonic secretions by lipooxygenase metabolites of arachidonic acid, *Science,* 217, 1255, 1982.
44. Rask-Madsen, J. and Bukhane, K., Inhibitors and gastrointestinal function, in *Prostaglandins and Related Lipids,* Vol. 1, Ramwell, P. W., Ed., Alan R. Liss, New York, 1980.
45. Hoult, J. R. S. and Moore, P. K., Sulphasalazine is a potent inhibitor of prostaglandin 15-hydroxy-dehydrogenase: possible basis for therapeutic action in ulcerative colitis, *Br. J. Pharmacol.,* 64, 6, 1978.
46. Flemstrom, G. and Garner, A., Gastroduodenal HCO_3 transport: characteristics and proposed role in acidity regulation and mucosal protection, *Am. J. Physiol.,* 242, G183, 1982.
47. Robert, A., Nezamis, J. E., Lancaster, C., and Hanchas, A. J., Prevention, through cytoprotection, of clindamycin-induced colitis in hamsters with 16,16-dimethyl PGE_2, *Gastroenterology,* 78, 1245, 1980.
48. Argenzio, R. A., Moon, H. W., Kemeny, L. J., and Whipp, S. C., Colonic compensation in transmissible gastroenteritis of swine, *Gastroenterology,* 86, 1501, 1984.
49. Allison, M. J. and Argenzio, R. A., Unpublished data.

Chapter 2

HEMORRHAGIC ENTERITIS OF TURKEYS

C. H. Domermuth and W. B. Gross

TABLE OF CONTENTS

I. INTRODUCTION

Hemorrhagic enteritis (HE) of turkeys is unique because it is an infectious disease which produces very high mortality due to intraintestinal bleeding from necrotic tips of villi. The physiological cause of bleeding associated with HE has not been elucidated.

HE was first reported in 1937.[1] From 1957[2] to the present, it has become epidemic in almost all states and foreign countries which have sizable turkey-producing industries. Prior to control of the disease by vaccination,[3] losses due to the disease exceeded $3 million/year.[4]

II. ETIOLOGY

HE is caused by an immunologically distinct group of adenoviruses designated "avian adenovirus group II".[5] The virus, a typical nonenveloped DNA virus,[4] is unique because it is replicated intranuclearly in cells of the reticuloendothelial system, primarily in the spleen.[6-12] Members of avian adenovirus group II also naturally infect pheasants and chickens. Isolates from these species, and from the turkey, have been classified only as to source. Pulmonary lesions, but not intraintestinal bleeding,[4] are produced in pheasants and chickens.

III. VIRUS PROPAGATION

Normally, the virus is isolated and propagated in vivo in turkey spleen cells. Briefly, this is accomplished by orally inoculating infectious tissues such as spleen, liver, blood, or serum, or by similarly inoculating infectious feces. Under these conditions, the virus is replicated and may be recovered from enlarged spleens of susceptible inoculated turkey poults 5 to 7 days after oral inoculation. More extensive descriptions of this process have been published.[4,13] The virus also has been recently replicated in lymphoblastoid B-cells of turkey origin, derived from a Mareks'-disease tumor.[15] At present, however, routine isolation and propagation are done in vivo in susceptible turkey poults.

IV. SIGNS, MORBIDITY, AND MORTALITY

The disease is characterized by depression, bloody droppings, and death. In individual poults, all signs of the disease occur within 24 hr.[14] Depressed poults die within a few hours or apparently recover completely. Field mortality has reached 60%, ranges between 10 to 15% in most outbreaks, but is usually less than 1% when caused by strains of low virulence. All, or nearly all, poults are infected.[16]

V. GROSS LESIONS

Poults that die due to HE infection appear pale because of anemia. Due to the acute nature of the disease, they are in good flesh and usually have feed in the crop. Dark red or brownish-colored blood frequently occurs on the skin of the vent and on the surrounding feathers, and blood may be expelled from the vent with moderate abdominally applied pressure. Intestines are dark in color, distended, and filled with blood. The jejunal mucosa is red and congested. Congestion also can be more extensive and may appear in all areas of the gut excluding the areas anterior to the duodenum. In poults which have died of the disease, spleens are slightly enlarged (1.5 to 2 ×) but are pale, due to exsanguination (Figure 1). Viremic, but otherwise normal penmates have

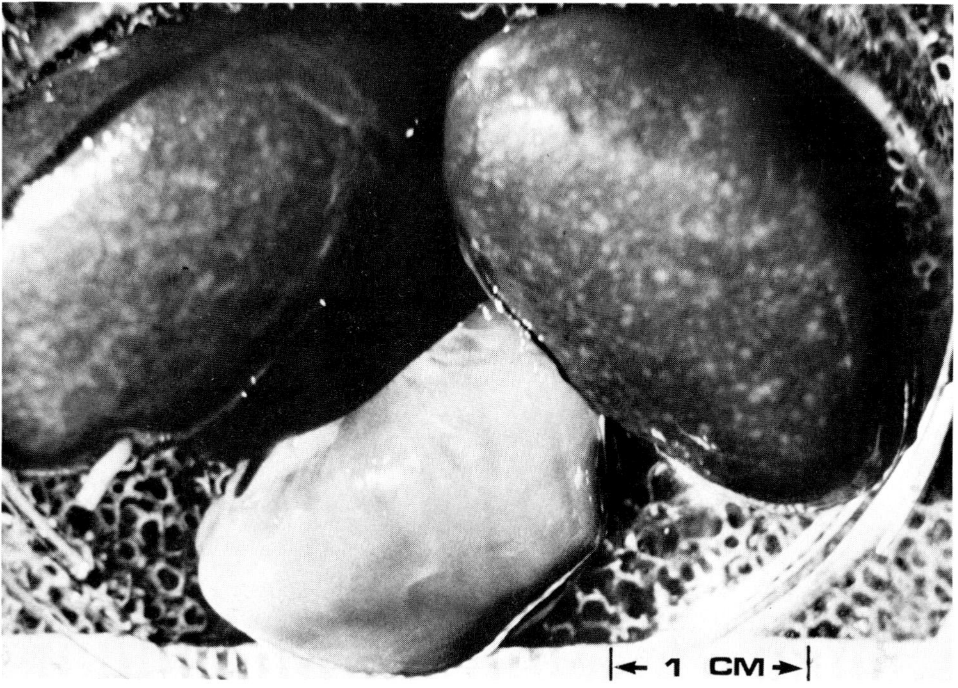

FIGURE 1.   Gross spleen lesions; the larger spleens showing "marbling". Birds were at the peak of viremia but with no other gross lesions. The two larger spleens were obtained after euthanization; the smaller spleen is from a bird that died due to massive virus-induced intraluminal bleeding. The typical, smaller size of the spleen is believed to be caused by blood loss.

enlarged (2 to 4 times) "marbled" spleens (Figure 1). Typical lesions also include congestion of lungs, pale vascular organs, enlarged livers, and petechial hemorrhages of various organs. More extensive descriptions, including atypical lesions, have been published elsewhere.[4]

VI. HISTOPATHOLOGY

Lesions that characterize the disease are found in the reticulothelial system and in the intestine. Splenic lesions include hyperplasia of the white pulp, necrosis of lymphoid cells, proliferation of enlarged endothelial and reticular cells, and virus-containing intranuclear inclusions (Figure 2) of reticular cells[8,9,17,18] (Figure 3). Inclusions are more frequent when death is imminent. Minor lesions of liver, thymus, bone marrow, kidney, lung, pancreas, and brain have also been reported,[8,9,17,19] as has a sequential study of HE-affected spleen cells.[18] Sequentially, intestinal lesions include severe mucosal congestion, degeneration and sloughing of the distal portion of the villi, and finally, hemorrhage into the lumen from disrupted capillaries of villi (Figure 4). In addition, the lamina propria contains increased numbers of reticular cells, plasma cells, and heterophils. Intranuclear inclusion bodies are also present in some reticular and endothelial cells. Histopathologic changes are most pronounced in the jejunum just posterior to the pancreatic ducts.[1,8,9,17,20]

VII. IMMUNITY

Poults that have recovered from natural or laboratory-induced infections apparently cannot be reinfected. Passive immunity can be conferred with less than 1.0 mℓ of

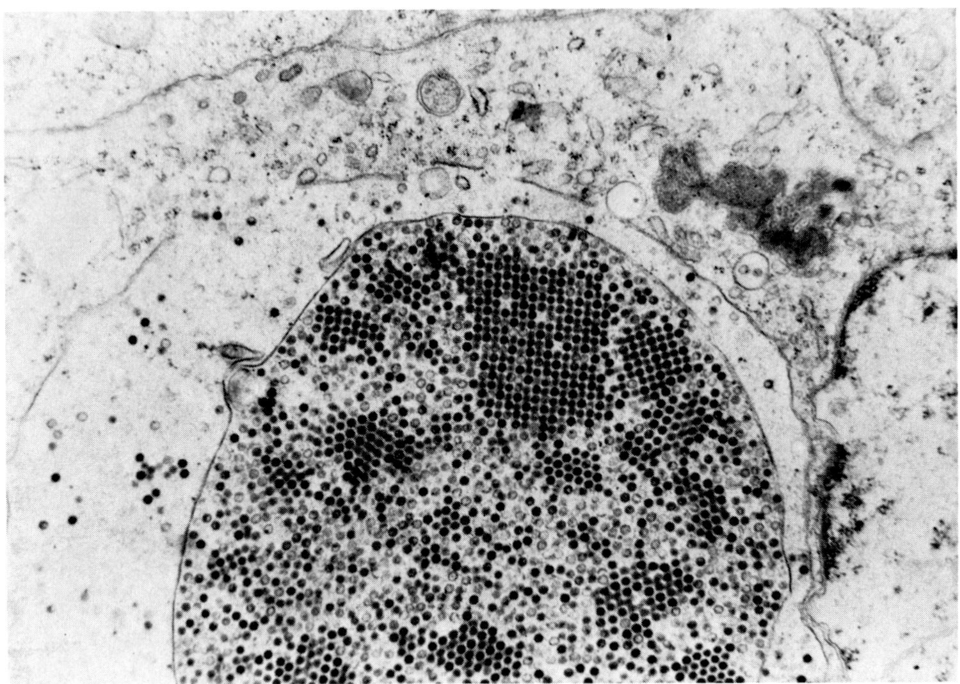

FIGURE 2.   The causal virus. Hemorrhagic enteritis is caused by an adenovirus as depicted in this figure.

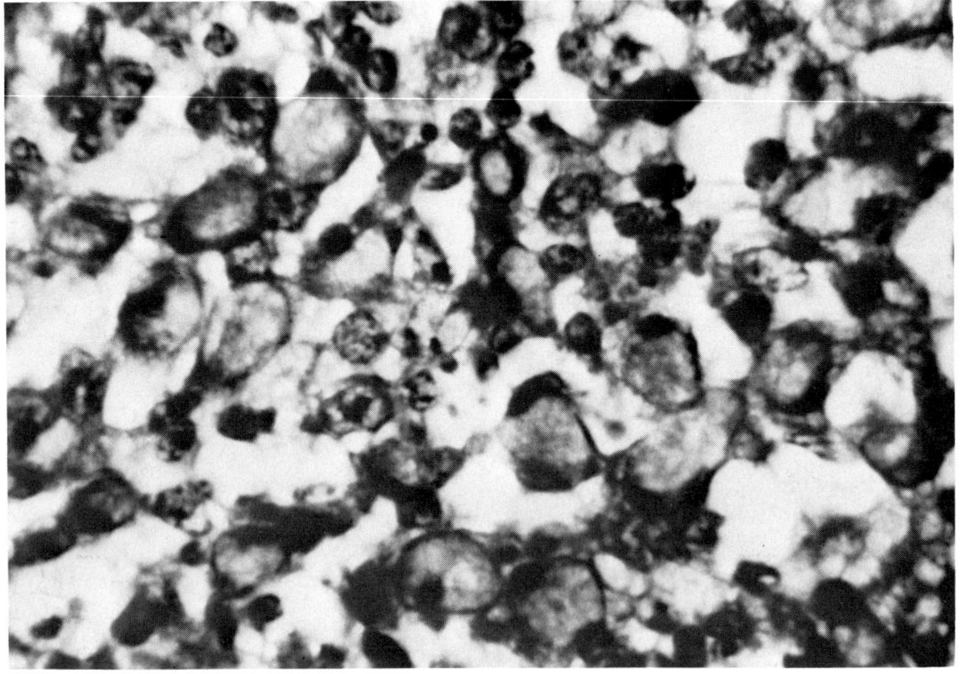

FIGURE 3.   Microscopic spleen lesions. This "typical" lesion may be observed in either the large or the smaller spleens depicted in Figure 1. Intranuclear inclusions, enlargement of reticular cells, and necrosis of lymphoid cells are considered typical for the acute stage of infection depicted.

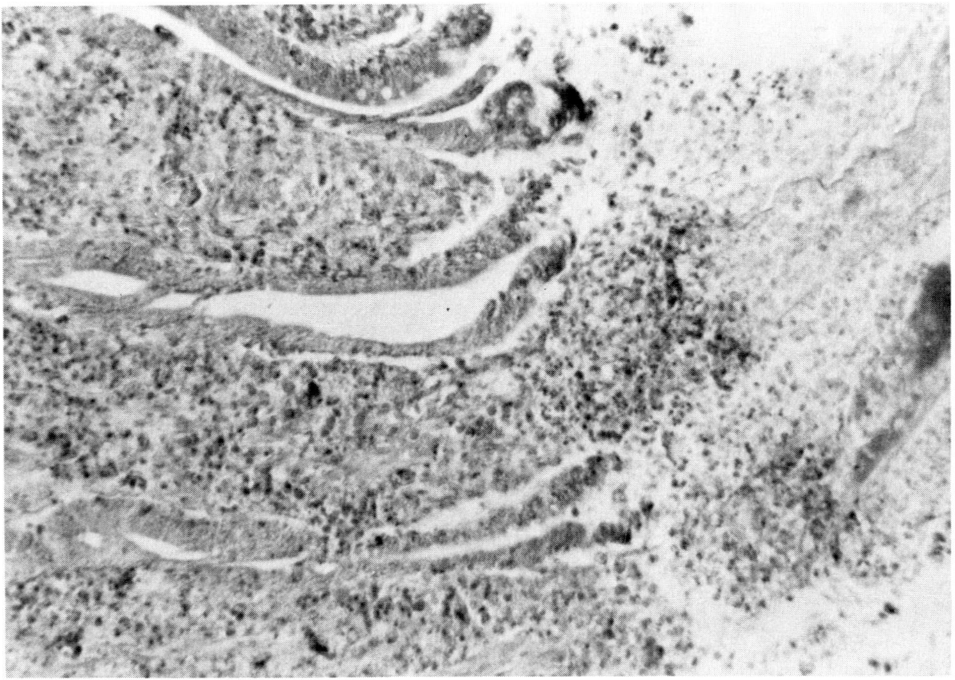

FIGURE 4. Microscopic intestinal lesions. Congestion, degeneration, and sloughing of distal epithelial cells of the villi and hemorrhage into lumen are evident.

convalescent antiserum. Immunity and precipitating antibody appears to last indefinitely. Indeed, convalescent antiserum is protective even if precipitating antibody is not detectable.[21] Protection does not seem to be virus strain specific, because infection with HE strains that produce little to no incidence of death produces solid immunity.[3]

VIII. SEROLOGY

An agar gel diffusion test has been developed using viral antigen extracted from virus-containing spleen. This reacts with convalescent antiserum in an agar gel test to produce a specific serologic reaction. To date, isolates of HE virus are serologically indistinguishable from each other.

IX. TREATMENT, PREVENTION, AND CONTROL

Hemorrhagic enteritis in the field has been treated by injection of convalescent antiserum when first signs of disease occur. Mortality within flocks ceases within 24 hr of such treatment.[22] Control of HE of turkeys has been achieved with a live, water-administered, turkey-spleen-propagated vaccine made from a strain (pheasant origin) of the avian adenovirus group II.[3] This strain is currently used to control the disease.[23]

X. OPPORTUNITIES

Additional research is needed to (1) elucidate the physiological cause of bleeding prior to death caused by HE virus infection of turkeys, (2) perfect and field-test a tissue-culture-propagated vaccine,[15] (3) investigate the reason for protection being conferred against HE by relatively miniscule quantities of antiserum, and (4) determine why mortality produced by HE strains varies from none to over 60%.

REFERENCES

1. Pomeroy, B. S. and Fenstermacher, R., Hemorrhagic enteritis in turkeys, *Poult. Sci.*, 16, 378, 1937.
2. Gale, C. and Wyne, J. W., Preliminary observations on hemorrhagic enteritis of turkeys, *Poult. Sci.*, 366, 1267, 1957.
3. Domermuth, C. H., Gross, W. B., Douglass, C. S., DuBose, R. T., Harris, J. R., and Davis, R. B., Vaccination for hemorrhagic enteritis of turkeys, *Avian Dis.*, 21, 557, 1977.
4. Domermuth, C. H. and Gross, W. B., Hemorrhagic enteritis, in *Diseases of Poultry,* 7th ed., Hofstad, M. S., Calnek, B. W., Helmboldt, C. F., Reid, W. M., and Yoder, H. W., Eds., Iowa State University Press, Ames, 1978, 590.
5. Domermuth, C. H., Weston, C. R., Cowen, B. S., Colwell, W. M., Gross, W. B., and DuBose, R. T., Incidents and distribution of "Avian adenovirus group II splenomegaly of chickens", *Avian Dis.*, 24, 591, 1980.
6. Wyand, D. S., Jakowski, R. M., and Burke, C. N., Marble spleen disease in ring-necked pheasants. Histology and ultrastructure, *Avian Dis.*, 16, 319, 1972.
7. Carlson, H. C., Pettit, J. R., Hemsley, R. V., and Mitchell, W. R., Marble spleen disease of pheasants in Ontario, *Can. J. Comp. Med.*, 37, 281, 1973.
8. Carlson, H. C., Al-Sheikhly, F., Pettit, J. R., and Seawright, G. L., Virus particles in spleens and intestines of turkeys with hemorrhagic enteritis, *Avian Dis.*, 18, 67, 1974.
9. Fujiwara, H., Tanaami, S., Yamaguchi, M., and Yoshino, T., Histopathology of hemorrhagic enteritis in turkeys, *Natl. Inst. Anim. Health Q.*, 15, 68, 1975.
10. Iltis, J. P., Ph.D. dissertation, University of Connecticut, Storrs, 1975.
11. Itakura, C. and Carlson, H. C., Electron microscopic findings of cells with inclusion bodies in experimental hemorrhagic enteritis of turkeys, *Can. J. Comp. Med.*, 39, 299, 1975.
12. Tolin, S. A. and Domermuth, C. H., Hemorrhagic enteritis of turkeys. Electron microscopy of the causal virus, *Avian Dis.*, 19, 118, 1975.
13. Domermuth, C. H. and Gross, W. B., Hemorrhagic enteritis of turkeys, in *Isolation and Identification of Avian Pathogens*, 2nd ed., Hitchner, S. B., Domermuth, C. H., Purchase, H. G., and Williams, J. E., Eds., Creative Printing, New York, 1980, 106.
14. Pomeroy, B. S., Hemorrhagic enteritis, in *Diseases of Poultry,* 6th ed., Hofstad, M. S., Calnek, B. W., Helmboldt, C. F., Reid, W. M., and Yoder, H. W., Jr., Eds., Iowa State University Press, Ames, 1972, 753.
15. Nazerian, K. and Fadley, A., Propagation of virulent and avirulent turkey hemorrhagic enteritis virus in cell culture, *Avian Dis.*, 26, 816, 1982.
16. Domermuth, C. H., Gross, W. B., DuBose, R. T., Douglass, C. S., and Reubush, C. B., Jr., Agar gel diffusion precipitin test for hemorrhagic enteritis of turkeys, *Avian Dis.*, 16, 852, 1972.
17. Itakura, C. and Carlson, H. C., Pathology of spontaneous hemorrhagic enteritis of turkeys, *Can. J. Comp. Med.*, 39, 310, 1975.
18. Gross, W. B. and Domermuth, C. H., Spleen lesions of hemorrhagic enteritis of turkeys, *Avian Dis.*, 20, 455, 1967.
19. Wilcock, B. P. and Thacker, H. L., Focal hepatic necrosis in turkeys with hemorrhagic enteritis, *Avian Dis.*, 20, 205, 1976.
20. Gross, W. B. and Moore, W. E. C., Hemorrhagic enteritis of turkeys, *Avian Dis.*, 11, 296, 1967.
21. Domermuth, C. H. and Gross, W. B., Hemorrhagic enteritis of turkeys. Antiserum — efficacy, preparation and use, *Avian Dis.*, 19, 657, 1975.
22. Gross, W. B., Unpublished data.
23. Domermuth, C. H., Harris, J. R., Thompson, C. T., and Gross, W. B., Vaccination for hemorrhagic enteritis — an update, *Avian Dis.*, in press.

Chapter 3

ESCHERICHIA COLI (STRAIN RDEC-1) DIARRHEA IN THE RABBIT: AN ANIMAL MODEL FOR ENTEROPATHOGENIC *E. COLI* (EPEC) INFECTION OF HUMAN INFANTS

Edgar C. Boedeker and Christopher P. Cheney*

TABLE OF CONTENTS

* The views expressed herein are those of the authors and not necessarily those of the U.S. Army or the Department of Defense.

I. INTRODUCTION/DISEASE DESCRIPTION

Escherichia coli strain-RDEC-1 was initially isolated in pure culture from the stools of a post-weaning rabbit with diarrhea by Dr. J. R. Cantey in his laboratory at the Medical University of South Carolina. Cantey was able to satisfy Koch's postulates and to establish RDEC-1 as a diarrheogenic agent in the rabbit by orogastrically inoculating young rabbits (0.7 to 1.1 kg) with a standard dose of 2×10^6 organisms.[1,2] In these animals diarrheal disease occurred in approximately 70%, with a mortality approaching 30%. Disease could be induced with similar frequency with as few as 1.5×10^2 organisms. Onset of diarrhea usually occurred 6 to 7 days postinoculation, lasted for approximately 4 days, but could recur. Intestinal colonization, as measured by a semiquantitative rectal swab culture technique,[3] reached a maximum at 3 to 4 days postinoculation, or 3 to 4 days before the onset of diarrhea, and did not begin to decrease until 15 days postinoculation. In surviving animals, RDEC-1 organisms were cleared from the stool by the 25th day postinoculation.

II. THE ORGANISM

RDEC-1 is an 015:K?:NM strain. This particular serotype has not specifically been recognized among those associated with diarrheal disease in other species; in particular, it is not one of the enteropathogenic *E. coli* (EPEC) serotypes specifically associated with epidemic childhood diarrhea.[4] The organism is not flagellated and therefore is nonmotile (H-). It has a negatively charged polysaccharide coat, as evidenced by ruthenium red staining, which has been identified morphologically as a "capsule",[5] but which is not a classical K antigen.[6] It better fits the Kauffman classification of a B antigen, a type of acidic lipopolysaccharide commonly found on classical EPEC serotypes.[7] There is some evidence that the organism expresses a negatively charged polysaccharide coat made up of repeating 0 antigen subunits.

Under appropriate growth conditions, the RDEC-1 organism can express at least two types of pili (or fimbriae). On serial passage of the surface-growing organisms from a variety of media, including Trypticase Soy Broth* and Brain Heart Infusion Broth*, the organisms express type 1, or common, pili[8] and will acquire the characteristic property of mannose-sensitive agglutination of guinea-pig red blood cells. The genetic locus for this, as for other type 1 pili, is located on the bacterial chromosome. In contrast, following overnight growth in Penassay Broth*, the organisms express a unique type of nonhemagglutinating pili (Figures 1 and 2) which we have designated AF/R1.[9] AF/R1 pili appear to function as an attachment factor (AF) for rabbit (R) ileal mucosae (the first *E. coli* attachment factor with this species specificity).[10] The RDEC-1 organism contains three large bacterial plasmids of approximately 85, 60, and 37 megadaltons[11] as well as a small 2.5-megadalton plasmid.[2] The 85-megadalton plasmid appears to encode the AF/R1 pili, as indicated by experiments involving transfer of the plasmid to other organisms.[11]

III. PATHOGENESIS

The striking pathological feature of diarrheal disease induced by RDEC-1 is the close adherence of the organisms to the mucosal surface of the distal intestine ileum, cecum, and colon.[1] As shown in Figure 3A, at the time of diarrheal disease there is a confluent layer of organisms over the mucosal surface of the cecum, with a more patchy but definite involvement of the distal ileum and proximal colon. Transmission electron

---

* Difco, Inc., Detroit, Mich.

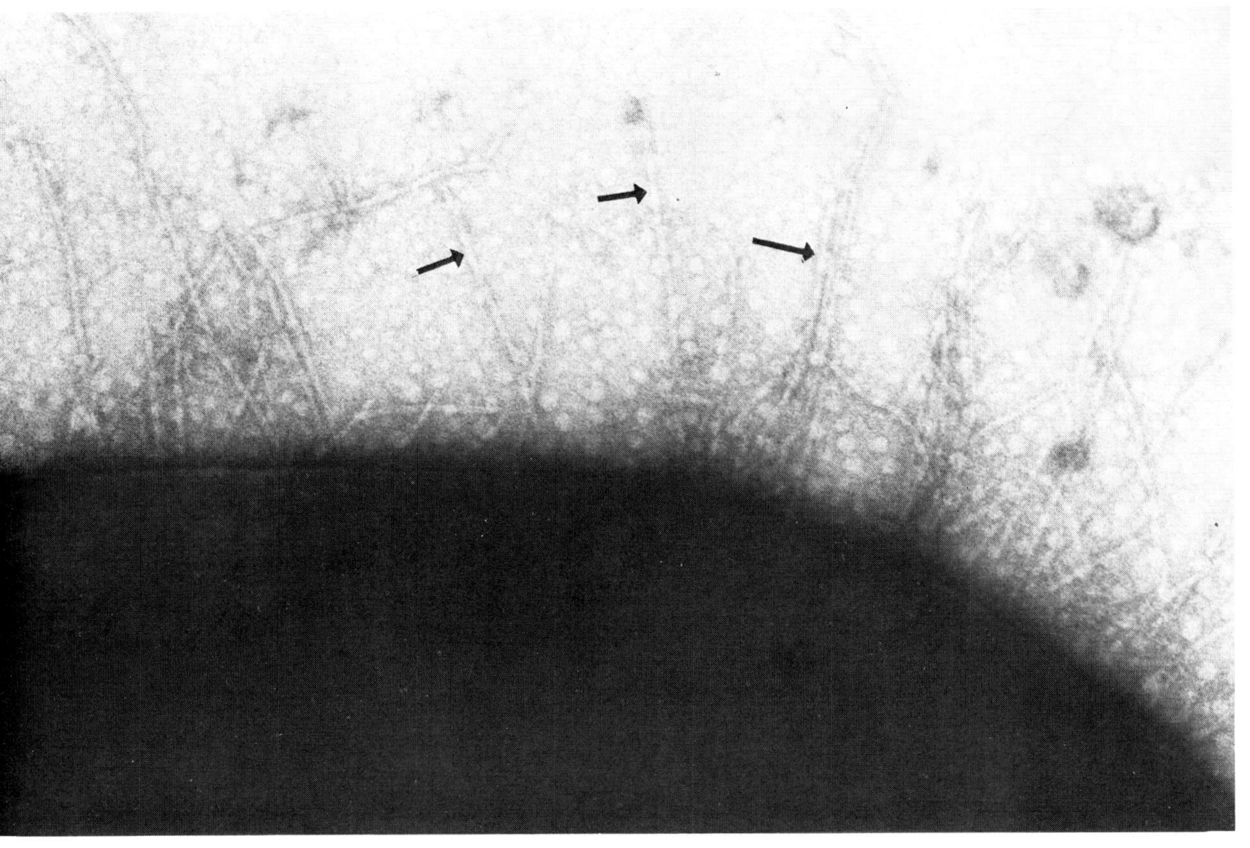

FIGURE 1.   Electron micrograph (× 80,000) of an RDEC-1 organism grown in Penassay broth, negatively stained with 1% phosphotungstic acid. Arrows identify individual AF/R1 pili.

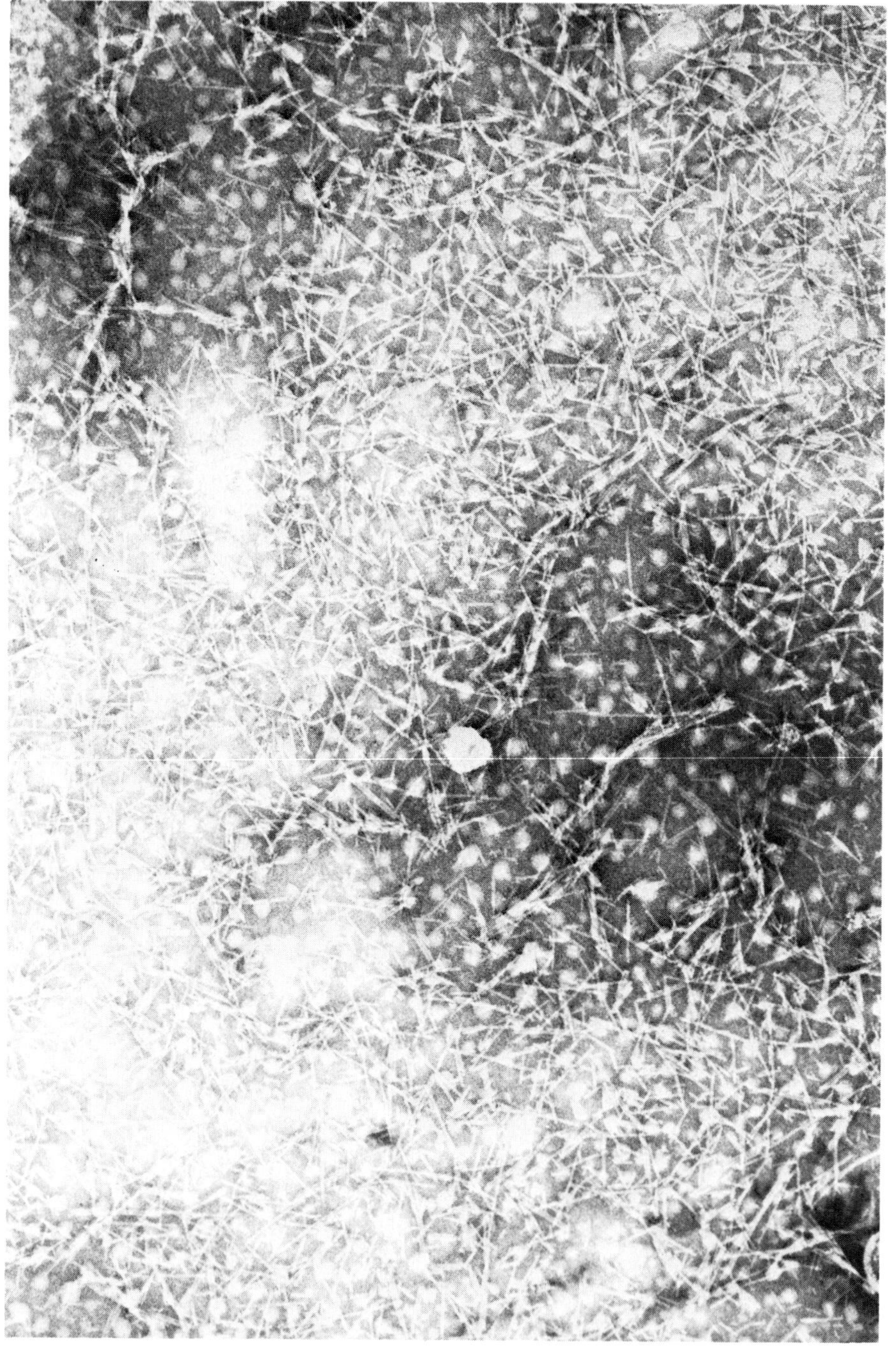

FIGURE 2.   Electron micrograph (× 55,000) of negatively stained (1% phosphotungstic acid) AF/R1 pili prepared from RDEC-1.

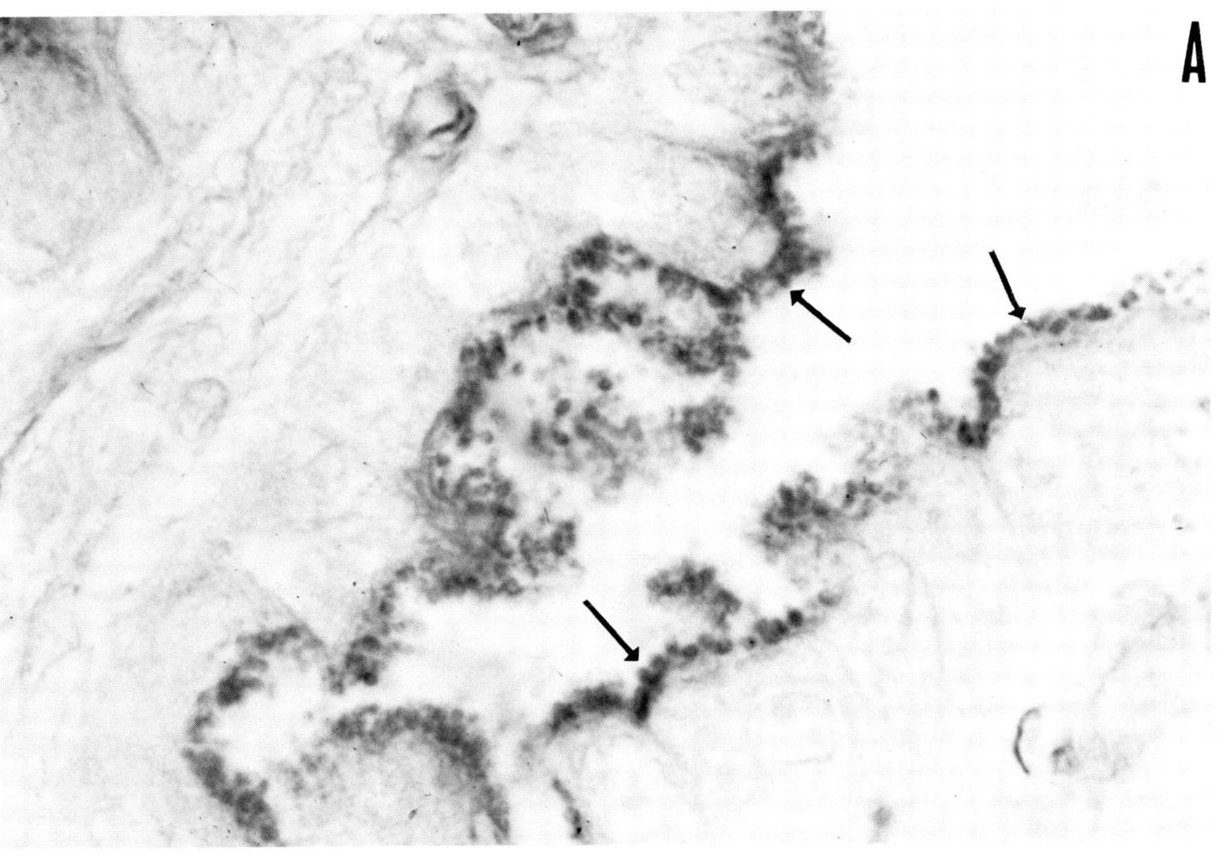

FIGURE 3A.   In vivo mucosal adherence of *E. coli* strain RDEC-1 during the course of infection. Giemsa-stained light micrograph of rabbit cecum ($\times$ 1000) demonstrating a confluent layer of RDEC-1 organisms (arrows) adhering to the apical surface of epithelial cells.

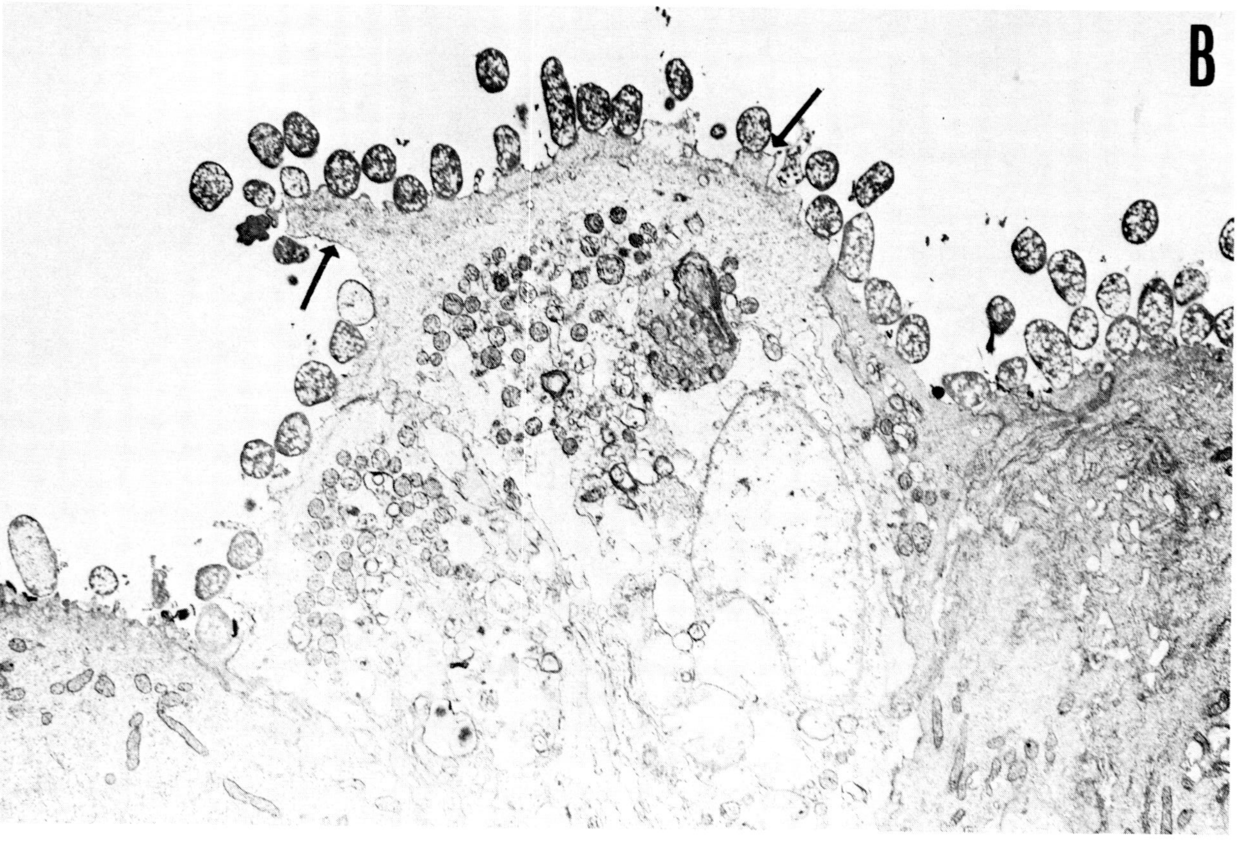

FIGURE 3B.   *In vivo* mucosal adherence of *E. coli* strain RDEC-1 during the course of infection. Electron micrograph of rabbit cecum (× 4000) demonstrating characteristic late stage, close attachment of RDEC-1 organisms to the apical surface of epithelial cells. Loss of apical microvilli, disruption of the apical cytoskeleton, and pedestal formation (arrows) are evident. (Electron micrograph courtesy of L. Inman and A. Takeuchi.)

microscopy reveals a characteristic appearance of involved areas (Figure 3B).[12] At the apical surface of the epithelial cells there is a loss of normal microvillar architecture that is related to a disruption of the cytoskeletal elements (bundled actin filaments). The plasma membrane remains intact, but it extends in characteristic cup-like or pedestal projections which partially surround adherent organisms. There is a loss of intestinal glycocalyx in these areas and only 11 μm separates the apical plasma membrane of the epithelial cell from the outer membrane of the bacterial cell.[2,6,12] This close adherence appears to be a late stage of the attachment progress, and other organisms can be seen more peripherally associated (50 to 100 mm) with epithelial cells with intact microvilli in a manner characteristic of the enterotoxigenic *E. coli*.[2,5,6] This peripheral adherence appears to be an early stage of RDEC-1 association with the mucosae. In addition, intermediate steps involved with elongation, budding, vesiculation, and shedding of microvilli have been observed.

A. Mechanisms of Adherence

In vitro studies in our laboratory have demonstrated that RDEC-1 organisms grown in Penassay broth adhere in a rapid, temperature-sensitive, and pH-dependent (pH optimum 7.4) manner to the mucosal surface of frozen sections of normal rabbit ileum (Figure 4A) as well as to isolated apical brush borders from rabbit ileum (Figure 4B).[13] These interactions are species-specific and appear to involve specific recognition between an adhesin on the bacterial cell and a receptor on the host epithelial cells.[10]

1. Bacterial Adhesins

In vitro interaction between RDEC-1 and host intestinal brush borders depends on the expression of pili designated AF/R1. Three lines of evidence have been developed to support this conclusion.[14] First, the phenotypic expression of AF/R1 pili can be suppressed by growth in enriched media and under these conditions in vitro adhesion is also eliminated.[11] Second, AF/R1 pili can be transferred, along with the 85-megadalton RDEC-1 plasmid, to other organisms. Organisms inheriting AF/R1 pili are adherent to rabbit brush borders.[11] Finally, isolated AF/R1 pili (Figure 2) adhere to the ileal mucosa with the same distribution and species specificity as do the whole organisms (Figure 5).[9] Thus AF/R1 pili appeared to mediate at least the early stage of association between RDEC-1 and the epithelial cell. The mechanisms whereby the bacterium continues its interaction with epithelial cells to produce late-stage or close adherence with cytoskeletal disruption are not clear, but may also involve AF/R1 pili.

2. Host Receptors

In vitro adherence to brush borders has been used to investigate the characteristics of host receptors for the AF/R1 adhesins. In vitro interactions of RDEC-1 bearing AF/R1 with brush borders are non-mannose-sensitive and cannot be inhibited by any of a series of membrane sugars or amino sugars.[13] Receptor activity can be released by papain digestion, suggesting that the receptors are expressed on extrinsic proteins or glycoproteins. Receptors are present on jejunal brush borders, but less densely than on ileal brush borders. Receptor activity is absent on brush borders prepared from animals less than 21 days of age,[15] which corresponds to the age of weaning in the rabbit. At this age there is also a marked change in the enzyme composition of the brush border, characterized by a shift from a predominance of lactase to a predominance of sucrase and isomaltase. In vivo experiments have confirmed the increased susceptibility of rabbits to colonization by RDEC-1 at the age (21 days) of first appearance of receptors.[16] This suggests that the particular susceptibility of weanling rabbits to RDEC-1 infection is related to the appearance of mucosal receptors as well as to the withdrawal of passive maternal immune protection via the milk.

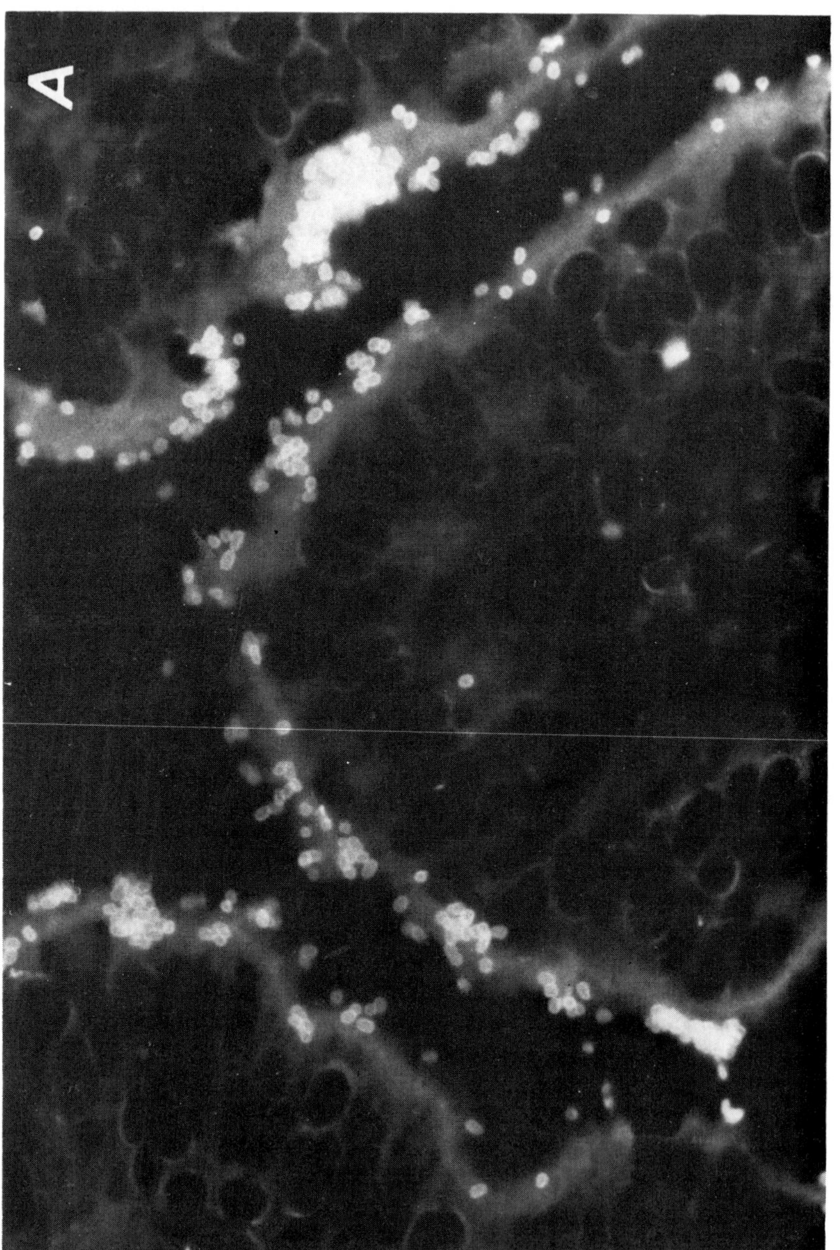

FIGURE 4. In vitro mucosal adherence of *E. coli* strain RDEC-1. (A) Light micrograph (× 1000) of a frozen section of normal rabbit ileum that was overlain with piliated RDEC-1 organisms. After washing, RDEC-1 organisms were stained with a fluorescent double antibody technique. Distribution of organisms is the same as that seen in Figure 3A. (B) Phase contrast light micrograph of RDEC-1 organisms adhering to isolated rabbit ileal brush borders (× 1200). Both in vitro interactions (A and B) are species-specific.

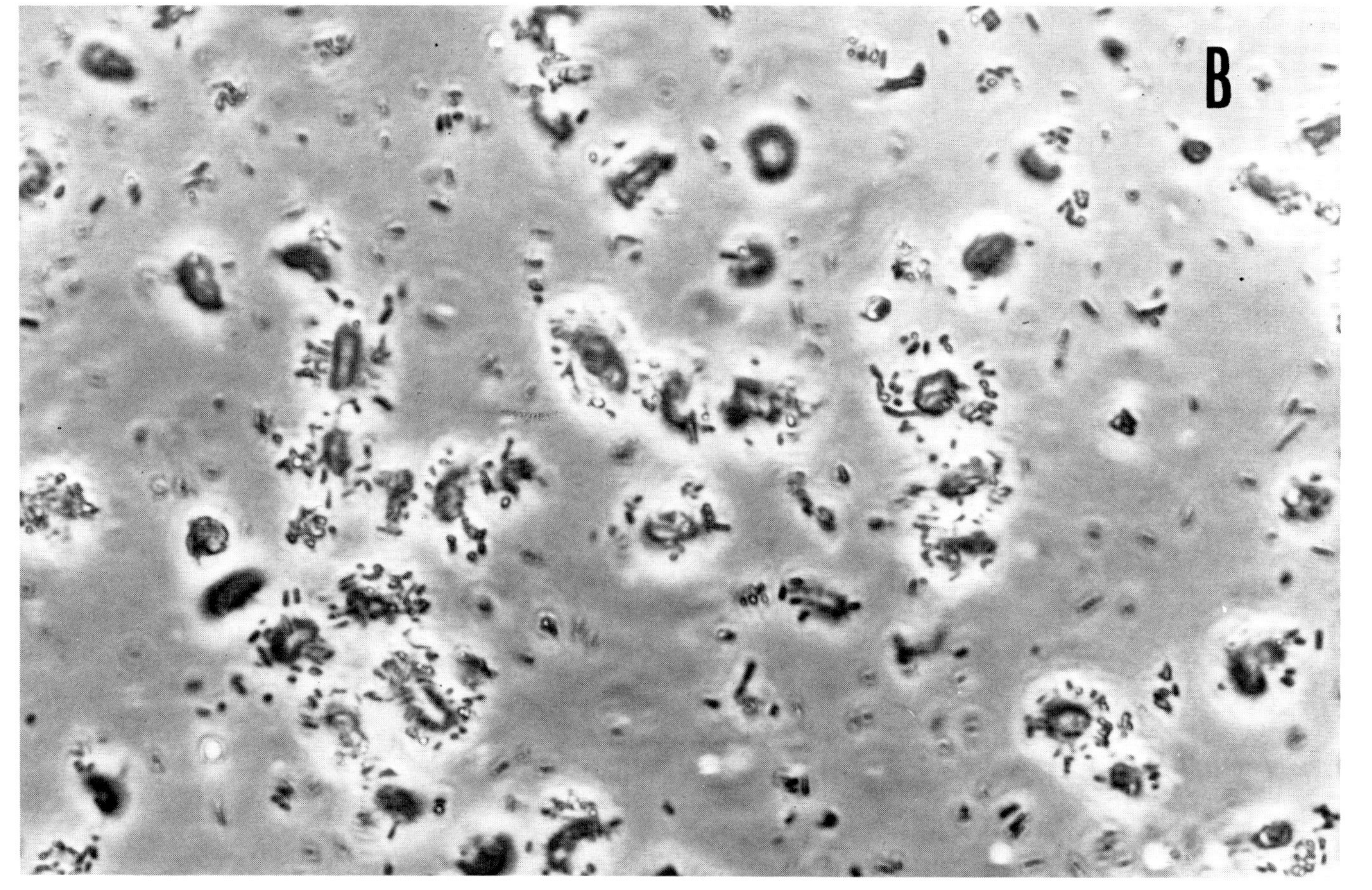

FIGURE 4B.

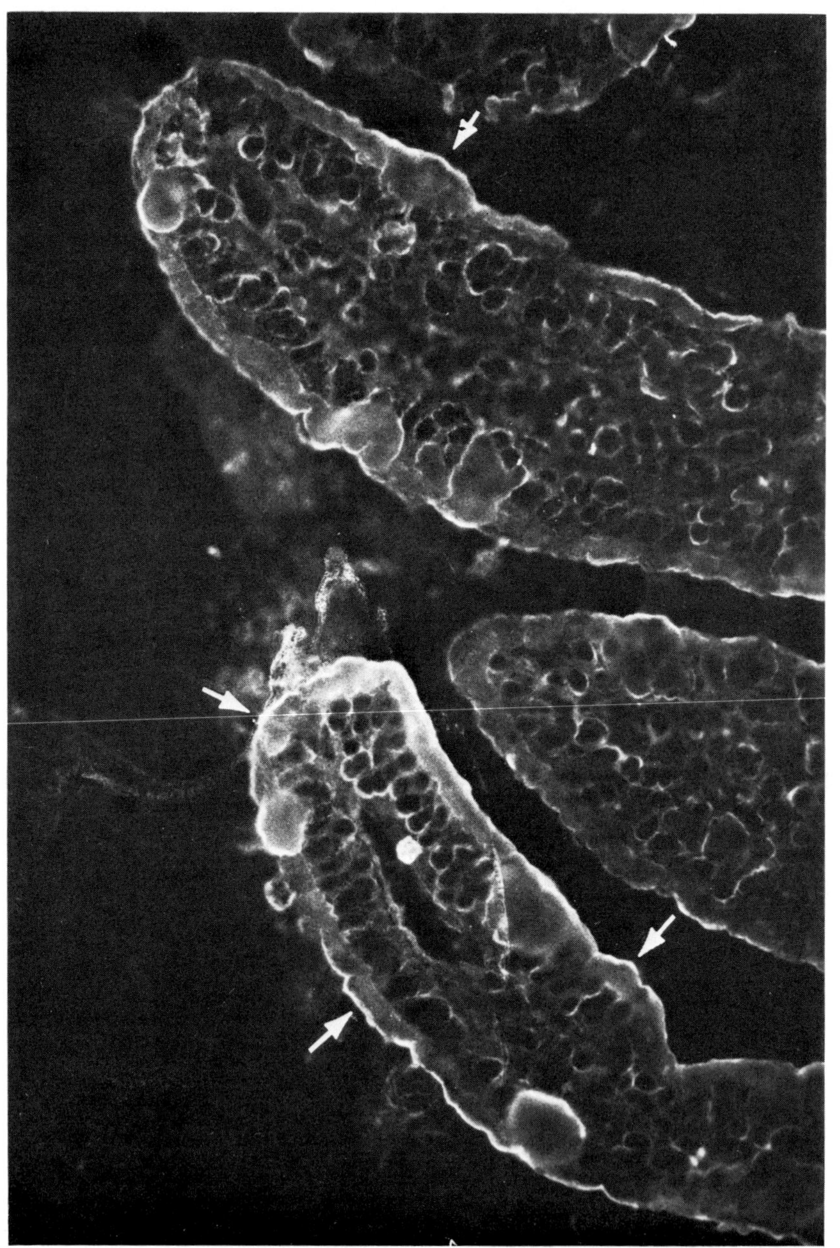

FIGURE 5.   Light photomicrograph (× 780) of a frozen section of a normal rabbit ileum incubated with AF/R1 pili and stained with a specific fluorescent double antibody technique. Linear fluorescence (arrows), demonstrating the affinity of AF/R1 for the mucosal surface, has the same distribution as that seen for whole organisms in Figure 4A.

B. Mechanism of Diarrhea Production

RDEC-1 organisms do not produce classical heat-labile (LT) or heat-stable (ST) *E. coli* enterotoxin, and they are not invasive. These observations led Cantey, in his original description of the disease,[1] to suggest that this organism caused diarrheal disease by a novel, if unspecified, mechanism distinct from the recognized mechanisms of LT production, ST production, and invasiveness. Mucosal adherence of these organisms correlates well with the occurrence of diarrhea, and the adherent organisms produce a profound alteration in the apical portion of the intestinal epithelial cells (Figure 3B). It is possible that surface membrane changes, including loss of surface area and/or changes in membrane permeability as well as disruption of the cytoskeletal elements, could cause diarrhea by interfering with the normal absorptive process or by the induction of a secretory state. The close apposition of the organisms would also place them in a favorable position for the transfer of a cytotonic or cytotoxic product directly to the epithelial cells. Recently O'Brien et al.[17] demonstrated and confirmed that RDEC-1 is among the group of *E. coli* strains, including a number of EPEC serotypes, that produces moderate levels of a toxin that is immunologically identical to Shigella dysenteria 1 toxin. This type of toxin has been shown to exert its effects through inhibition of protein synthesis at the ribosomal level. In addition, using perfusion techniques, Mullaney and Cantey[18] have demonstrated the presence of enterotoxin activity in whole-cell lysates of RDEC-1 organisms. Thus, it seems likely, although it is not definitely established, that toxin production by the adherent organisms will prove to be an important part of the pathogenesis of this disease. It should be noted that the 7-day interval between oral inoculation of RDEC-1 and the development of diarrhea is relatively long compared to the incubation period of 2 to 3 days for classical enterotoxigenic *E. coli* strains. It is possible that toxin production by luminal organisms may serve to prepare the host mucosa for RDEC-1 adherence either by altering the mucus coat or by causing alterations in intestinal motility. These topics are currently subjects for ongoing investigation.

C. Relation to the Immune System/Clearance

Although RDEC-1 diarrhea can recur shortly after the initial clearance of the organism (a phenomenon which may be related to coprophagia in the rabbit), recovery from RDEC-1 diarrhea provides protection against subsequent challenge with the organism. Presumably, this protection is related to the development of a local secretory immunoglobulin A response to RDEC-1 in the intestine. Cantey[20] has demonstrated that the feeding of immune secretory IgA, obtained from the milk of pregnant rabbits who had recovered from RDEC-1 infection, protected animals against challenge with RDEC-1. This same IgA preparation[34] can prevent and reverse the attachment of RDEC-1 to rabbit ileal brush borders in vitro.

Recently, Cantey and Inman and Inman and Cantey[21,22] have shown that RDEC-1 has a unique relation to the intestinal immune system in that during the course of experimental infection, RDEC-1 organisms are first found adhering to the lymphoepithelial tissue overlying Peyer's patches. This adherence occurs at a time when the organisms are not adherent to adjacent absorptive epithelial cells. Moreover the attached organism divide on the surface of the Peyer's patch to develop microcolonies. The interaction of RDEC-1 with the lymphoepithelium appears to first involve the M (microfold or membranous) cells overlying the Peyer's patch.[22] These M cells are specialized epithelia cells felt to be involved in sampling luminal antigens for presentation to the gut mucosal immune system. This interaction of RDEC-1 with the lymphoepithelium presumably leads to the development of a local immune response that is related to the initial clearing of the infection. In addition, since the organisms are found associated and dividing over the lymphoepithelium prior to interaction with the absorptive cells, Cantey has postulated that RDEC-1 organisms may differentiate in this area to develop the particular surface properties (such as AF/R1 pilus adhesins) necessary for subsequent interaction with the absorptive epithelial cells.

IV. RELATION TO HUMAN ENTEROPATHOGENIC *E. COLI* (EPEC) DISEASE

RDEC-1 infection of rabbits has come to be recognized as the best available animal model for diarrhea caused by EPEC strains in humans.[23,24] This limited group of serotypes responsible for epidemic outbreaks of infantile enteritis has been recognized since the 1940s,[4,25] but the pathogenic mechanisms whereby they induce diarrheal disease are only beginning to be defined. Organisms of the EPEC serotypes rarely produce classical *E. coli* LT and ST, and yet their ability to produce diarrheal disease in volunteers has been firmly established[26] in the absence of the ability to produce LT or ST. Klipstein et al.[27] have demonstrated the production of enterotoxic substances by EPEC strains using perfusion techniques. Recently, EPEC strains have been shown to produce intermediate levels of Shigella dysenteria 1 toxin,[17] a property they share with the RDEC-1 strain. This toxin is likely to prove to be of importance in the pathogenesis of this type of diarrheal disease as described above for RDEC-1.

A second major similarity between EPEC strains and RDEC-1 is their characteristic enteroadherence. Ulshen and Rollo[28] were the first to describe the enteroadherence of an EPEC strain to the small-bowel mucosa of an infant with diarrhea. Their important report documents a transmission electron microscopic appearance of close attachment of the organisms to the apical surface of intestinal epithelial cells which is entirely analogous to that previously described by Takeuchi et al.[12] for RDEC-1 (Figure 3B). Subsequent reports of similar enteroadherence of EPEC strains, involving the colon as well as the small intestine have been published by Rothbaum et al.,[29] Clausen and Christie,[30] and Philips.[31] Thus, it now seems to be firmly established that EPEC organisms adhere to the intestinal mucosa in a manner that is entirely analogous to that of RDEC-1. The report by Moon et al.,[32] demonstrating similar effacing adherence to pig and rabbit intestine by both RDEC-1 and EPEC isolates, has emphasized this analogy. In their report, Clausen and Christie[20] demonstrated that EPEC 0111 and 0119 isolates adhere to HEPII cells in tissue cultures. Although the EPEC adhesins expressed on the bacterial surface have not been defined, Baldini et al.,[33] using tissue culture adherence assays, have recently demonstrated that the enteroadherence of EPEC strains is mediated by a large-molecular-weight plasmid, reminiscent of the plasmid associated with in vitro adherence of RDEC-1 and with AF/R1 pilus expression. If the analogy between EPEC strains and RDEC-1 is complete, EPEC strains may ultimately be shown to express pilus adhesins under the appropriate growth conditions.

The availability of an animal model for EPEC-induced diarrhea should be of particular importance in studying methods of therapy, in particular active and passive immunotherapy, for this important group of diseases.

REFERENCES

1. Cantey, J. R. and Blake, R. K., Diarrhea due to *Escherichia coli* in the rabbit: a novel mechanism, *J. Infect. Dis.*, 135, 454, 1977.
2. Cantey, J. R., The rabbit model of *Escherichia coli* (strain RDEC-1) diarrhea, in *Attachment of Microorganisms to the Gut Mucosa*, Vol. 1, Boedeker, E. C., Ed., CRC Press, Boca Raton, Fla., 1984.

3. Cantey, J. R. and Hosterman, D. S., Characterization of colonization of the rabbit gastrointestinal tract by *Escherichia coli* RDEC-1, *Infect. Immunol.*, 26, 1099, 1979.
4. Gangarosa, E. J. and Merson, M. H., Epidemiologic assessment of the relevance of the so-called enteropathogenic serogroups of *Escherichia coli* diarrhea, *N. Engl. J. Med.*, 296, 1211, 1977.
5. Cantey, J. R., Lushbaugh, W. B., and Inman, L. R., Attachment of bacteria to intestinal epithelial cells in diarrhea caused by *Escherichia coli* strain RDEC-1 in the rabbit: stages and role of the capsule, *J. Infect. Dis.*, 143, 219, 1981.
6. Cantey, J. R. and Inman, L. R., Role of the negatively charged surface polysaccharide in the adherence of *Escherichia coli* strain RDEC-1 to gut epithelial cells in the rabbit, in *Attachment of Microorganisms to the Gut Mucosa*, Vol. 1, Boedeker, E. C., Ed., CRC Press, Boca Raton, Fla., 1984.
7. Jann, K. and Jann, B., The K antigens of *Escherichia coli*, in *Progress in Allergy*, Vol. 33, Hanson, L. A., Kallos, P., and Westphal, O., Eds., S. Karger, Basel, 1983, 53.
8. Brinton, C. C., The piliation phase syndrome and the uses of purified pili in disease control, in Proc. 13th Jt. Conf. Cholera, Publ. (NIH)78-1590, Department of Health, Education and Welfare, Washington, D.C., 1978, 34.
9. Berendson, R., Cheney, C. P., Schad, P. A., and Boedeker, E. C., Species-specific binding of purified pili (AF/R1) from the *Escherichia coli* RDEC-1 to rabbit intestinal mucosa, *Gastroenterology*, 85, 837, 1983.
10. Cheney, C. P., Schad, P. A., Formal, S. B., and Boedeker, E. C., Species specificity of in vitro *Escherichia coli* adherence to host intestinal cell membranes and its correlation with in vivo colonization and infectivity, *Infect. Immunol.*, 28, 1019, 1980.
11. Cheney, C. P., Formal, S. B., Schad, P. A., and Boedeker, E. C., Genetic transfer of a mucosal adherence factor (R1) from an enteropathogenic *Escherichia coli* strain into a *Shigella flexneri* strain and the phenotypic suppression of this adherence factor, *J. Infect. Dis.*, 147, 711, 1983.
12. Takeuchi, A., Inman, L. R., O'Hanley, P. D., Cantey, J. R., and Lushbaugh, W. B., Scanning and transmission electron microscopic study of *Escherichia coli* 015 (RDEC-1) enteric infection in rabbits, *Infect. Immunol.*, 19, 686, 1978.
13. Cheney, C. P., Boedeker, E. C., and Formal, S. B., Quantitation of the adherence of an enteropathogenic *Escherichia coli* to isolated rabbit intestinal brush borders, *Infect. Immunol.*, 26, 736, 1979.
14. Boedeker, E. C. and Cheney, C. P., Pili as adherence factors in *Escherichia coli* strain RDEC-1, in *Attachment of Microorganisms to the Gut Mucosa*, Vol. 1, Boedeker, E. C., Ed., CRC Press, Boca Raton, Fla., 1984.
15. Cheney, C. P. and Boedeker, E. C., Appearance of host intestinal receptors for pathogenic *E. coli* with age, in *Attachment of Microorganisms to the Gut Mucosa*, Vol. 2, Boedeker, E. C., Ed., CRC Press, Boca Raton, Fla., 1984.
16. Shoham, H. H., Kelly, E. P., Finlay, P. G., Cheney, C. P., and Boedeker, E. C., Appearance of mucosal receptors for pathogenic *E. coli* with age: in vivo studies of RDEC-1 enteroadherence and colonization in infant rabbit, in *Proc. 4th Int. Symp. Neonatal Diarrhea*, Acres, S. D., Ed., VIDO, Saskatoon, Canada, 1983.
17. O'Brien, A. D., LaVeck, G. D., Thompson, M. R., and Formal, S. B., Production of *Shigella dysenteriae* type 1-like toxin by *Escherichia coli*, *J. Infect. Dis.*, 146, 763, 1972.
18. Mullaney, D. T. and Cantey, J. R., Detection of enterotoxin-like activity in the whole cell lysate of an enteroadherent *Escherichia coli* (strain RDEC-1), *Clin. Res.*, 30, 374A, 1982.
19. Guerrant, R. L., Yet another pathogenic mechanisms for *Escherichia coli* diarrhea, *N. Engl. J. Med.*, 302, 113, 1980.
20. Cantey, J. R., Prevention of bacterial infections of mucosal surfaces by immune secretory IgA, in *Advances in Experimental Medicine and Biology*, Vol. 107, McGhee, J. R., Mestecky, J., and Babb, J. F., Eds., Plenum Press, New York, 1978, 461.
21. Cantey, J. R. and Inman, L. R., Diarrhea due to *Escherichia coli* strain DEC-1 in the rabbit: the Peyer's patch as the initial site of attachment and colonization, *J. Infect. Dis.*, 143, 440, 1981.
22. Inman, L. R. and Cantey, J. R., Specific adherence of *Escherichia coli* (strain RDEC-1) to membranous (M) cells of the Peyer's patch in *Escherichia coli* diarrhea in the rabbit, *J. Clin. Invest.*, 71, 1, 1983.
23. Boedeker, E. C. and Cheney, C. P., RDEC-1 enteric infection of rabbits: a model for epidemic infantile diarrhea caused by enteropathogenic *Escherichia coli* (EPEC) strains, in *Experimental Bacterial and Parasitic Infections*, Keusch, J. and Wadstrom, T., Eds., Elsevier, New York, 1983, 203.
24. Anon., Mechanisms in enteropathogenic *Escherichia coli* diarrhea (editorial), *Lancet*, 1, 1254, 1983.
25. Bray, J., Isolation of antigenically homogeneous strains of *Bact. coli Neapolitanum* from summer diarrhea of infants, *J. Pathol. Bacteriol.*, 57, 239, 1945.
26. Levine, M. M., Berquist, E. J., Nalin, D. R., Waterman, D. H., Hornick, R. B., Young, C. R., and Sotsman, S., *Escherichia coli* strains that cause diarrhea but do not produce heat-labile or heat stable enterotoxins and are noninvasive, *Lancet*, 1, 1119, 1978.

27. Klipstein, F. A., Rowe, B., Engert, R. F., Short, H. B., and Gross, R. J., Enterotoxicity of entero-pathogenic serotypes of *Escherichia coli* isolated from infants with epidemic diarrhea, *Infect. Immunol.*, 21, 171, 1978.
28. Ulshen, M. H. and Rollo, J. L., Pathogenesis of *Escherichia coli* gastroenteritis in man—another mechanism, *N. Engl. J. Med.*, 302, 99, 1980.
29. Rothbaum, R. J., McAdams, A. J., Giannella, R. A., and Partin, J. C., A clinicopathologic study of enterocyte adherent *Escherichia coli:* a cause of protracted diarrhea in infants, *Gastroenterology,* 83, 441, 1982.
30. Clausen, C. R. and Christie, D. L., Chronic diarrhea in infants caused by adherent enteropathogenic *Escherichia coli, J. Pediatr.,* 100, 358, 1982.
31. Phillips, A. D., Small intestine mucosa in childhood in health and disease, *Scand. J. Gastroenterol.,* 16, 65, 1981.
32. Moon, H. W., Whipp, S. C., Argenzio, R. G., Levine, M. M., and Giannella, R. A., Attaching and effacing activities of rabbit and human enteropathogenic *Escherichia coli* in pig and rabbit intestines, *Infect. Immunol.,* 41, 1340, 1983.
33. Baldini, M., Kaper, J. B., Levine, M. M., Candy, D. C. A., and Moon, H. W., Plasmid mediated adhesion in enteropathogenic *Escherichia coli, J. Pediatr. Gastroenterol. Nutr.,* 2, 534, 1983.
34. Boedeker, E. C. and Cheney, C. P., Unpublished observations.

Chapter 4

ENTERIC PATHOPHYSIOLOGY OF BOVINE COLIBACILLOSIS

James C. Keith, Jr. and Carl J. Pfeiffer

TABLE OF CONTENTS

I. INTRODUCTION

Acute enteric infection causing diarrhea and dysentery is one of the leading causes of infant deaths in underdeveloped countries and contribute to one of the greatest economic losses associated with death and morbidity of domestic food animals. Bovine colibacillosis, caused by enterotoxigenic strains of *Escherichia coli,* is a leading cause of death in the U.S., accounting for the majority of calf losses, which approach $100 million yearly. It can, therefore, be anticipated that the study of animal models of such entities will contribute to a better understanding of both human and animal disease mechanisms. It has been established that there are many principles in common between human and animal intestinal reactions to bacterial, viral, and toxic agents responsible for acute hemorrhagic diarrhea or dysentery, and that these diatheses frequently represent a common clinical manifestation of several concurrent events. The latter condition may include infection with pathogenic microbial strains, impaired or undeveloped immune status of the host, malnutrition, environmental stress, and filthy or crowded living conditions.

It is frequently some combination of the above factors that allows infection and colonization of the proximal small intestine with a virulent microbial organism. In some instances more than one pathogenic microbial species may be present and viral and bacterial infections may be concurrent. Diarrhea observed in newborn calves may be caused by *Escherichia coli,* Salmonellae, *Pseudomonas* sp., Chlamydiae, and various viruses, and in the foal by an even greater spectrum of organisms. In the piglet, *E. coli, Clostridium perfringens* Type C, and transmissible gastroenteritis (TGE) virus may be pathogenic for this malady. Infection in the newborn animal is usually associated with deficient immunity, resulting from inadequate transfer of maternal immunity via colostrum, or lack of maternal immunity to a new, virulent strain. In humans, acute diarrheal diseases are frequently caused by enteropathogenic *E. coli, Salmonella, Shigella,* or other bacteria or intestinal parasites. There seem to be great similarities in the animal and human intestinal responses to *E. coli* infections, and both artificial animal models (e.g., rabbit model) and spontaneous animal models (e.g., bovine colibacillosis) offer opportunities to investigate the mechanisms of this disease. The secretory diarrhea produced in bovine colibacillosis closely parallels certain types of *E. coli* diarrhea in human neonates (e.g., infantile diarrhea), and also resembles the diarrhea of human cholera. Conversely, further elucidation of human colibacillosis might be expected to contribute to the therapy and/or prevention of this problem in veterinary medicine.

II. CHARACTERISTICS OF THE BOVINE GUT

The bovine neonatal gastrointestinal tract closely resembles that of a simple, monogastric species such as the human being. Several weeks elapse before ruminant stomach development occurs. *E. coli* are normally present within the distal portions of the gut, with the highest concentrations occurring in the colon, cecum, and distal ileum.[1]

The immune status of the neonatal calf is of crucial importance in regard to the calf's ability to deal with *E. coli* infection. Few, if any, immunoglobulins cross the bovine placenta and thus it is of great importance that the calf ingest adequate amounts of colostrum as soon after birth as possible. The colostrum is rich in IgG and IgM, and these immunoglobulins are rapidly absorbed in the bovine intestine during the first 24 hr post partum.[2] After 24 hr, little if any colostrum crosses the intestinal barrier and reaches the bloodstream.

III. PATHOGENIC CHARACTERISTICS OF *E. COLI*

Bovine diarrhea may be caused by a variety of pathogenetic mechanisms associated with *E. coli* infection. Indeed, in very recent years the multiplicity of mechanisms involved in the pathogenesis of colibacillosis of several species, the variations in response to different virulent strains of *E. coli,* and the species-specific character of the host-animal reactions to strains of *E. coli* have been reported. Earlier studies of a decade ago had established two different pathogenetic mechanisms. These included the direct invasion of the intestinal epithelial cells, the lamina propria, and the bloodstream by *E. coli,* as well as the production of heat-stable or heat-labile types of enterotoxins.[3-6]

Later evidence that the diarrhea observed in some species infected with *E. coli* of strains did not produce enterotoxins and were not invasive, suggested that other mechanisms must be operable.[7] One of the available animal models for experimental colibacillosis — the rabbit infected with *E. coli* 015 (RDEC-1) — provided morphologic evidence of another mechanism for the pathogenesis.[6] It was observed that intestinal epithelial cell microvilli were damaged by adhering bacteria during the absence of enterotoxin production or invasion. As discussed by Brasitus,[8] this brush border damage in rabbits was very similar to that seen in human infants with chronic diarrhea and *E. coli* overgrowth in the upper small intestine. Brush border damage and villus shortening have been seen in bovine colibacillosis. However, on closer examination, concurrent infection with rota or corona virus was detected.[9] The adherence of enteropathogenic bacteria to the epithelial surface represents a general mechanism by which the organisms can colonize the proximal small intestine and replicate without being cleared by normal intestinal peristalsis. Data have now established that this mechanism is a key determinant of infectivity, and comparison of strains of *E. coli* with greater or lesser virulence have indicated enhanced adherence properties with the more virulent strains.

The RDEC-1 strain of *E. coli* used in the rabbit model described above colonizes the mucosal surface of the ileum and cecum, though in bovine and human *E. coli* infections adherence is seen more proximally in the small intestine. The adherence of *E. coli* to the gut wall is dependent upon the presence of surface pili on the bacteria — fine hairlike structures that can be seen by electron microscopy (Figure 1). Animal studies with enterotoxigenic *E. coli* have identified pilus-like surface antigens of porcine origin (K88 and 987P) and of strains pathogenic for calves and lambs (K99 and F41). In the RDEC-1 strain of *E. coli,* environmental conditions which reduce the development of pili upon the bacterial surface are also associated with reduced adherence.[8,10] Pili have been characterized according to type. Type 1 pili are commonly found on both non-pathogenic and pathogenic strains of *E. coli* and these pili have the ability to facilitate adherence to, and hemagglutination of, guinea pig erythrocytes.

Production of pili and enterotoxin is plasmid-mediated in animals and humans. It is interesting to note, however, that the enterotoxin genes are easily lost in the *E. coli* strains isolated from human infections, while the enterotoxin genes from bovine isolates are quite stable. Many times, both the enterotoxin genes and the pili genes are lost concurrently from human *E. coli* isolates.[11] This instability of plasmid-mediated traits from *E. coli* strains affecting humans could account for the marked variability in finding enterotoxigenic strains in outbreaks of human diarrheal disease caused by *E. coli.*[12] The pili observed on RDEC-1 strain *E. coli* were not Type 1 pili and do not hemagglutinate erythrocytes.

Berendson and co-workers[13] have recently studied the species specificity of binding properties, i.e., adherence, of purified pili from REDC-1 strain *E. coli.* They reported that purified pili incubated with post-frozen sections of rabbit ileum attached from the crypts to the villus tips, but sections from rat, guinea pig, and human small intestine did not bind with RDEC-1-extracted pili, as determined by an indirect immunofluorescence technique. Nonpiliated RDEC-1 intact organisms did not significantly attach to the rabbit ileum. These studies confirm the important role of pili to the bacterial adherence of *E. coli* and the species specificity of the binding phenomenon.

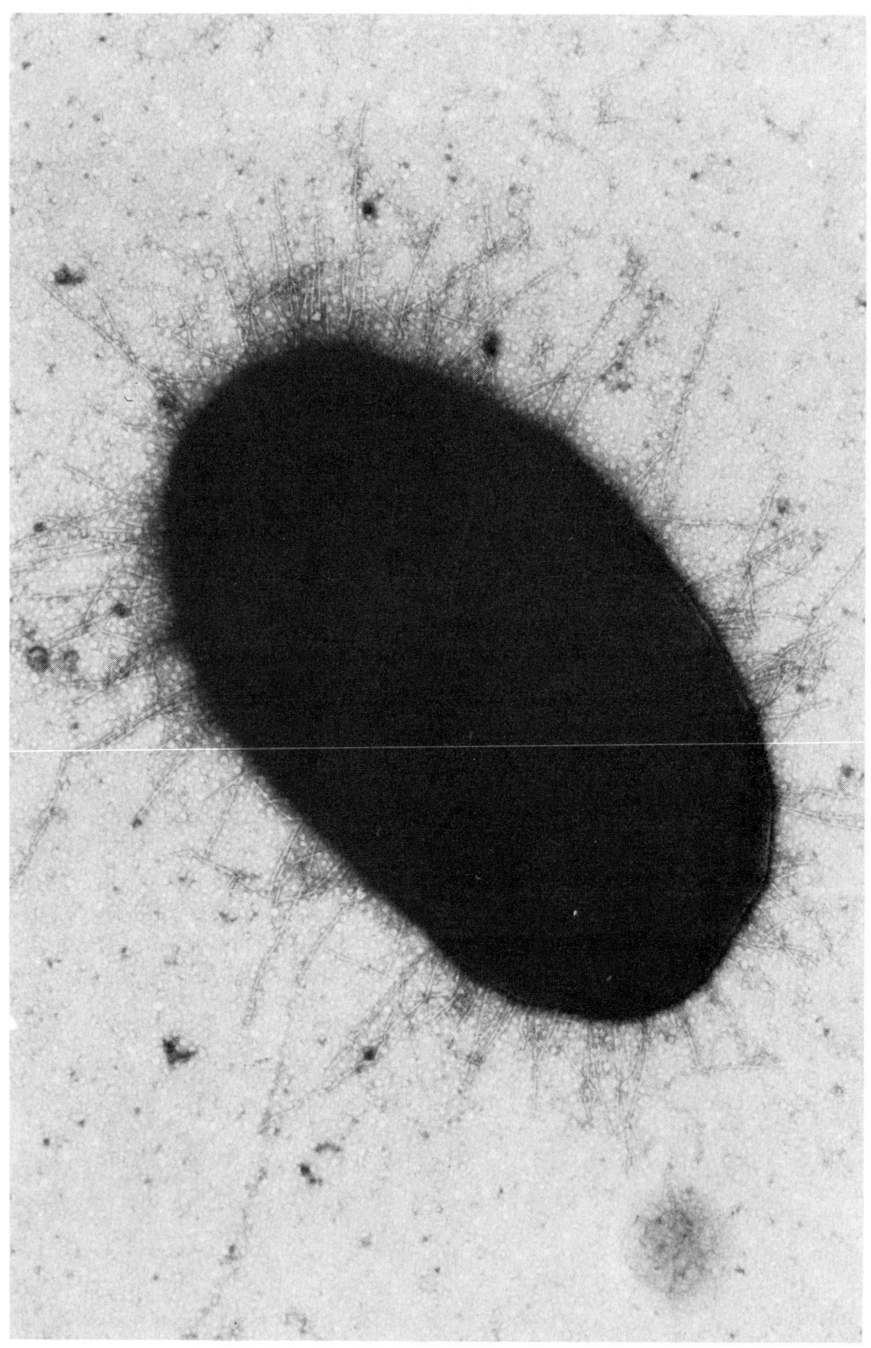

FIGURE 1.   Negatively stained (1% phosphotungstic acid, PTA) RDEC-1 organism, showing numerous pili extending from the surface. (Magnification × 32,800.) (Prepared through courtesy of Drs. E. C. Boedeker and C. P. Cheney.)

Detailed studies on the specificity of the *E. coli* strains causing bovine colibacillosis, with respect to comparative binding with other mammalian species, have not yet been reported. Data on adherence of human enterotoxigenic *E. coli* H10407 have shown that this virulent strain binds with terminal ileal brush borders,[14] but that a genetically nonpiliated mutant of *E. coli* H10407 does not colonize the human intestine.[15-18] The role of mucosal adherence of enteropathogenic *E. coli* strains has also recently been emphasized in reports of infantile diarrhea by Rothbaum and co-workers[19] and Ulshen and Rollo.[20]

IV. BOVINE CLINICAL SYNDROME

Bovine colibacillosis in colostrum-fed calves is characterized by colonization of the proximal small intestine by enterotoxigenic *E. coli.* The most common source of the *E. coli* is the feces from another infected animal. Therefore, those animals housed in close confinement and subjected to substandard sanitation practices are most likely to be exposed to the infectious agent. This is followed by the production of both heat-stable and heat-labile enterotoxins. The heat-stable toxin is a low-molecular-weight compound that stimulates water and electrolyte secretion via activation of guanylate cyclase.[21] The heat-labile toxin is of high molecular weight and shares partial antigenic identity with the enterotoxin of *Vibrio cholerae.*[22] The heat-labile toxin causes increased secretion of fluid and electrolytes, primarily HCO_3^-,[23] by activating adenyl cyclase.

The response to the heat-labile toxin appears to be delayed in onset but lasts longer than the heat-stable enterotoxin.[22] If the infected calf is colostrum fed but less than 24 hr old when infected, a severe and often fatal diarrhea ensues.[24] Barring concurrent viral infections, little, if any, intestinal villus damage occurs and the diarrhea is purely secretory in nature. Therefore, in this instance it closely resembles the diarrhea produced by *Vibrio cholerae.*

Since the basic pathophysiologies are very similar, the treatments also closely resemble one another. The absorptive unit of the gut is still intact and if the disease is detected early (before severe dehydration occurs), oral electrolyte and fluid replacement are the therapies of choice. The key, of course, is to administer enough volume to offset the net secretion of fluid that is occurring due to enterotoxin-mediated mechanisms. However, if the disease is not detected early, a profound dehydration occurs that quickly leads to severe metabolic acidosis, prerenal renal failure, and hypovolemic shock.[25] In these animals, intensive intravenous fluid and electrolyte therapy is required to prevent death. Cardiac dysrhythmias, sinus bradycardia, or sinus arrest are typically present due to hyperkalemia produced by acute renal failure and metabolic acidosis.[26] Mortality often exceeds 50% when these clinical signs are present, and if the animals become recumbent and coma occurs mortality rates approach 90%.

Recent experimental studies by Wise et al.[27] with in vivo intestinal loops of 1- to 5-day-old calves have demonstrated that intravenous infusion of sodium salicylate afforded significant protection, i.e., reduced intestinal water and electrolyte secretion, against the secretory diarrhea caused by administered *E. coli* heat-stable enterotoxin. Thus, this finding suggests a novel mode of clinical therapy for calves with this diathesis. This possible mode of therapy warrants exploration with other species as well, since bovine enterotoxigenic *E. coli* (ETEC) shares several features with porcine class 2 ETEC, such as possession of 0 group antigens 8, 9, 20, and 101, presence of K99 pili, production of heat-stable enterotoxin, and other features.[28]

In colostrum-fed calves which are older than 24 hr when first infected, the diarrhea is less severe, but more chronic in its clinical course. The degree of dehydration is less severe and in most cases tachydysrhythmias occur, due primarily to the modest dehydration. In these animals, oral electrolyte and fluid therapy is all that is required.

However, these animals tend to remain ill for longer periods of time and will be slower to grow and gain weight.[29]

The third form of bovine colibacillosis occurs in animals infected before they have ingested adequate amounts of colostrum. In these animals, *E. coli* attach to the intestinal epithelium, invade the cells and the lamina propria, and are readily detected in the bloodstream. These animals become septicemic, endotoxemic, and often die within 4 to 6 hr. In this peracute form of colibacillosis, they often die before the onset of diarrhea.[30]

V. OTHER MECHANISMS

Another mechanism by which *E. coli* produce bloody diarrhea, distinct from invasion of the mucosa or production of enterotoxins, has recently been identified. In both Canada[31] and the U.S.,[32] outbreaks of human hemorrhagic colitis have lately been reported in association with *E. coli* strain 0157:H7 — a strain which is not invasive or enterotoxigenic. It was hypothesized[31,33] that this strain produced a Vero cell cytotoxin, such as described earlier,[34] but it has not been documented that the Shiga-like toxin produced by *E. coli* and the Vero cytotoxin are identical.[35-37] Recently, O'Brien and co-workers[38] examined 13 strains of *E. coli* implicated in cases of diarrhea in humans, for the in vitro production of a toxin such as the *Shigella dysenteriae* Type 1. They found that 11 of these 13 strains produced a Shiga-like cytotoxin. Trace levels were produced by only two of the strains that had elicited minimal virulence. The other strains produced high levels of Shiga-like toxin that were enterotoxic for rabbits and inhibitory toward HeLa cell protein synthesis. Thus far, these types of *E. coli* have not been found in bovine *E. coli* infections.

In summary, bovine colibacillosis resembles certain aspects of human *E. coli* and *Vibrio cholera* infections and may be useful to study selected aspects of the pathogenesis of both of these human diarrheal syndromes. Additionally, due to the ease which human pathogenic *E. coli* strains lose plasmid-mediated enterotoxin genes, caution should be exercised when stating that human colibacillosis frequently is not due to enterotoxin production.

REFERENCES

1. Moon, H. W., Isaacson, R. E., and Pohlenz, J., Mechanisms of association of enteropathogenic *Escherichia coli* with intestinal epithelium, *Am. J. Clin. Nutr.,* 32, 119, 1979.
2. Blood, D. C., Henderson, J. A., and Radostits,O. M., *Veterinary Medicine,* 5th ed., Lea & Febiger, Philadelphia, 1979, 463.
3. DuPont, H. L., Formal, S. B., Hornick, R. B., Synder, M. J., Libonati, J. P., Sheahan, D. G., LaBrec, E. H., and Kalas, J. P., Pathogenesis of *Escherichia coli* diarrhea, *N. Engl. J. Med.,* 285, 1, 1971.
4. Guerrant, R. L., Moore, R. A., Kirschenfeld, P. M., and Sande, M. A., Role of toxigenic and invasive bacteria in acute diarrhea of childhood, *N. Engl. J. Med.,* 293, 567, 1975.
5. Ryder, R. W., Wachsmuth, I. K., Buxton, A. E., Evans, D. G., DuPont, H. L., Mason, E., and Barrett, F. F., Infantile diarrhea produced by heat-stable enterotoxigenic *Escherichia coli*, *N. Engl. J. Med.,* 295, 849, 1976.
6. Cantey, J. R., O'Hanley, P. D., and Blake, R. K., A rabbit model of diarrhea due to invasive *Escherichia coli*, *J. Infect. Dis.,* 136, 640, 1977.
7. Levine, M. M., Bergquist, E. J., Nalin, D. R., Waterman, D. H., Hormick, R. B., Young, C. R., and Sotman, S., *Escherichia coli* strains that cause diarrhea but do not produce heat-labile or heat-stable enterotoxins and are non-invasive, *Lancet,* 1, 1119, 1978.

8. Brasitus, T. A., Another mechanism by which *Escherichia coli* causes diarrhea, *Gastroenterology*, 85, 972, 1983.

9. Moon, H. W., McClurkin, A. W., Isaacson, R. E. et al., Pathogenic relationships of *rotavirus*, *Escherichia coli* and other agents in mixed infection in calves, *J. Am. Vet. Med. Assoc.*, 173, 577, 1978.

10. Cantey, J. R. and Blake, R. K., Diarrhea due to *Escherichia coli* in the rabbit: a novel mechanism, *J. Infect. Dis.*, 135, 454, 1977.

11. Gyles, C. L., Comments on detection and importance of enteropathogenic *Escherichia coli* in diarrheal disease of human beings, *J. Am. Vet. Med. Assoc.*, 173, 598, 1979.

12. Thorne, G. M. and Gorbach, S. L., Enterotoxigenic *Escherichia coli* detection and importance in diarrheal disease of children, *J. Am. Vet. Med. Assoc.*, 173, 592, 1978.

13. Berendson, R., Cheney, C. P., Schad, P. A., and Boedeker, E. C., Species-specific binding of purified pili (AF/R1) from the *Escherichia coli* RDEC-1 to rabbit intestinal mucosa, *Gastroenterology*, 85, 837, 1983.

14. Cheney, C. P., Schad, P. A., Formal, S. B., and Boedeker, E. C., Species specificity of in vitro *Escherichia coli* adherence to host intestinal cell membranes and its correlation with in vitro colonization and infectivity, *Infect. Immunol.*, 28, 1019, 1980.

15. Cheney, C. P. and Boedeker, E. C., Adherence of an enterotoxigenic *Escherichia coli*, serotype 078:H11 to purified human brush borders, *Infect. Immunol.*, 39, 1280, 1983.

16. Evans, D. G., Satterwhite, T. K., Evans, D. J., and Dupont, H. L., Differences in serological responses and excretion patterns of volunteers challenged with enterotoxigenic *Escherichia coli* with and without the colonization factor antigen, *Infect. Immunol.*, 18, 883, 1978.

17. Satterwhite, T. K., DuPont, H. L., Evans, D. G., and Evans, D. J., Role of *Escherichia coli* colonization factor antigen in acute diarrhea, *Lancet*, 2, 181, 1978.

18. Evans, D. G., Silver, R. P., Evans, D. J., Chase, D. G., and Gorbach, S. L., Plasmid-controlled colonization factor associated with virulence in *Escherichia coli* enterotoxigenicity for humans, *Infect. Immunol.*, 12, 656, 1975.

19. Rothbaum, R., McAdams, A. J., Giannella, R., and Partin, J. C., A clinico-pathologic study of enterocyte-adherence *Escherichia coli*: a cause of protracted diarrhea in infants, *Gastroenterology*, 83, 441, 1982.

20. Ulshen, M. H. and Rollo, J. L., Pathogenesis of *Escherichia coli* gastroenteritis in man — another mechanism, *N. Engl. J. Med.*, 302, 99, 1980.

21. Laird, W. J., Gill, D. M., Field, M. et al., Purification and mode of action of heat-stable enterotoxin of *E. coli* (abstr.), 13th Jt. Conf. Cholera, U.S.-Jpn. Coop. Med. Sci. Prog., Atlanta, 1977, 29.

22. Gyles, C. L., Heat labile and heat stable forms of the enterotoxin from *E. coli* strains enteropathogenic for pigs, *Ann. N.Y. Acad. Sci.*, 176, 314, 1971.

23. Moon, H. W., Mechanisms in the pathogenesis of diarrhea: a review, *J. Am. Vet. Med. Assoc.*, 172, 443, 1978.

24. Smith, H. W., and Halls, S., Observations by the ligated intestinal segment and oral inoculation methods on *Escherichia coli* infection in pigs, calves, lambs and rabbits, *J. Pathol. Bacteriol.*, 93, 499, 1967.

25. Tennant, B., Harrold, D., and Reina-Guerra, M., Physiologic and metabolic factors in the pathogenesis of neonatal enteric infections in calves, *J. Am. Vet. Med. Assoc.*, 161, 993, 1972.

26. Fisher, E. W., Hydrogen ion and electrolyte disturbances in neonatal calf diarrhea, *Ann. N.Y. Acad. Sci.*, 176, 223, 1971.

27. Wise, C. M., Knight, A. P., Lucas, M. J., Morris, C. J., Ellis, R. P., and Phillips, R. W., Effect of salicylates on intestinal secretion in calves given (intestinal loops) *Escherichia coli* heat-stable enterotoxin, *Am. J. Vet. Res.*, 44, 2221, 1983.

28. Harnett, N. M. and Gyles, C. L., Enterotoxigenicity of bovine and porcine *Escherichia coli* of O groups 8, 9, 20, 64, 101, and X46, *Am. J. Vet. Res.*, 44, 1210, 1983.

29. Boyd, J. W., Baker, J. R., and Leyland, A., Neonatal diarrhea in calves, *Vet. Rec.*, 95, 310, 1974.

30. Moon, H. W., Pathogenesis of enteric diseases caused by *Escherichia coli*, *Adv. Vet. Sci. Comp. Med.*, 18, 179, 1974.

31. Johnson, W. M., Lior, H., and Bezanson, G. S., Cytotoxic *Escherichia coli* 0157:H7 associated with hemorrhagic colitis in Canada, *Lancet*, 1, 76, 1983.

32. Riley, L. W., Remis, R. S., Helgerson, S. D., McGee, H. B., Wells, J. G., Davis, B. R., Herbert, R. J., Olcott, E. S., Johnson, L. M., Hargrett, N. T., Blake, P. A., and Cohen, M. L., Hemorrhagic colitis associated with a rare *Escherichia coli* serotype, *N. Engl. J. Med.*, 308, 61, 1983.

33. Wade, W. G., Thom, B. T., and Evans, N., Cytotoxic enteropathogenic *Escherichia coli*, *Lancet*, 2, 1235, 1979.

34. Konowalchuk, J., Speirs, J. I., and Stavric, S., Vero response to a cytotoxin of *Escherichia coli*, *Infect. Immunol.*, 18, 775, 1977.

35. O'Brien, A. D., LaVeck, G. D., Griffin, D. E., and Thompson, M. R., Characterization of *Shigella dysenteriae* 1 (Shiga) toxin purified by anti-Shiga toxin affinity chromatography, *Infect. Immunol.*, 30, 170, 1980.
36. O'Brien, A. D., Laveck, G. D., Thompson, M. R., and Formal, S. B., Production of *Shigella dysenteriae* type 1-like cytotoxin by *Escherichia coli*, *J. Infect. Dis.*, 146, 763, 1982.
37. O'Brien, A. D., Lively, T. A., Chen, M. E., Rothman, S. W., and Formal, S. B., *Escherichia coli* 0157:H7 strains associated with haemorrhagic colitis in the United States produces a *Shigella dysenteriae* 1 (Shiga)-like cytotoxin, *Lancet*, 1, 702, 1983.
38. O'Brien, A. O., LaVeck, G. D., Thompson, M. R., and Formal, S. B., Production of *Shigella dysenteriae* type 1-like cytotoxin by *Escherichia coli*, *J. Infect. Dis.*, 146, 763, 1982.

Chapter 5

YERSINIOSIS

Philip B. Carter and Brian D. Perry

TABLE OF CONTENTS

I. INTRODUCTION AND HISTORY

Yersinia pseudotuberculosis has long been recognized as a cause of mesenteric lymphadenitis in animals and humans. It has only been in the last two decades that increasing attention has been directed toward *Y. enterocolitica* as an etiologic agent in human ileitis, mesenteric lymphadenitis, and septicemia, as well as possible sequelae of the enteric infection: arthritis, Reiter's syndrome, and erythema nodosum. As recently as 1970, the causative role of *Y. enterocolitica* in acute ileitis was still being questioned.[1] A serious weakness in establishing a case for a causal relationship between *Y. enterocolitica* and acute ileitis and mesenteric lymphadenitis had been the inability to confirm an early report[2] of the pathogenicity of human isolates for laboratory animals.[3,4] In recent years, however, human isolates of *Y. enterocolitica* have been shown to be virulent for laboratory animals, reproducing in them the basic characteristics of the human disease.[5-7] It is the function of this chapter to review the work which has been done on animal models of human *Yersinia* enteritis, to evaluate models for assessing the virulence of *Y. enterocolitica* for humans, and to discuss present knowledge of virulence mechanisms.

II. EPIDEMIOLOGY

A. Global Distribution of Organisms and Diseases

Both *Y. enterocolitica* and *Y. pseudotuberculosis* are extremely widely distributed in the world, and where they are encountered, they are usually present in a variety of host species.

Probably the most widespread of the two organisms is *Y. enterocolitica*, and its reported distribution is illustrated in Figure 1. Since first being recognized in 1934,[8] albeit under a variety of names until the currently used nomenclature was adopted by Frederiksen,[9] it has been recorded in North, Central, and South America; west, central, and eastern Europe; parts of the Middle East; North, West, central, and southern Africa; Japan; and Australia. However, the organism is much more widespread than the reported clinical manifestations of its presence in a host. While disease causally associated with *Y. enterocolitica* has been identified in all of the areas indicated above, many of the isolations have been from animals or humans without clinical disease, or from animal sources such as water or foodstuffs.

Disease entities associated with *Y. enterocolitica* have been recorded principally in man, and the majority of cases have occurred in northern Europe, North America, South Africa, and Japan. However, given the variety of clinical manifestations associated with *Yersinia* infections, and the need for special laboratory isolation procedures, it is likely that clinical yersiniosis is much more widespread than is reported.

Approximately 34 serotypes of *Y. enterocolitica* have been identified,[10] and of these, four are "classically" associated with human disease.[11] These are serotypes 0:3, 27, 0:8, and 0:9. These serotypes have generally not been isolated from sources other than clinically ill humans. *Y. enterocolitica* isolations from healthy humans, domestic and wild animals, and environmental sources are usually serologically distinct from the "classic" strains; many are not serologically typeable. The exception to this is isolates of porcine origin, which have been predominantly serotype 0:3 both in Europe and Canada.[12-14]

The distinct geographic distribution of the classic strains isolated from man is also illustrated in Figure 1. Serotype 0:3 is the predominant human strain isolated throughout the reported distribution, with the exception of the U.S. and western Canada, where a variety of serotypes have been identified, with serotype 0:8 predominant.[15]

Further epidemiological division of the serotypes has been achieved by biotyping and

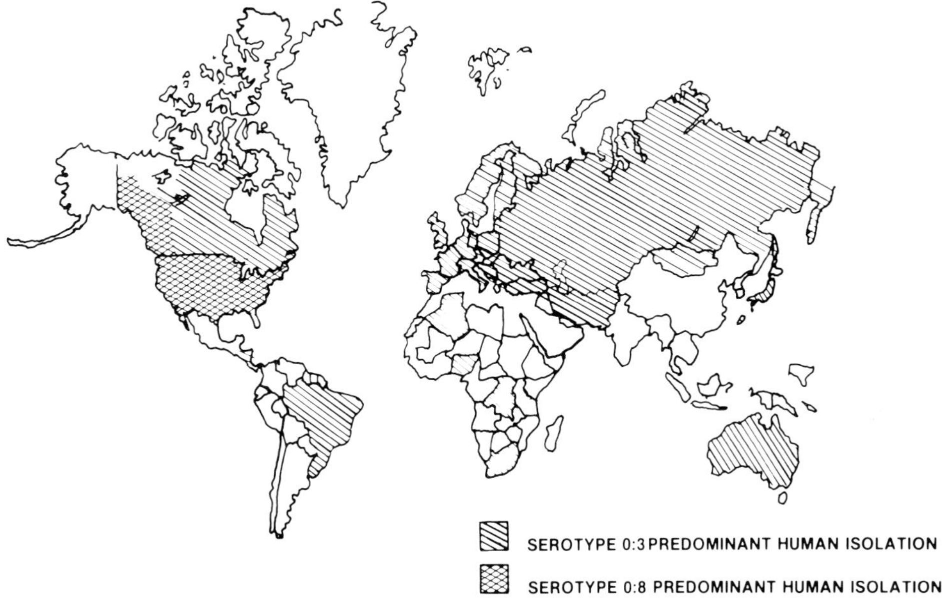

FIGURE 1.   Reported world distribution of *Y. enterocolitica*.

phage typing, and the latter technique has distinguished between human *Y. enterocolitica* isolates from Europe (serotype 0:3, biotype 4, phage type 8), Canada (serotype 0:3, biotype 4, phage type 9B), and South Africa (serotype 0:3, biotype 4, phage type 9A).[16]

Y. pseudotuberculosis is also widely distributed geographically and in nature, and has been recorded as occurring worldwide.[10,17] However, until recently it has, like *Y. enterocolitica*, been identified predominantly from northern Europe. Mair[18] reported the hypothesis of Mollaret that the European distribution of *Y. pseudotuberculosis* coincides roughly with the boundaries reached by plague during the second pandemic. As infection with *Y. pseudotuberculosis* imparts protective immunity to *Y. pestis*, it was suggested that the development of an endemic state to *Y. pseudotuberculosis* may not only have contributed to the extinction of the pandemic, but may have prevented its establishment during the third pandemic. The hypothesis attributes the occurrence of *Y. pseudotuberculosis* elsewhere in the world to the importation of infected animals from Europe. The current reported distribution is somewhat similar to that of *Y. enterocolitica*, and includes Europe, North America, North Africa, Japan, and Australia.

Unlike *Y. enterocolitica*, disease entities are widely reported in these geographic areas from animals as well as man. In the U.S., isolations from diseased and healthy domestic mammals, wild mammals, and birds were reported by Hubbert;[19] Mair[18] reported isolations in Britain from 6 species of wild mammals, 21 species of birds and numerous farm animals, domestic pets, and experimental animals.

While there is a diversity of serotypes of *Y. pseudotuberculosis* recognized, there does not appear to be the geographical variation in distribution reported with *Y. enterocolitica*. Of the six serotypes recognized, the serotype usually responsible for disease in man, serotype I, is the most prevalent of the positive identification of *Y. pseudotuberculosis* from all the regions recording this organism. However, like *Y. enterocolitica*, it has recently been shown that serotypes that are not responsible for human disease can be widely distributed in other species. Mair et al.[20] reported that *Y. pseu-*

Table 1

SPECIES OF ANIMALS RECORDED WITH *Y. ENTEROCOLITICA* INFECTION[26]

Mammals						
Domestic pets	Livestock	Laboratory animals	Wild mammals	Birds	Fish	Other
Dog	Cattle	Monkey	Fox	Chicken	Trout	Snail
Cat	Sheep	Guinea pig	Raccoon	Goose	Perch	Frog
	Goat	Rabbit	Deer	Duck	Roach	Oyster
	Horse		Elk	Pigeon		Flea
	Pig		Rabbit	Sparrow		Mussels
	Camel		Hare	Goldfinch		
	Chinchilla		Ocelot	Canary		
			Wild rodents	Grouse		
				Bunting		
				Finch		
				Lapwing		
				Seagull		

Table 2

INANIMATE SOURCES OF *Y. ENTEROCOLITICA*[26]

Meat & meat products		Milk & milk products	Vegetables	Environmental
Beef[a]	Pig tongue	Raw milk	Carrots	Soil
Pork	Hare	Pasteurized milk	Tomatoes	Wall
Lamb[a]	Meat pate	Chocolate milk	Green salads	Milking machine
Chicken	Black pudding	Cream	Coarse salads	Rivers, ponds
		Ice cream	Beetroot	Sewers
			Mushrooms	Drinking water

[a]   Raw and vacuum packed.

dotuberculosis serotype III, which is rarely reported as a cause of yersiniosis in man, is the predominant serotype isolated from healthy pigs in the U.K. The consistency of this in other geographical regions has yet to be confirmed, but similar findings to these have been recorded from Canada and Japan.[21,22]

B. Life Cycles

The life cycles of *Y. enterocolitica* and *Y. pseudotuberculosis* have been the subject of much conjecture, but the epidemiology of these diseases remains obscure. With the enteropathogenic behavior of *Yersinia*[23,24] and the frequent simultaneous isolation of enteropathic *Escherichia coli* and *Salmonella* spp.,[25] it is generally considered that infection of humans and other animals is by ingestion. Furthermore, the catholic nature of *Y. enterocolitica* in respect to host range (Table 1) and its isolation from a number of foodstuffs and environmental sources (Table 2) suggests at first glance that a wide variety of wild mammals may act as a reservoir of infection for man, who might be infected directly, or indirectly by the contamination of fomites.

However, serotyping and biotyping procedures have indicated that with the exception of the strains isolated from healthy pigs, most of the strains isolated from pets, domestic and wild animals, foodstuffs, water, and other environmental sources are antigenically distinct from the strains isolated from human patients with *Yersinia*-associated clinical manifestations. Nevertheless, these sources have been circumstantially

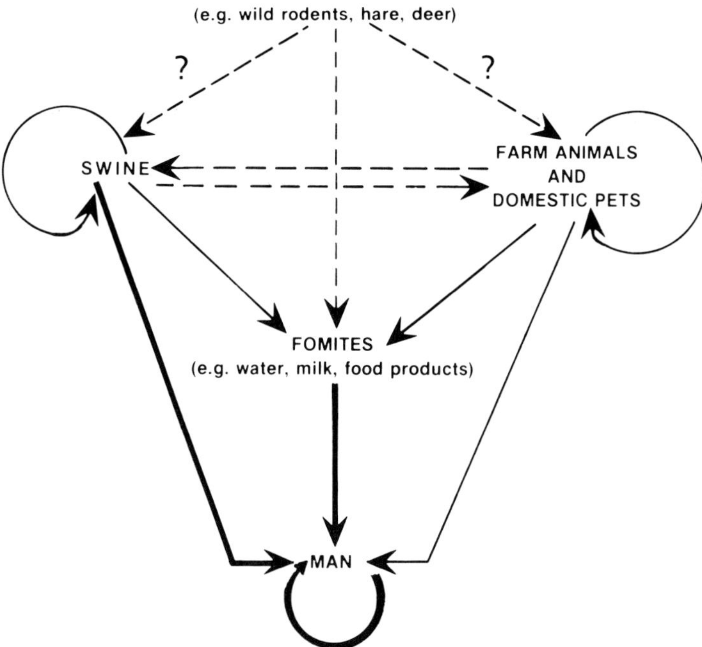

FIGURE 2.   Cycle of *Y. enterocolitica* indicating potential sources of human infection.

incriminated as the origin of human infections on occasion,[27,28] but bacteriological confirmation has rarely been made.[29-31] The long-awaited proof of the existence of food-borne yersiniosis was made in the autumn of 1976 when Black et al.[32] confirmed the presence of serotype 0:8 in chocolate milk drunk by children, from whom the same serotype had been isolated. Since then, two other food-associated outbreaks have been confirmed in the U.S. One, affecting 87 individuals and associated with consumption of commercial tofu (soybean curd), was thought to be caused by a classical 0:8 serotype,[33] while another, in which milk was the vehicle was caused by *Y. enterocolitica* 0:13 and involved several thousand persons, the largest reported outbreak of the disease.[34]

During the last decade, numerous authors have described the isolation of *Y. enterocolitica* from healthy pigs in Europe,[14,35-38] Canada,[13,21] South Africa,[39] and Japan.[22,40] A high proportion of these isolates belong to the serotypes commonly associated with infections in man, principally serotype 0:3. This has led to the presumption that swine may act as the principal reservoir of *Y. enterocolitica* for man. The evidence that *Y. enterocolitica* serotype 0:3 is a normal inhabitant of the oral cavity of pigs in endemic regions suggests that there is a direct relationship between human *Y. enterocolitica* infections and healthy pigs and their food products. Furthermore, it seems likely in the light of available evidence that this relationship is stronger than other interspecies infection routes which have been postulated.

However, with the strong circumstantial evidence that some human infections may originate from other animals and environmental sources, one may speculate that swine populations may have become infected from wildlife sources, particularly the wild rodents (which serve as primary hosts for all the *Yersinia species*), and these swine have served as an amplifier host of those serotypes pathogenic to man. The probable life-cycle of *Y. enterocolitica* is illustrated in Figure 2.

Once the infection is established in man, he may serve as a reservoir of infection to

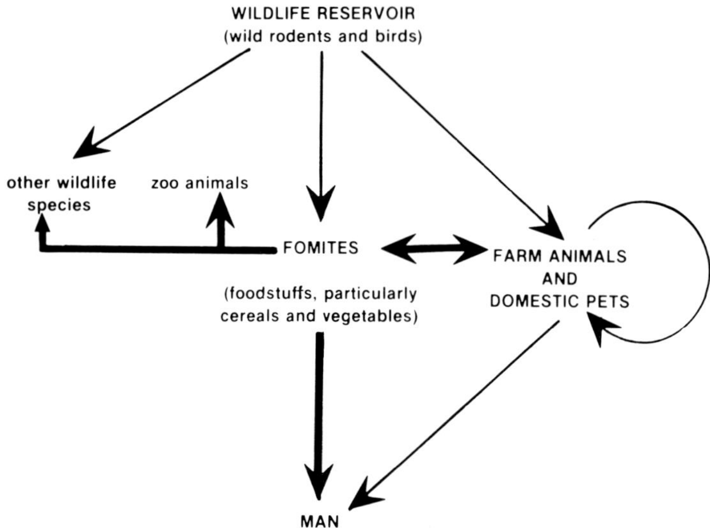

FIGURE 3.   Cycle of *Y. pseudotuberculosis.*

his fellow humans both during active infection, as is seen with familial outbreaks of disease,[29,41-45] and as a healthy carrier of the organism.[46]

While considerable attention has been paid to the epidemiology of *Y. pseudotuberculosis* during the last 15 years, investigational work into this organism has recently been overshadowed by that of *Y. enterocolitica,* due principally to the greater significance of the latter organism as a human pathogen. *Y. pseudotuberculosis* has like *Y. enterocolitica,* been isolated from a great variety of wild animals[18,19,47] and wild rodents serve as the principal reservoir of infection to other species.[18] However, unlike *Y. enterocolitica,* wild birds appear to act as important reservoirs of the organism,[18] and wood pigeons have been incriminated in both direct transmission to other animals, and indirect transmission by contamination of green crops such as kale, cabbage, and brussel sprouts with huge numbers of viable organisms.[48] It is possibly in this way that infection has been introduced to laboratory animal colonies, where epidemics have been reported in North America and Europe.[18,49-53]

Mair[18] considers that contaminated foods also offer a significant source of infection for both domestic and farm animals, and for animals confined in zoological parks. The probable cycle of infection of *Y. pseudotuberculosis* is illustrated in Figure 3.

Infection of humans is probably acquired from direct contact with animals, or indirect contact by means of contaminated fomites, although as pointed out by Bottone,[10] this argument is speculative in nature. The principal serotype responsible for human disease, serotype I, is also the predominant serotype isolated from other animal sources.[19]

The possibility of vector-borne transmission has been considered by some workers, and infected *Ixodes ricinus* ticks have been collected from cattle.[54] However, transmission of the organism to guinea pigs by the flea *Xenopsylla cheopsis* was unsuccessful, although the fleas remained carriers for up to 35 days.[55]

C. Epidemic and Endemic Behavior

There is considerable variation in the epidemic and endemic behavior of *Yersinia* infections, dependent upon many factors which have as yet not been elucidated. Some of the recognized influences are recorded below.

1. Strain

Considerable variations in disease pattern and manifestation occur with different strains of both *Y. enterocolitica* and *Y. pseudotuberculosis.* The serotypes of *Y. enterocolitica* isolated from clinically ill humans have greater invasive qualities to serotypes commonly isolated from other sources, and this subject is covered under pathogenic mechanisms.

2. Host Species

There is considerable variation in species susceptibility reported between the two organisms. *Y. enterocolitica* is generally considered nonpathogenic or of low pathogenicity to wildlife, although infections are possibly relatively frequent. Disease in wildlife has been reported principally in species kept in captivity.[7,56] With the exception of the pig, very little is known of infection rates in domestic pets and farm animals, but clinical disease is relatively rare and has been recorded principally in swine,[26] dogs,[57] goats,[26] and house rats.[57] Similarly, the organism is rarely recorded from avian hosts.

Yersinia pseudotuberculosis contrasts sharply in behavioral characteristics, and is a relatively common infection of a wide range of wild and domestic animals and birds, where it can cause serious disease. In humans, however, the disease is uncommon and manifested usually as a localized mesenteric form and rarely as a generalized septicemic form.[17] Mollaret[11] hypothesized that *Y. enterocolitica,* in contrast to *Y. pseudotuberculosis,* is still evolving with respect to its host adaptation characteristics, and can be considered as comprising two groups. The first group is host adapted, produces "typical" clinical manifestations, and contains the serotypes 0:3, 0:5, 27, 0:8, and 0:9, while the second group contains the diverse atypical serotypes which are of restricted pathogenic potential. Bottone[10] suggests that these latter strains may, when host adapted, ultimately contribute to the expanding spectrum of yersiniosis. The interrelationship between host species and the serotype of isolated *Y. enterocolitica* is not restricted to man and pigs. Isolates from hares and goats are usually serotypes 2a, 2b, or 3, while those from chinchillas are commonly 1; 1, 2a or 1, 2a, 3.[26]

a. Age

Data on the age distribution of *Yersinia* infections in animals are scarce, but in man Vandepitte and Wauters[46] reported that although *Y. enterocolitica* was diagnosed in a wide range of patients in Belgium during the years 1963—1975, almost 80% of the patients were under 10 years of age. When age incidence was examined with respect to the type of clinical manifestation, 80% of all patients with gastroenteritis were under 5 years of age, whereas patients with the pseudo-appendicular syndrome reached their highest frequency among older children and young adults. Similar observations have been reported by Van Noyen et al.[25]

b. Sex

In humans, the frequency of *Y. enterocolitica* infection appears almost identical in the two sexes.[25]

c. Season

Numerous authors have observed an increase in the frequency of *Y. enterocolitica* and *Y. pseudotuberculosis* infections during the autumn and winter.[46,59-61] The reasons for this apparent seasonal incidence are speculative, but documented suggestions have included the stress of cold and starvation in animals,[17] the increase in survival time of *Yersinia* in the environment at low temperatures, and the increase of the domestic slaughter of pigs in households during the festive occasion of that time of year.

III. PATHOGENICITY OF *Y. ENTEROCOLITICA* AND *Y. PSEUDOTUBERCULOSIS* FOR LABORATORY ANIMALS

A. Studies in Guinea Pigs and Rabbits

Guinea pigs have long been known to be extremely susceptible to infection with *Y. pseudotuberculosis*. Infections with this organism are epizootic in guinea pig populations, often with high mortality rates; they are enzootic in rabbits.

The first attempts to infect laboratory animals with *Y. enterocolitica* were made at the New York State Department of Health Laboratories in 1933. A single paragraph in their 1933 Annual Report[62] describes pathology in guinea pigs following injection with two different human isolates of the same serotype submitted in 1923 and 1932. The route of inoculation was not indicated in the report, but it is likely to be intraperitoneal. The isolates were from superficial lesions of the face and may not have been *Y. enterocolitica*. However, later studies by Schleifstein and Coleman[2] demonstrated that these two early isolates were serologically and physiologically identical to three additional isolates from patients with enteritis. All five isolates studied by Schleifstein and Coleman produced disease in intraperitoneally infected guinea pigs, but were nonpathogenic when given either subcutaneously or in food. More recent work[5] has shown that isolates of *Y. enterocolitica*, highly pathogenic in mice, are virtually nonpathogenic for guinea pigs. The susceptibility of guinea pigs to *Y. enterocolitica* is the reverse of that found for *Y. pseudotuberculosis* and thus the guinea pig is rarely used any longer in the study of the pathogenesis of *Y. enterocolitica* infections.

Schleifstein and Coleman[2] report no ill effects in rabbits following intraperitoneal injection of *Y. enterocolitica* isolated from humans. However, Une[63] has recently been able to induce disease in rabbits by injecting human isolates of the 0:3 and 0:9 serotypes intraduodenally. Such infection gives rise to an acute diarrhea 2 to 3 days after infection, thus resembling human gastroenteritis caused by the 0:3 serotype of *Y. enterocolitica.*

Une[63] and Une and Zen-Yoji[24] have demonstrated that *Y. enterocolitica* isolates from human patients are pathogenic for rabbits when injected intraduodenally. They observed penetration of the mucosal epithelium with subsequent invasion of the draining lymphoid tissues. Unlike the mouse model in which abscess formation is commonly observed, a granulomatous response was often seen. Granulomas, characterized by an infiltrate of mononuclear phagocytes, develop in the appendix, mesenteric lymph nodes, liver, and spleen of rabbits as early as 7 days postinfection. Une and Zen-Yoji[24] showed that virulent *Y. enterocolitica* would actually multiply in rabbit macrophages in vitro whereas avirulent strains would be phagocytized and killed.

Rabbits that survived an intraduodenal infection with 0:3 and 0:9 serotypes of *Y. enterocolitica* were found to excrete the infecting organisms in their feces for as long as 40 days postinfection.[63] It was not determined whether the infecting agents actually colonized the intestinal tract for this period of time, or whether the organisms present in the feces issued from mucosal ulcerations of the gut-associated lymphoid tissue. The latter would be consistent with the pathology described.

B. Studies in Mice and Rats

Primarily for economic reasons, most laboratory studies done in vivo with *Y. enterocolitica* have employed mice. Fortunately, studies in the last decade have demonstrated that the major pathological features of *Y. enterocolitica* infections in humans are also reproduced in naturally infected mice. Schleifstein and Coleman[2] were the first to employ the mouse in virulence studies on *Y. enterocolitica*, at that time only an unidentified microorganism resembling *Y. pseudotuberculosis* and *Actinobacillus lignierisii*. Their studies showed that mice were particularly susceptible to infection by the human isolates used, more so than guinea pigs, rabbits, and rats, and most interestingly could be infected via contaminated food. These workers[2] mentioned that the isolates attenuated quickly and attempted to maintain the virulence of the microorganisms by mouse-to-mouse passage. It was this attenuation[5] and inability to confirm[3,4] the early New York State work on virulence that led to the skepticism that the early work was perhaps performed using an organism different from what is presently recognized as *Yersinia enterocolitica.* Recent studies in many laboratories have since confirmed the early work using both the New York serotype and biotype (0:8)[5,64] and the European 0:3 serotype.[65-67]

The pathogen-free mouse has proven to be an excellent model for the type of human infection in the U.S. associated with the 0:8 serotype, i.e., acute ileitis, mesenteric lymphadenitis, and rarely, enteric fever.[68] Oral infection of mice with virulent human isolates of *Y. enterocolitica* causes a suppurative infection of the Peyer's patches and mesenteric lymph nodes.[69] With a high challenge dose, the microorganisms can proceed past the draining lymph nodes to cause a systemic infection of the lungs, liver, and spleen. In orally infected pathogen-free mice, a neutrophil infiltrate appears early after infection in the Peyer's patches of the distal ileum. The Peyer's patches develop abscesses and the surrounding mucosa becomes inflamed. The infection extends to the mesenteric lymph nodes where abscesses develop, and from there to the systemic reticuloendothelial organs. A leukocytosis ensues and specific antibodies appear in the serum after 1 week. Diarrhea or loose stools are not common features of yersiniosis in mice infected with the 0:8 serotype. Again, this reflects the human infection in which fever and abdominal pain without diarrhea are the common clinical manifestations of the disease.[32]

As stated above, human infection with serotype 0:8 is rare in Europe and Canada; most human isolates are serotype 0:3. Diarrhea, abdominal pain, but rare systemic involvement are associated with infections by these serotypes. Although mice can be infected with *Yersinia enterocolitica* serotypes 0:9 and 0:3[65,70] and *Y. pseudotuberculosis* IVA,[70] and excrete the microorganisms in their feces for long periods,[70-73] diarrhea has not been reported in such mice. Therefore, it may be that the laboratory mouse does not represent a suitable model for gastroenteritis caused by *Y. enterocolitica* serotype 0:3.

Rats have not commonly been used in experimental studies involving *Y. enterocolitica.* McGregor and Carter (unpublished) showed that it was possible to infect inbred rats parenterally with *Y. enterocolitica* strain WA. However, the rats were able to withstand a much higher challenge dose than mice and there was great variation in the severity of the disease within groups, an undesirable feature for a model system. Attempts at oral infection failed to produce disease.

C. Studies in Monkeys

In 1973, Maruyama[6] reported the establishment of an experimental *Y. enterocolitica* infection in *Macaca irus* monkeys. Oral infection with an 0:3 serotype of human origin resulted in an acute infection of less than 2 weeks duration with minimal pathological changes.[74]

Naturally occurring *Y. enterocolitica* infections have been reported in two monkey colonies in the U.S. In 1971, McClure et al.[75] reported an outbreak in which two vervet monkeys *(Cerophithecus aethiops)* and one mangabey *(Cercocebus torquatus)* died of a pseudotuberculosis-like disease in which *Y. enterocolitica* was isolated. Two of the monkeys exhibited a granulocytosis and had lesions in the intestine (Peyer's patches), liver, and spleen. Attempts to parenterally infect six pigtailed macaque monkeys *(Macaca memestrina)* were unsuccessful. In 1976, a large outbreak occurred in a colony of owl monkeys *(Aotus trivirgatus)* in which 20 of the animals died.[76] Typical pseudotuberculosis-like lesions in the intestine, spleen, and liver were observed in the 29 animals dying of the spontaneous disease. Two of four monkeys experimentally infected orally with the *Y. enterocolitica* strain isolated during the outbreak developed yersiniosis and one died. The serotype responsible for either of these outbreaks was not reported.

D. In Vitro Correlates

The need to develop a means for testing the virulence of environmental isolates of *Y. enterocolitica* has led to the examination of possible in vitro correlates of the animal infection. The most popular has been the ability of an isolate to invade HeLa cells, a method used successfully by LaBrec et al.[77] to study invasiveness of *Shigella* and by Giannella et al.[78] to assess invasiveness of salmonellae. In both systems, the ability of the strains to infect HeLa cells in culture correlated directly with the ability to penetrate the intestinal mucosal epithelium of laboratory animals.

Lee et al.[79] and Une[80] were the first to correlate HeLa cell invasiveness by *Y. enterocolitica* with animal pathogenicity. A number of laboratories have since confirmed that human isolates of *Y. enterocolitica* serotypes 0:8, 0:3, 0:9, and others are HeLa cell invasive;[81-84] atypical forms of *Y. enterocolitica* obtained from the environment or foodstuffs are exclusively noninvasive.[82] Even so, the ability to invade HeLa cells may not mean that the isolate is capable of causing disease in mammals. Such invasion occurs in the absence of the 42-mdal "virulence" plasmid,[33] discussed in detail below, and the organism does not multiply inside the HeLa cell,[85] an unlikely characteristic for a virulent microbe. The ability of *Y. enterocolitica* isolates to invade HeLa cells is temperature-dependent.[79,82] The microorganisms are most invasive when grown at 22°C, less invasive if cultured at 30°C, and some strains are almost completely noninvasive when grown at 36°C.[79]

IV. PATHOGENIC MECHANISMS

A. Temperature and Virulence

The incidence of human disease caused by *Y. enterocolitica* peaks during the cold months of the year,[45] just the reverse of what is observed for *Salmonella* infections. It was, therefore, quite interesting when a temperature-dependent differential in the mouse virulence of a single *Y. enterocolitica* strain was observed.[64] Whether administered orally or parenterally, a marked lowering of the virulence of *Y. enterocolitica* WA for mice was consistently observed if the challenge inoculum was cultured at temperatures exceeding 28°C. When cultured at temperatures below 25°C to as low as 5°C, *Y. enterocolitica* WA was optimally virulent. The less virulent organisms were cleared more quickly from the blood of infected animals and destroyed more rapidly by phagocytes.[64]

Y. pseudotuberculosis is nonmotile at 37°C and indole production and motility are absent in *Y. enterocolitica* at this temperature; it is unlikely that these characteristics have any relation to virulence. Rather, the temperature-dependent differential in virulence may be related to the presence of a higher proportion of VW antigen-negative *Y. enterocolitica* in challenge inocula grown at 37°C[86] and a differential production of outer membrane proteins (OMP).[87,88]

B. Attachment Factors and Invasiveness

As already mentioned, several different serotypes of *Y. enterocolitica* have been shown to possess invasive properties similar to those described for *Salmonella* and *Shigella*. In addition to HeLa cell invasiveness, pathogenic *Y. enterocolitica* and *Y. pseudotuberculosis* are capable of producing a positive Sereny reaction (conjunctivitis in the guinea pig)[89,90] and penetration of the rabbit[24,63,91] and mouse[68,92] ileal mucosa.

These properties require attachment as a first step; factors necessary for attachment may be contained among the novel OMP produced when *Y. enterocolitica* or *Y. pseudotuberculosis* are cultivated at 37°C.[87,88,93,94] Such a property can account for the *Salmonella*-like gastroenteritis commonly caused by the 0:8 serotype of *Y. enterocolitica*, but for the acute diarrhea often associated with 0:3 serotypes, a different virulence mechanism was sought.

C. Enterotoxin

At a meeting in 1977, Feeley et al.[89] and Robins-Browne et al.[91] reported the independent discovery of a heat-stable enterotoxin in human isolates of *Y. enterocolitica*. Enterotoxin was demonstrable only in the infant mouse assay (heat-stable toxin[95]) and not in the Y-1 adrenal cell assay (heat-labile toxin). Heat-stable enterotoxin has been found in a large number of *Y. enterocolitica* serotypes and biotypes, but is most prevalent among those that are associated with human gastrointestinal disease.[96] The heat-stable enterotoxin produced by isolates of *Y. enterocolitica* is identical in its physical, chemical, and physiological characteristics to that produced by *Escherichia coli*,[97-99] Production of enterotoxin in vitro is temperature dependent; it is not produced when culture temperatures exceed 30°C.[89,91,97] Since the enterotoxin is only produced at lower temperatures, and an enterotoxin-negative *Y. enterocolitica* 0:3, capable of producing diarrhea in mice has been described,[100] its role in the pathogenesis of diarrheal disease remains a mystery and must be documented by in vivo studies.

D. VW Antigens and Calcium Dependence

The high rate of attenuation of human isolates of *Y. enterocolitica* led to the suspicion that a plasmid was involved in the virulence of this organism. The existence of a plasmid approximately 42 mdal in size (i.e., 72 kilobases) was subsequently demonstrated by Zink et al.[101] and Gemski et al.[102] in virulent strains of *Y. enterocolitica* 0:8 and shortly thereafter, in *Y. pseudotuberculosis* as well.[103]

Further similarity between *Y. enterocolitica* and other species in the genus *Yersinia* has recently been demonstrated by the finding of V and W antigens in virulent forms of *Y. enterocolitica* 0:8[86] identical to the antigens previously associated with virulence in *Y. pestis*[104] and *Y. pseudotuberculosis*.[105] The presence of V and W antigens in *Y. enterocolitica* was demonstrated by immunochemical and biochemical means[86] and directly correlates with virulence for mice. These antigens are probably encoded by the 42 mdal plasmid since *Escherichia coli* minicells containing the plasmid from *Y. pestis* exhibit the V antigen.[106] The plasmid has thus been referred to as "Vwa". The possession of common virulence antigens in all species of the genus *Yersinia* may account for the resistance against plague observed in mice experimentally infected with *Y. enterocolitica*.[107]

The presence of such plasmid-mediated virulence factors in pathogenic *Y. enterocolitica* 0:3 serotypes remains to be clarified. The Vwa plasmid has been found in those *Yersinia* capable of producing systemic infections (predominately 0:8) as well as 0:3 and other serotypes,[87] but may not be necessary for the production of diarrheal diseases typical of 0:3 strains of *Y. enterocolitica*. Parental Vwa+ *Y. enterocolitica* WA is both invasive and enterotoxigenic while Vwa− derivatives of this strain are noninvasive but still produce a heat-stable enterotoxin.[86,102]

Although the capability of isolates to produce the V and W antigens is directly related to their pathogenicity in mice, proof that virulence depends upon possession of the V antigen has been lacking. Recently, Portnoy et al.[106] have described a number of virulence plasmid mutants in *Y. pestis* produced by transposon Tn5 insertions which suggest that virulence is not V-dependent in that species. Only those mutants that abolished calcium dependency became avirulent for mice; plasmid mutants with insertions that resulted in diminished production of V antigen but which retained calcium dependence remained fully virulent.

Calcium dependency refers to the phenomenon observed in all *Yersinia* species[86] in which highly virulent strains demonstrate an in vitro growth requirement for calcium at 37 but not at 25°C.[108-110] This dependency, also related to magnesium concentration,[111] results in a rapid shift to avirulence since culture at 37°C without calcium (<2.0 m*M*) permits the outgrowth of organisms lacking the 42 mdal plasmid and capacity to produce V antigen.[86,112] Thus, in vitro conditions for near optimal production of V antigen is aeration at 37°C in an enriched medium that lacks calcium but contains at least 20 m*M* magnesium.[109] These conditions are almost bacteriostatic for Vwa+, but not Vwa− organisms; growth of Vwa+ yersiniae does occur at 37°C if that amount of Ca^{2+} present in mammalian plasma (2.5 m*M*) is added to the medium, otherwise colonies of *Y. enterocolitica* and *Y. pseudotuberculosis* are minute. This calcium requirement does not exist at 25°C where V antigen is not produced.

Associated with the above culture conditions that mimic the mammalian intracellular environment, is the production of the novel OMP mentioned earlier.[88,93,94,113] These novel OMP are encoded by the plasmid present in all three species of *Yersinia*,[88] but are only expressed in *Y. pseudotuberculosis* and *Y. enterocolitica,* a fact that can be teleologically associated with their respective life histories: *Y. enterocolitica* and *Y. pseudotuberculosis,* being intestinal pathogens, may depend upon expression of these OMP for attachment, whereas such attachment factors need not be expressed in *Y. pestis* which is vector-borne. Autoagglutination, which occurs in *Y. pseudotuberculosis*[114] and *Y. enterocolitica,*[115] but not in *Y. pestis,*[87] loosely correlates with the expression of these OMP. The novel OMP, and a non-VW protein associated with virulence, WA-SAA (which may be one of these OMP[116]), are temperature and not Ca^{2+} dependent.[87,116] A similar correlation with temperature is observed in regard to sensitivity to normal human serum.[87,117] Avirulent *Y. enterocolitica* are usually killed by incubation in 10% normal human serum at 37°C whereas virulent organisms are resistant to this treatment.[117] Serum resistance is independent of the ability to produce pVwa-encoded virulence antigens in both *Y. pseudotuberculosis*[87] and *Y. enterocolitica,*[118,119] but may be related to the presence of a larger (82 mdal) plasmid associated with virulence.[120]

E. Iron Dependence

Epidemiological studies in a South African black population led Rabson et al.[121] to suggest that iron may enhance virulence of *Y. enterocolitica* serotype 0:3. Robins-Browne et al.[122] have shown that iron, in the form of ferric ammonium citrate, interferes with the natural bactericidal activity of fresh human serum. The ability of fresh human serum to kill as many as 106 *Y. enterocolitica* 0:3 per milliliter in 4 hr is completely ablated by either heat inactivation (56°C/30 min) or by saturation with iron. Intraperitoneal inoculation of mice with graded doses of ferric ammonium citrate increased their susceptibility to subsequent intraperitoneal challenge with *Y. enterocolitica* 0:3,[122] 0:8,[123] and 0:9.[124] The iron overload did not reduce the survival time of infected mice, rather it increased the number of mice that succumbed.[123] It remains to be determined whether any of the OMP present in virulent yersiniae are iron-binding proteins that facilitate this effect in the normal host.

REFERENCES

1. Knapp, W., Fahrlander, H., and Hartweg, H., Zur Atiologie der akuten regionaren Enteritis (Ileitis), *Schweiz. Med. Wochenschr.*, 100, 364, 1970.
2. Schleifstein, J. I. and Coleman, M. B., An unidentified microorganism resembling *B. lignieri and P. pseudotuberculosis*, and pathogenic for man, *N. Y. State J. Med.*, 39, 1749, 1939.
3. Knapp, W. and Thal, E., Untersuchungen uber die kulturellgbiochemischen, serologischen, tierexperimentellen and immunologishen Eigenschaften einer vorlaufig "Pasteurella X" benannter Bakterienart, *Zentralbl. Bakteriol. Parisitenkd. Infektionskr. Hyg. Abt. 1: Orig. Reihe B:*, 190, 472, 1963.
4. Mollaret, H. H. and Guillon, J. C., Contribution l'etude d'un nouveau group de germes proches du bacille de Mallassez et Viginal. I. Caracteres culturaux et biochimique, *Ann. Inst. Pasteur Paris,* 109, 608, 1965.
5. Carter, P. B., Varga, C. F. and Keet, E. E., A new strain of *Yersinia enterocolitica* pathogenic for rodents, *Appl. Microbiol.,* 26, 1016, 1973.
6. Maruyama, T., Studies on biological characteristics and pathogenicity of *Yersinia enterocolitica*. II. Experimental infections in monkeys (in Japanese), *Jpn. J. Bacteriol.,* 28, 413, 1973.
7. Quan, T. J., Meek, J. L., Tsuchiya, K. R., Hudson, B. W., and Barnes, A. M., Experimental pathogenicity of recent North American isolates of *Yersinia enterocolitica, J. Infect. Dis.,* 129, 341, 1974.
8. McIver, M. A. and Pike, R. M., Chronic glanders-like infection of face caused by an organism resembling *Flavobacterium pseudomallei*, in *Clinical Miscellany*, Vol. 1, Mary Imogene Bassett Hospital, Cooperstown, N.Y., 1934, 16.
9. Frederiksen, W., A study of some *Yersinia pseudotuberculosis*-like bacteria ("Bacterium enterocoliticum" and "Pasteurella X"), *Proc. 14th Scand. Congr. Pathol. Microbiol.,* Oslo, 1964, 103.
10. Bottone, E. J., *Yersinia enterocolitica* and *Yersinia pseudotuberculosis,* in *The Prokaryotes,* Vol. 2, Starr, M. P., Stolp, H., Truper, H. G., Balow, A., and Schlegel, H. C., Eds., Springer-Verlag, Berlin, 1981, 1225.
11. Mollaret, H. H., Contribution a l'etude epidemiologique des infections a *Yersinia enterocolitica.* II. Bilan provisoire des connaissances, *Med. Malad. Infect.,* 6, 442, 1976.
12. Hurvell, B., Glatthard, V., and Thal, E., Isolation of *Yersinia enterocolitica* from Swine at an abattoir in Sweden, in *Contributions to Microbiology and Immunology,* Vol. 5, Carter, P. B., Lafleur, L., and Toma, S., Eds., S. Karger, Basel, 1979, 243.
13. Toma, S., Lafleur, L., and Diedrick, V. R., Canadian experience with *Yersinia enterocolitica (1966-1977),* in *Contributions to Microbiology and Immunology,* Vol. 5, Carter, P. B., Lafleur, L., and Toma, S., Eds., S. Karger, Basel, 1979, 144.
14. Wauters, G., Carriage of *Yersinia enterocolitica* serotype 3 by pigs as a source of human infection, in *Contributions to Microbiology and Immunology,* Vol. 5, Carter, P. B., Lafleur, L., and Toma, S., Eds., S. Karger, Basel, 1979, 249.
15. Quan, T. J., Biotypic and serotypic profiles of 367 *Yersinia enterocolitica* cultures of human and environmental origin in the United States, in *Contributions to Microbiology and Immunology,* Vol. 5, Carter, P. B., Lafleur, L., and Toma, S., Eds., S. Karger, Basel, 1979, 83.
16. Mollaret, H. H., *Yersinia enterocolitica* infection: A new problem in pathology (editorial translation), *Ann. Biol. Clin.,* 30, 1, 1972.
17. Obwolo, M. J., A review of Yersiniosis *(Yersinia pseudotuberculosis)* infection, *Vet. Bull.,* 46, 167, 1976.
18. Mair, N. S., Yersiniosis in wildlife and its public health implications, *J. Wildl. Dis.,* 9, 64, 1973.
19. Hubbert, W. T., Yersiniosis in mammals and birds in the United States. Case reports and a review, *Am. J. Trop. Med. Hyg.,* 21, 458, 1972.
20. Mair, N. S., Fox, E., and Thal, E., Biochemical, Pathogenicity and Toxicity Studies of Type III Strains of *Yersinia pseudotuberculosis* isolated from the cecal contents of pigs, in *Contributions to Microbiology and Immunology,* Vol. 5, Carter, P. B., Lafleur, L., and Toma, S., Eds., S. Karger, Basel, 1979, 359.
21. Toma, S. and Diedrick, V. R., Isolation of *Yersinia enterocolitica* from swine, *J. Clin. Microbiol.,* 2, 478, 1975.
22. Zen-Yoji, H., Sakai, S., Maruyama, T., and Yanagawa, Y., Isolation of *Yersinia enterocolitica* and *Yersinia pseudotuberculosis* from swine, cattle and rats at an abattoir, *Jpn. J. Microbiol.,* 18, 103, 1974.
23. Une, T., Studies on the pathogenecity of *Yersinia enterocolitica.* III. Comparative studies between *Y. enterocolitica* and *Y. pseudotuberculosis, Microbiol. Immunol.,* 21, 505, 1977.
24. Une, T. and Zen-Yoji, H., Investigations on the pathogenicity of *Yersinia enterocolitica* by experimental infection in rabbits and cultured cells, in *Contributions to Microbiology and Immunology,* Vol. 5, Carter, P. B., Lafleur, L., and Toma, S., Eds., S. Karger, Basel, 1979, 304.

25. Van Noyen, R., Vandepitte, J., and Selderslaghs, R., Human gastrointestinal infections by *Yersinia enterocolitica*, in *Contributions to Microbiology and Immunology*, Vol. 5, Carter, P. B., Lafleur, L., and Toma, S., Eds., S. Karger, Basel, 1979, 283.

26. Mollaret, H. H., Bercovier, H., and Alonso, J. M., Summary of the data received at the WHO Reference Center for *Yersinia enterocolitica*, in *Contributions to Microbiology and Immunology*, Vol. 5, Carter, P. B., Lafleur, L., and Toma, S., Eds., S. Karger, Basel, 1979, 174.

27. Anon., Multistate outbreak of Yersiniosis, *Morbidity Mortality Wkly. Rep.*, 31, 505, 1982.

28. Asakawa, Y., Akahane, S., Kagata, N., Noguchi, M., Sakazaki, R., and Tamura, K., Two community outbreaks of human infection with *Yersinia enterocolitica*, *J. Hyg. (Cambridge)*, 71, 715, 1973.

29. Martin, T., Kasian, G. F., and Stead, S., Family outbreak of Yersiniosis, *J. Clin. Microbiol.*, 16, 622, 1982.

30. Shayegani, M., Morse, D., DeForge, I., Root, T., Parsons, L. M., and Maupin, P., Foodborne outbreak of *Yersinia enterocolitica* in Sullivan County, New York, with pathologic studies of the isolates, Abstr. *Annu. Meet. Am. Soc. Microbiol.*, C175, 1982.

31. Keet, E. E., *Yersinia enterocolitica* septicemia. Source of infection and incubation period identified, *N. Y. State J. Med.*, 74, 2226, 1974.

32. Black, R. E., Jackson, R. J., Tsai, T., Medevesky, M., Shayegani, M., Feeley, J. C., MacLeod, K. I. E., and Wakelee, A. M., Epidemic *Yersinia enterocolitica* infection due to contaminated chocolate milk, *N. Engl. J. Med.*, 298, 76, 1978.

33. Aulisio, C. C. G., Stanfield, J. T., Weagant, S. D., and Hill, W. E., Yersiniosis associated with tofu consumption: serological, biochemical and pathogenicity studies of *Yersinia enterocolitica* isolates, *J. Food Prod.*, 46, 226, 1983.

34. Aulisio, C. C. G., Lanier, J. M., and Chappel, M. A., *Yersinia enterocolitica* 0:13 associated with outbreaks in three southern states, *J. Food Prot.*, 45, 1263, 1982.

35. Essereld, H. and Goudzwaart, C., On the epidemiology of *Y. enterocilitica* infections: pigs as the source of infections in man, in *Contributions to Microbiology and Immunology*, Vol. 2, Winblad, S., Ed., Karger, Basel, 1973, 99.

36. Narucka, U. and Westendoorp, Y. F., Een onderzoek noar het voorhomen van *Yersinia enterocolitica* en *Yersinia pseudotuberculosis* bij Klinisch normale varkens, *Tijdschr. Diergeneeskd.*, 102, 299, 1977.

37. Pedersen, K. B., Isolation of *Yersinia enterocolitica* from Danish swine and dogs, *Acta Pathol. Microbiol. Scand. Sect. B.*, 84, 317, 1976.

38. Pedersen, K. B., Occurrence of *Yersinia enterocolitica* in the throat of swine, in *Contributions to Microbiology and Immunology*, Vol. 5, Carter, P. B., Lafleur, L., and Toma, S., Eds., S. Karger, Basel, 1979, 253.

39. Rabson, A. R. and Koornhof, H. J., *Yersinia enterocolitica* infections in South Africa, in *Contributions to Microbiology and Immunology*, Vol. 2, Winblad, S., Ed., S. Karger, Basel, 1973, 102.

40. Tsubokura, M., Otsuki, K., and Hagaki, K., Studies on *Yersinia enterocolitica* I. Isolation of *Y. enterocolitica* from swine, *Jpn. J. Vet. Sci.*, 35, 419, 1973.

41. Ahvonen, P. and Rossi, T., Familial occurrence of *Yersinia enterocolitica* infection and acute arthritis, *Acta Paediatr. Scand. Suppl.*, 206, 121, 1970.

42. Ahvonen, P., Human yersiniosis in Finland. II. Clinical features, *Ann. Clin. Res.*, 4, 39, 1972.

43. Delorme, J., Laverdiere, M., Martineau, B., and Lafleur, L., Yersiniosis in children, *Can. Med. Assoc. J.*, 110, 281, 1974.

44. Gutman, L. T., Ottesen, E. A., Quan, T. J., Noce, P. S., and Katz, S. L., An inter-familial outbreak of *Yersinia enterocolitica* enteritis, *N. Engl. J. Med.*, 288, 1372, 1973.

45. Mollaret, H. H., L'infection humaine a *Yersinia enterocolitica* en 1970, a la lumiere de 642 cas recents: aspects clinique et perspectives epidemiologiques, *Pathol. Biol. (Paris)*, 19, 189, 1971.

46. Vandepitte, J. and Wauters, G., Epidemiological and clinical aspects of human *Yersinia enterocolitica* infections in Belgium, in *Contributions to Microbiology and Immunology*, Vol. 5, Carter, P. B., Lafleur, L., and Toma, S., Eds., S. Karger, Basel, 1979, 150.

47. Mair, N. S., Sources and serological classification of 177 strains of *Pasteurella pseudotuberculosis* isolated in Great Britain, *J. Pathol. Bacteriol.*, 90, 275, 1965.

48. Paterson, J. S. and Cook, R., A method for the recovery of *Pasteurella pseudotuberculosis* from faeces, *J. Pathol. Bacteriol.*, 85, 241, 1963.

49. Biship, L. M., Study of an outbreak of pseudotuberculosis in guinea pigs (cavies) due to *P. pseudotuberculosis rodentium*, *Cornell Vet.*, 22, 1, 1932.

50. Branch, A., Spontaneous infections of guinea pigs. Pneumococcus, Friedlander bacillus and pseudotuberculosis (Eberthella caviae), *J. Infect. Dis.*, 40, 533, 1948.

51. Chapman, M. P., *Pseudotuberculosis redentium* in Chinchilla. A field case, *North Am. Vet.*, 29, 493, 1948.

52. Gomez, A. K., An infectious disease of guinea pigs, *J. Am. Vet. Med. Assoc.*, 53, 511, 1918.

53. Leader, R. W. and Baker, G. A., A report of two cases of *Pasteurella pseudotuberculosis* infection in the chinchilla, *Cornell Vet.*, 44, 262, 1954.

54. Mollaret, H. H. and Placidi, L., Le bacille de Malassez et Vignal chez le monton et la chevre, *Rec. Med. Vet.*, 140, 515, 1964.
55. Blanc, G. and Baltazard, M., Contribution a l'etude du comportement des microbes pathogene chez les insect hematophage, *Arch. Inst. Pasteur Maroc.*, 3, 21, 1944.
56. Baggs, R. B., Hunt, R. D., Garcia, F. G., Hajema, E. M., Blake, B. J., and Fraser, C. E. O., Pseudotuberculosis *(Yersinia enterocolitica)* in the owl monkey *(Aotus trivirgatus)*, *Lab. Anim. Sci.*, 26, 1079, 1976.
57. Wilson, H. D., McCormick, J. B., and Feeley, J. C., *Yersinia enterocolitica* infection in a four month infant associated with infection in household dogs, *J. Pediatr.*, 89, 767, 1976.
58. Kaneko, K., Hamada, S., Kasai, Y., and Kato, E., Occurrence of *Yersinia enterocolitica* in house rats, *Appl. Environ. Microbiol.*, 36, 314, 1978.
59. Vandepitte, J., Van Noyen, R., and Isebaert, A., *Yersinia enterocolitica:* its incidence in patients with infectious diarrhea. A report of 100 cases, *Proc. 5th Int. Congr. Infect. Dis. Vienna*, Vol. 3, 1970, 119.
60. Bergstrand, C. G. and Winblad, S., Clinical manifestations of infection with *Yersinia enterocolitica* in children, *Acta Paediat. Scand.*, 63, 875, 1974.
61. Dominowska, C. and Mallottke, R., Survival of *Yersinia* in water samples originating from various sources, *Bull. Inst. Marine Trop. Med.*, 22, 173, 1971.
62. Gilbert, R., Interesting Cases and Unusual Specimens, Ann. Rep. Div. Lab. Res., N.Y. State Department of Health, Albany, 1933, 57.
63. Une, T., Studies on the pathogenicity of *Yersinia enterocolitica*. I. Experimental infection in rabbits, *Microbiol. Immunol.*, 21, 349, 1977.
64. Carter, P. B. and Collins, F. M., Experimental *Yersinia enterocolitica* infection in mice: kinetics of growth, *Infect. Immunol.*, 9, 851, 1974.
65. Alonso, J. M., Bercovier, H., Destombes, P., and Mollaret, H. H., Pouvoir pathogene experimental de *Yersinia enterocolitica* chez la souris athymique (nude), *Ann. Microbiol. (Inst. Pasteur)*, 126B, 187, 1975.
66. Bercovier, H., Alonso, J. M., Destombes, P., and Mollaret, H. H., Infection experimentale de souris axeniques par *Yersinia enterocolitica, Ann. Microbiol. (Inst. Pasteur)*, 127A, 493, 1976.
67. Alonso, J. M., Mazigh, D., Bercovier, H., and Mollaret, H. H., Infection experimentale de la souris par *Yersinia enterocolitica* (souche du chimiotype 4, du serogroupe 0:3, du lysotype VIII): devenir de l'inoculum chez des souris athymiques ou traitees par le cyclophosphamide, *Ann. Microbiol. (Inst. Pasteur)*, 129B, 27, 1978.
68. Carter, P. B., Animal model: oral *Yersinia enterocolitica* infection of mice, *Am. J. Pathol.*, 81, 703, 1975.
69. Carter, P. B., Pathogenicity of *Yersinia enterocolitica* for mice, *Infect. Immunol.*, 11, 164, 1975.
70. Kaneko, K. and Hashimoto, N., Fecal excretion associated with Ca$^+$ dependency of *Yersinia enterocolitica* 03 and 09 and *Yersinia pseudotuberculosis* in mice, *Microbiol. Immunol.*, 27, 199, 1983.
71. Uchida, I., Kaneko, K., and Hashimoto, N., Cross-protection against fecal excretion of *Yersinia enterocolitica* and *Yersinia pseudotuberculosis* in mice by oral vaccination of viable cells, *Infect. Immunol.*, 36, 837, 1982.
72. Ricciardi, I. D., Pearson, A. D., Suckling, W. G., and Klein, C., Long-term fecal excretion and resistance induced in mice infected with *Yersinia enterocolitica, Infect. Immunol.*, 21, 342, 1978.
73. Pearson, A. D., Ricciardi, I. D., Wright, D. H., and Suckling, W. G., An experimental study of the pathology and ecology of *Yersinia enterocolitica* infection in mice, in *Contributions to Microbiology and Immunology*, Vol. 5, Carter, P. B., Lafleur, L., and Toma, S., Eds., S. Karger, Basel, 1979, 336.
74. Fukai, K. and Maruyama, T., Histopathological studies on experimental *Yersinia enterocolitica* infection in animals, in *Contributions to Microbiology and Immunology,* Vol. 5, Carter, P. B., Lafleur, L., and Toma, S., Eds., S. Karger, Basel, 1979, 310.
75. McClure, H. M., Weaver, R. E., and Kaufmann, A. F., Pseudotuberculosis in nonhuman primates: infection with organisms of the *Yersinia enterocolitica* group, *Lab. Anim. Sci.*, 21, 376, 1971.
76. Baggs, R. B., Hunt, R. D., Garcia, F. G., Hajema, E. M., Blake, B. J., and Fraser, C. E. O., Pseudotuberculosis *(Yersinia enterocolitica)* in owl monkey, *(Aotus trivirgatus)*, *Lab. Anim. Sci.*, 26, 1079, 1976.
77. LaBrec, E. H., Schneider, H., Magnani, T. J., and Formal, S. B., Epithelial cell penetration as an essential step in the pathogenesis of bacillary dysentery, *J. Bacteriol.*, 88, 1503, 1964.
78. Giannella, R. A., Washington, O., Gemski, P., and Formal, S. B., Invasion of HeLa cells by *Salmonella typhimurium:* a model for study of invasiveness of *Salmonella, J. Infect. Dis.*, 128, 69, 1973.
79. Lee, W. H., McGrath, P. P., Carter, P. H., and Eide, E. L., The ability of some *Yersinia enterocolitica* strains to invade HeLa cells, *Can. J. Microbiol.*, 23, 1714, 1977.
80. Une, T., Studies on the pathogenicity of *Yersinia enterocolitica*. II. Interaction with cultured cells *in vitro, Microbiol. Immunol.*, 21, 365, 1977.

81. Une, T., Zen-Yoji, H., Maruyama, T., and Yanagawa, Y., Correlation between epithelial cell infectivity in vitro and O-antigen groups of *Yersinia enterocolitica, Microbiol. Immunol.,* 21, 727, 1977.
82. Lee, W. H., Testing for the recovery of *Yersinia enterocolitica* in foods and their ability to invade HeLa cells, in *Contributions to Microbiology and Immunology,* Vol. 5, Carter, P. B., Lafleur, L., and Toma, S., Eds., S. Karger, Basel, 1979, 229.
83. Maruyama, T., Une, T., and Zen-Yoji, H., Observations on the correlation between pathogenicity and serovars of *Yersinia enterocolitica* by the assay applying cell culture system and experimental mouse infection, in *Contributions to Microbiology and Immunology,* Vol. 5, Carter, P. B., Lafleur, L., and Toma, S., Eds., S. Karger, Basel, 1979, 318.
84. Schiemann, D. A. and Devenish, J. A., Relationship of HeLa cell infectivity to biochemical, serological, and virulence characteristics of *Yersinia enterocolitica, Infect. Immunol.,* 35, 497, 1982.
85. Devenish, J. A. and Schiemann, D. A., HeLa cell infection by *Yersinia enterocolitica:* evidence for lack of intracellular multiplication and development of a new procedure for quantitative expression of infectivity, *Infect. Immunol.,* 32, 48, 1981.
86. Carter, P. B., Zahorchak, R. J., and Brubaker, R. R., Plaque virulence antigens from *Yersinia enterocolitica, Infect. Immunol.,* 28, 638, 1980.
87. Perry, R. D. and Brubaker, R. R., Vwa⁺ phenotype of *Yersinia enterocolitica, Infect. Immunol.,* 40, 166, 1983.
88. Portnoy, D. A., Wolf-Watz, H., Bolin, I., Beeder, A. B., and Falkow, S., Characterization of common virulence plasmids in *Yersinia* and their role in the expression of outer membrane proteins, *Infect. Immunol.,* 43, 108, 1984.
89. Feeley, J. C., Wells, J. G., Tsai, T. F., and Puhr, N. D., Detection of enterotoxigenic and invasive strains of *Yersinia enterocolitica,* in *Contributions to Microbiology and Immunology,* Vol. 5, Carter, P. B., Lafleur, L., and Toma, S., Eds., S. Karger, Basel, 1979, 329.
90. Schiemann, D. A. and Devenish, J. A., Virulence of *Yersinia enterocolitica* determined by lethality in Mongolian gerbils and by the Sereny test, *Infect. Immunol.,* 29, 500, 1980.
91. Robins-Browne, R. M., van Vuuren, C. J. J., Still, C. S., Miliotis, M. D., and Koornhof, H. J., The pathogenesis of *Yersinia enterocolitica* gastroenteritis, in *Contributions to Microbiology and Immunology,* Vol. 5, Carter, P. B., Lafleur, L., and Toma, S., Eds., S. Karger, Basel, 1979, 324.
92. Aulisio, C. C. G., Hill, W. E., Stanfield, J. T., and Sellers, R. L., Jr., Evaluation of virulence factor testing and characteristics of pathogenicity in *Yersinia enterocolitica, Infect. Immunol.,* 40, 330, 1983.
93. Straley, S. C. and Brubaker, R. R., Cytoplasmic and membrane proteins of yersiniae cultivated under conditions simulating mammalian intracellular environment, *Proc. Natl. Acad. Sci. U.S.A.,* 78, 1224, 1981.
94. Martinez, R. F., Plasmid-mediated and temperature-regulated surface properties of *Yersinia enterocolitica, Infect. Immunol.,* 41, 921, 1983.
95. Sack, R. B., Human diarrheal disease caused by enterotoxigenic *Escherichia coli, Annu. Rev. Microbiol.,* 29, 33, 1975.
96. Pai, C. H., Mors, V., and Toma, S., Prevalence of enterotoxigenicity in human and nonhuman isolates of *Yersinia enterocolitica, Infect. Immunol.,* 22, 334, 1978.
97. Pai, C. H. and Mors, V., Production of enterotoxin by *Yersinia enterocolitica, Infect. Immunol.,* 19, 908, 1978.
98. Boyce, J. M., Evans, D. J., Jr., Evans, D. G., and Dupont, H. L., Production of heat-stable, methanol-soluble enterotoxin by *Yersinia enterocolitica, Infect. Immunol.,* 25, 532, 1979.
99. Robins-Browne, R. M., Still, C. S., Miliotis, M. D., and Koornhof, H. J., Mechanism of action of *Yersinia enterocolitica* enterotoxin, *Infect. Immunol.,* 25, 680, 1979.
100. Schiemann, D. A., An enterotoxin-negative strain of *Yersinia enterocolitica* serotype 0:3 is capable of producing diarrhea in mice, *Infect. Immunol.,* 32, 571, 1981.
101. Zink, D. L., Feeley, J. C., Wells, J. G., Vanderzant, C., Vickery, J. C., and O'Donovan, G. A., Possible plasmid-mediated virulence in *Yersinia enterocolitica, Trans. Gulf Coast Mol. Biol. Conf.,* 3, 155, 1978.
102. Gemski, P., Lazere, J. R., and Casey, T., A plasmid associated with pathogenicity and calcium dependency of *Yersinia enterocolitica, Infect. Immunol.,* 27, 682, 1980.
103. Gemski, P., Lazere, J. R., Casey, T., and Wohlhieter, J. A., Presence of a virulence-associated plasmid in *Yersinia pseudotuberculosis, Infect. Immunol.,* 28, 1044, 1980.
104. Burrows, T. W. and Bacon, G. A., The basis of virulence in *Pasteurella pestis:* an antigen determining virulence, *Br. J. Exp. Pathol.,* 37, 481, 1956.
105. Burrows, T. W. and Bacon, G. A., V and W antigens in strains of *Pasteurella pseudotuberculosis, Br. J. Exp. Pathol.,* 39, 278, 1960.
106. Portnoy, D. A., Blank, H. F., Kingsbury, D. T., and Falkow, S., Genetic analysis of essential plasmid determinants of pathogenicity in *Yersinia pestis, J. Infect. Dis.,* 148, 297, 1983.

107. Alonso, J. M., Joseph-Francois, A., Mazigh, D., Bercovier, H., and Mollaret, H. H., Resistance a la peste de souris experimentalement infectees par *Yersinia enterocolitica, Ann. Microbiol. (Inst. Pasteur)*, 129B, 203, 1978.

108. Higuchi, K., Kupferberg, L. L., and Smith, J. L., Studies on the nutrition and physiology of *Pasteurella pestis*. III. Effects of calcium ions on the growth of virulent and avirulent strains of *Pasteurella pestis, J. Bacteriol.*, 77, 317, 1959.

109. Brubaker, R. R., The genus *Yersinia:* biochemistry and genetics of virulence, *Curr. Top. Microbiol. Immunol.*, 57, 111, 1972.

110. Berche, P. A. and Carter, P. B., Calcium requirement and virulence of *Yersinia enterocolitica, J. Med. Microbiol.*, 15, 277, 1982.

111. Brubaker, R. R. and Surgalla, M. J., The effect of Ca^{++} and Mg^{++} on lysis, growth, and production of virulence antigens by *Pasteurella pestis, J. Infect. Dis.*, 114, 13, 1964.

112. Portnoy, D. A. and Falkow, S., Virulence-associated plasmids from *Yersinia enterocolitica* and *Yersinia pestis, J. Bacteriol.*, 148, 877, 1981.

113. Portnoy, D. A., Moseley, S. L., and Falkow, S., Characterization of plasmids and plasmid-associated determinants of *Yersinia enterocolitica* pathogenesis, *Infect. Immunol.*, 31, 775, 1981.

114. Brubaker, R. R., Growth of *Pasteurella pseudotuberculosis* in simulated intracellular and extracellular environments, *J. Infect. Dis.*, 117, 403, 1967.

115. Laird, W. J. and Cavanaugh, D. C., Correlation of autoagglutination and virulence of yersiniae, *J. Clin. Microbiol.*, 11, 430, 1980.

116. Doyle, M. P., Hugdahl, M. B., Chang, M. T., and Beery, J. T., Serological relatedness of mouse-virulent *Yersinia enterocolitica, Infect. Immunol.*, 37, 1234, 1982.

117. Pai, C. H. and DeStephano, L., Serum resistance associated with virulence in *Yersinia enterocolitica, Infect. Immunol.*, 35, 605, 1982.

118. Chiesa, C. and Bottone, E. J., Serum resistance of *Yersinia enterocolitica* expressed in the absence of other virulence markers, *Infect. Immunol.*, 39, 469, 1983.

119. Une, T., and Brubaker, R. R., *In vivo* comparison of avirulent Vwa− and Pgm− or Pstr phenotypes of yersiniae, *Infect. Immunol.*, 43, 895, 1984.

120. Kay, B. A., Wachsmuth, K., and Gemski, P., New virulence-associated plasmid in *Yersinia enterocolitica, J. Clin. Microbiol.*, 15, 1161, 1982.

121. Rabson, A. R., Hallet, A. F., and Koornhof, H. J., Generalized *Yersinia enterocolitica* infection, *J. Infect. Dis.*, 131, 447, 1975.

122. Robins-Browne, R. M., Rabson, A. R., and Koornhof, H. J., Generalized infection with *Yersinia enterocolitica* and the role of iron, in *Contributions to Microbiology and Immunology*, Vol. 5, Carter, P. B., Lafleur, L., and Toma, S., Eds., S. Karger, Basel, 1979, 277.

123. van Vuuren, C. J. J., The Pathogenic Mechanisms of *Yersinia enterocolitica* Disease, Doctoral dissertation, University of the Witwatersrand, Witwatersrand, South Africa, 1982.

124. Smith, R. E., Carey, A. M., Damare, J. M., Hetrick, F. M., Johnston, R. W., and Lee, W. H., Evaluation of iron dextran and mucin for enhancement of the virulence of *Yersinia enterocolitica* serotype 0:3 in mice, *Infect. Immunol.*, 34, 550, 1981.

Part II
*Spontaneous or Induced Cancers or Chronic
Inflammatory Conditions of the Intestinal
Tract*

Chapter 6

ADENOCARCINOMA OF THE COLON AND CHRONIC COLITIS IN *SAGUINUS OEDIPUS:* A POSSIBLE MODEL FOR ANALOGOUS HUMAN DISEASE*

Laura V. Chalifoux, Ronald D. Hunt, and Norval W. King, Jr.

TABLE OF CONTENTS

* This work supported by Division of Research Resources (NIH) grant #RR00168 to the New England Regional Primate Research Center.

I. INTRODUCTION

Colonic adenocarcinoma in the cotton-top tamarin *(Saguinus oedipus)* is the most common neoplastic disease of nonhuman primates. The incidence and total number of cases of this cancer that have been seen in two colonies of tamarins[1,2] is rivaled only by the occurrence of malignant lymphoma in *Macaca* species.[3] The association of this neoplasm with a chronic colitis in these monkeys resembles that of colon cancer and inflammatory bowel disease as described in human beings.[4,5]

Various naturally occurring and experimentally induced enteric maladies of animals have been described that have similarities to inflammatory bowel disease in humans. These include canine histiocytic ulcerative colitis in the boxer[6,7] and cocker spaniel[8] breeds of dogs, ulcerative colitis induced in guinea pigs by degraded carrageenans,[9,10] and proliferative ileitis and colitis of hamsters[11,12] and mice.[13] Bacterial colitis in some species has also been suggested as a model of certain human large-bowel diseases by some investigators. Most of these models, however, have shortcomings in their resemblance to the human disease and in none has neoplasia been associated with chronicity.

Although colonic adenocarcinoma occurs occasionally as a spontaneous disease in dogs, cats, and other domestic animals, it is not seen with sufficient regularity to be used in experimental studies. The most commonly studied models of colonic cancer are those induced by the chemical carcinogens, dimethylhydrazine, methylazoxymethanol acetate, or azoxymethane, usually in rats.

Previously we described 15 cases of colonic adenocarcinoma in *Saguinus oedipus* associated with chronic colitis[2] that occurred in our colony between August 1977 and August 1980. Five additional cases were observed between August and December 1980. During 1981, no further colon cancers were diagnosed although colitis was seen with regularity in rectal biopsy specimens. Between June 1982 and January 1983, 4 additional tamarins died with colon cancer, bringing the total to 24. The four most recent cases were old monkeys (>6 years) in which colitis had been previously confirmed by rectal biopsy. This chapter will review our experience with this disease and will include a discussion of the most recent cases.

II. CLINICAL OBSERVATIONS

The general husbandry practices and diet for this colony have been described previously.[14,15] The animals are maintained in accordance with the guidelines of the Committee on Animals of the Harvard Medical School and those prepared by the Committee on Care and Use of Laboratory Animals of the Institute of Laboratory Animal Resources, National Research Council (DHEW Publ. No. NIH 78-23, revised 1978).

Clinically, this colitis in tamarins is characterized by diarrhea which may range from soft, bulky stools to profuse, explosive, and watery diarrhea. There is usually no gross evidence of hemorrhage; however, the mucosa is frequently friable and clinical manipulations such as proctoscopy or swabbing easily induce bleeding. Anorexia, dehydration, and extreme weight loss are observed, and if the animal is not treated death ensues quickly. Advanced cases of colonic cancer may be palpable through the abdominal wall and obstruction of the colon, resulting in constipation, can be an additional indication of neoplasia.

III. PATHOLOGY

At necropsy, the gross appearance of the colonic mucosa varies from essentially normal to congested and thickened with focal areas of hemorrhage and ulceration. The lumen may be empty or contain watery or mucoid contents that are occasionally blood tinged. Adjacent colonic lymph nodes are large and edematous.

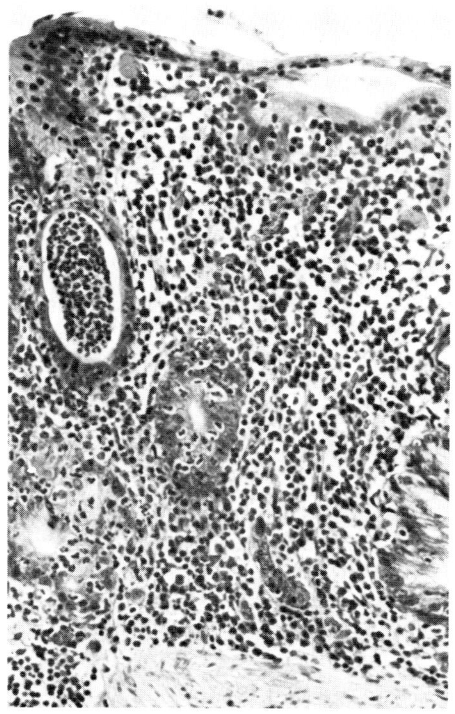

FIGURE 1. Active colitis with neutrophils in crypt epithelium and lumen of the crypt as well as the lamina propria. Rectal biopsy from tamarin #661-76 taken 28 months before death. (H.E.; magnification × 280.)

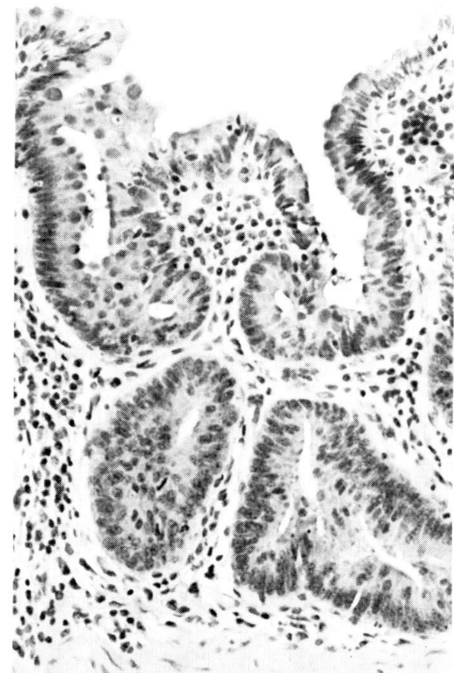

FIGURE 2. Chronic colitis with distorted and branched crypts and mononuclear cell infiltrate in lamina propria. Tamarin #688-76 at necropsy. (Periodic acid-Schiff; magnification × 280.)

Thickened areas in the colonic wall may indicate early neoplastic invasion. Extensive invasion accompanied by fibrosis, often with partial occlusion of the lumen and dilation of that portion of the colon proximal to the lesion, is a frequent observation. Adhesions of the colon to portions of small intestine or to parietal peritoneum may also be present. Occasionally, peritonitis associated with transmural invasion is seen. Enlarged, often firm and white colonic lymph nodes, ileocecolic nodes, and sometimes pancreatic nodes are frequent findings.

Examination of more than 200 necropsies and sequential rectal biopsies taken from approximately 100 animals at various intervals over a period of 2 years has resulted in the recognition of several patterns of the colonic disease. What is believed to be the earliest lesion, usually seen in punch biopsies taken from the rectum rather than at necropsy, is characterized by a few polymorphonuclear neutrophils in the lamina propria with mild congestion of the mucosa. Subsequently, neutrophils are more prevalent within the epithelial layer of crypts and then appear in the crypt lumens (Figure 1). Affected crypts become dilated with flattened epithelium and microulcerations that may coalesce to form larger mucosal ulcers. There is a decrease in the number of goblet cells. The number of mitotic figures in the crypt epithelium increases, sometimes extending more than halfway up the length of the crypt. Large numbers of Paneth cells in the bases of crypts are found in some colons. Areas where crypts have been destroyed are often replaced by foci of regenerating epithelial cells.

In other examples there is little purulent inflammation, but the lamina propria is infiltrated by inflammatory cells consisting predominantly of lymphocytes and plasma cells (Figure 2). Crypts in these colons are usually distorted and contain very few goblet

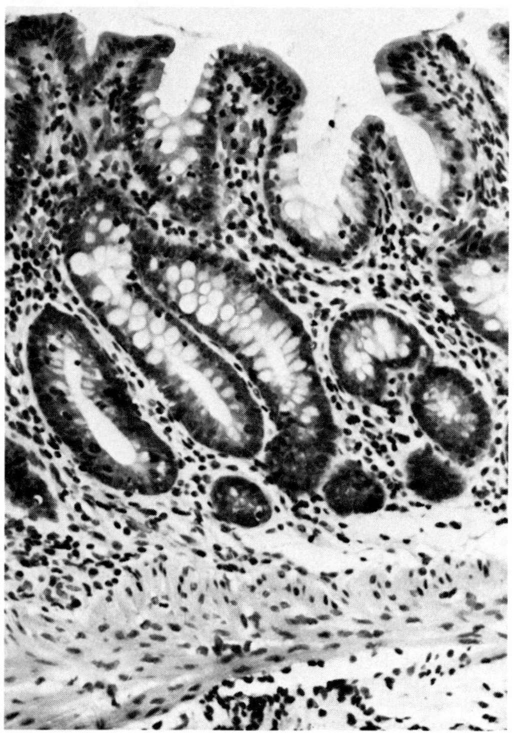

FIGURE 3.   Colitis in remission. Active inflammation is gone and goblet cells are present, but crypts remain distorted. Rectal biopsy from tamarin #661-76, 24 months before death, and after 6 weeks of treatment with sulfasalazine. Compare with Figure 1 taken before treatment. (H.E.; magnification × 280.)

cells. In most colonic mucosae there is a mixture of both chronic and acute inflammatory cellular infiltrates as well as changes indicative of preexisting colitis.

Some specimens have a histologic appearance suggestive of remission, based upon the presence of residual lesions indicative of previous mucosal damage. In such cases, purulent inflammation is no longer present and goblet cells are evident, but scattered crypts are obliterated or markedly distorted in shape (Figure 3). Mononuclear cells are present in smaller numbers. Remnants of undermined mucosa persist in the form of irregular tags, bridges, and polyps, and prior ulceration is evidenced by microherniation of large numbers of crypts into the submucosa with occasional disruption of the muscularis mucosae. Areas of mild to severe mucosal atrophy are also seen.

The inflammatory process, which is diffuse and involves the cecum, colon, and rectum, tends to be limited to the mucosa, except for the occasional crypt herniations into the submucosa, mentioned earlier. Rarely does the mononuclear infiltrate extend into the submucosa.

In the presence of severe active inflammation, most pathologists are reluctant to evaluate dysplasia in human inflammatory bowel disease. The same problem exists in evaluating the colons of these monkeys. There is certainly proliferation and regeneration of the inflamed crypt epithelium. Also, the surface epithelium is often piled up, resembling pseudostratified epithelium. In some crypts in which there is no evidence of inflammation, there is, however, evidence of dysplasia characterized by epithelial cells with hyperchromatic, pleomorphic nuclei that have lost their normal orientation

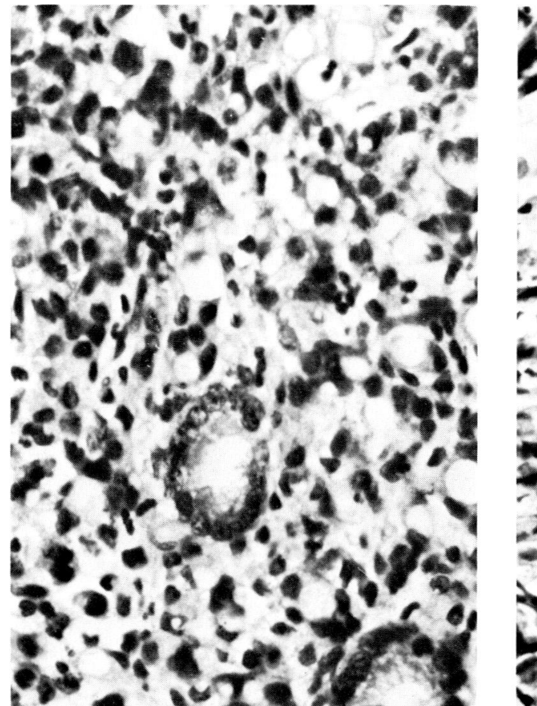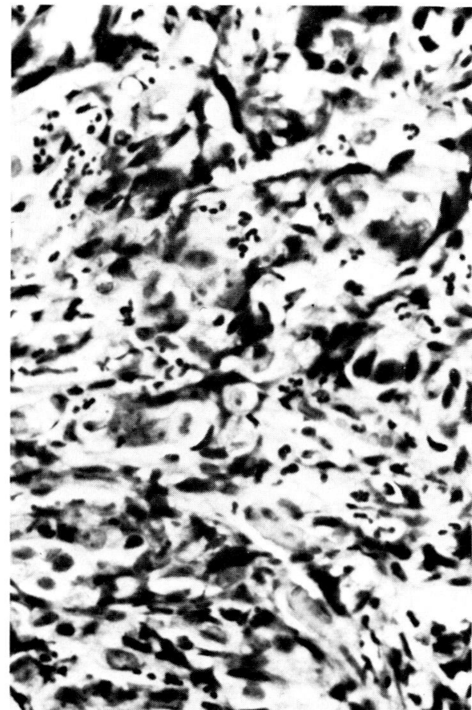

FIGURE 4. Adenocarcinoma in colonic mucosa. Some cells are arranged in a glandular pattern. Tamarin #347-76 at necropsy. (H.E.; magnification × 600.)

FIGURE 5. Poorly differentiated adenocarcinoma in biopsy of rectal mucosa. Tamarin #347-76, 22 months before death. (H.E.; magnification × 600.)

with respect to the basement membrane. Small numbers of crypts that exhibit back-to-back orientation may be found among the distorted and branched forms.

Foci of intramucosal adenocarcinoma are seen in colons with and without invasive carcinoma. They are often multifocal and occur in flat mucosae near the bases of crypts. Some of the neoplastic cells are arranged in poorly differentiated glands with or without a lumen (Figure 4). Others have no distinctive pattern of growth and simply appear as sheets of cells with pale pink cytoplasm (Figure 5). Periodic acid Schiff (PAS) stains demonstrate diffuse positive material in the cytoplasm of these cells. Signet ring cells containing PAS-positive mucin may be present in the neoplastic infiltrates.

The invasive carcinomas are either limited to only a few cells infiltrating through the muscularis mucosae or they may extend through the entire muscularis involving the serosa and be accompanied by extensive fibrosis. The invading cells have hyperchromatic nuclei, scant cytoplasm, and either form glands (Figure 6) or are present in large mucin-filled lakes (Figure 7). Identification of neoplastic cells within the large pools of mucin located within the muscularis may be difficult in these instances.

Metastases are frequently found in regional lymph nodes where the cells are present either in ill-defined nests or sheets, or arranged in glandular structures containing goblet cells. Metastases beyond the regional lymph nodes were observed in only one case and these were widely distributed throughout the lung (Figure 8).

IV. EPIDEMIOLOGY AND PATHOGENESIS

Table 1 lists cases of adenocarcinoma in the chronological order in which they were

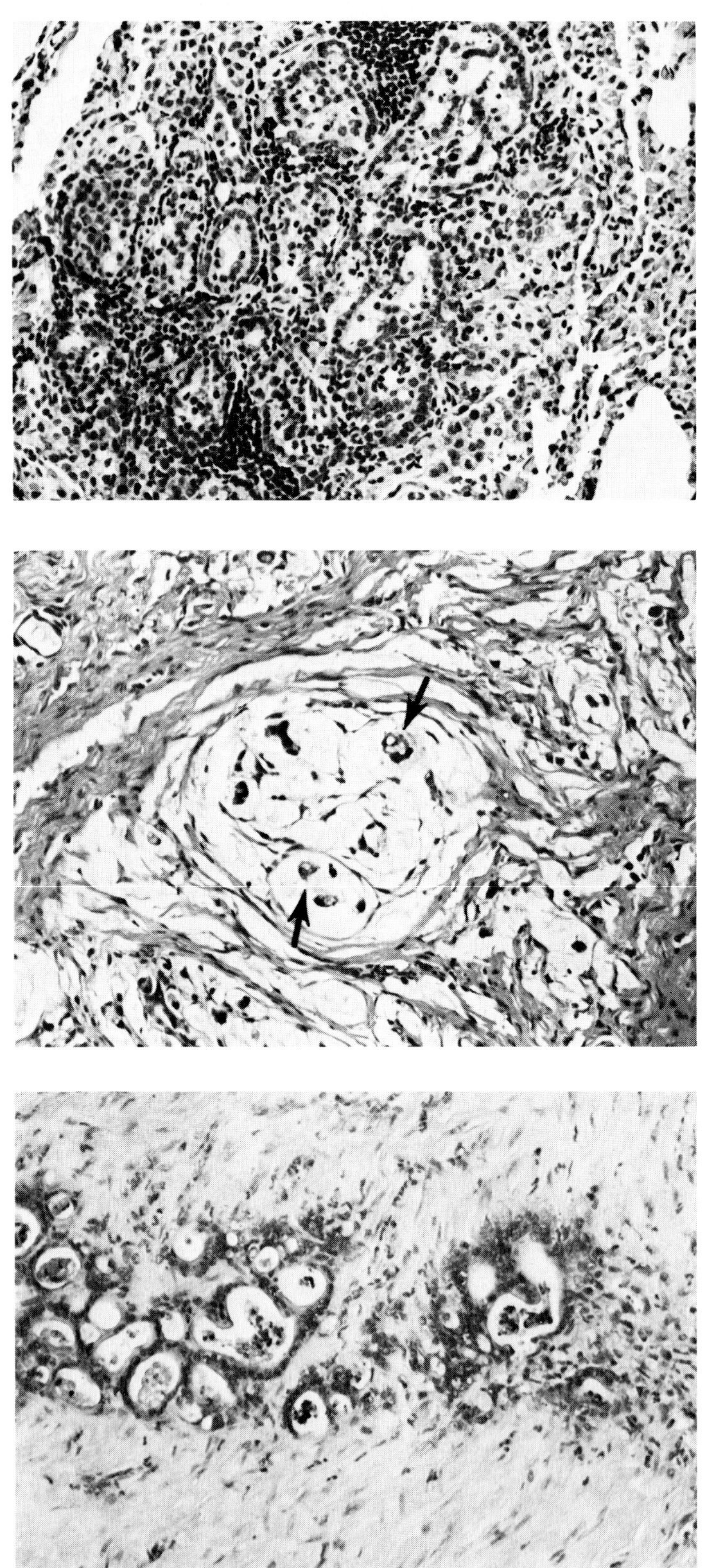

FIGURE 6.   Invasive adenocarcinoma in muscularis. Cells have hyperchromatic nuclei, scant cytoplasm, and are forming glands. Tamarin #347-76 at necropsy. (H.E.; magnification × 280.)

FIGURE 7.   Mucin-filled lake within muscularis. A few signet ring cells are seen (arrows). Tamarin #347-76 at necropsy. (H.E.; magnification × 280.)

FIGURE 8.   Pulmonary metastasis. Tamarin #661-76. (H.E.; magnification × 280.)

Table 1
SEQUENCE OF DEATHS OF *SAGUINUS OEDIPUS* FROM COLONIC ADENOCARCINOMA

Date of death	Animal #	Age	Sex	Origin	Time at PRC (months)	Intramucosal carcinoma	Invasive carcinoma	Metastasis
Aug 77	223-75	A[a]	F	Importer #1	27	S[b]	M	LN[d]
Jun 78	722-76	A	M	Importer #2	19	M[c]	—	—
Mar 79	688-76	A	M	Importer #2	32	M	M	LN
Apr 79	718-76	A	M	Importer #2	29	—	M	LN
Oct 79	789-76	A	F	Importer #2	35	M	M	LN
Nov 79	607-76	A	F	Importer #2	36	M	M	LN
Nov 79	693-76	A	M	Importer #2	36	M	M	—
Jan 80	708-76	A	F	Importer #2	38	—	S	LN
Jan 80	219-75	A	F	Importer #1	56	—	S	—
Feb 80	406-76	A	M	Importer #2	43	S	—	—
Feb 80	410-76	A	M	Importer #2	43	—	S	LN
Mar 80	740-76	A	M	Importer #2	40	—	M	LN
Jun 80	459-76	A	F	Importer #2	46	S	M	LN
Jul 80	107-75	A	F	Importer #1	64	M	S	LN
Aug 80	710-76	A	M	Importer #2	45	—	M	—
Oct 80	30-79	20 mo.	M	PRC	20	—	M	—
Nov 80	632-76	A	M	Importer #2	48	—	S	—
Nov 80	697-76	A	M	Importer #2	48	S	M	Lymphatics
Dec 80	244-78	31 mo.	M	PRC	31	S	M	LN
Dec 80	758-76	A	F	Importer #2	49	M	M	LN
Jun 82	347-76	A	M	Importer #2	71	—	S	LN
Dec 82	609-76	A	M	Importer #2	73	S	S	LN
Dec 82	661-76	A	M	Importer #2	73	—	S	Lung, LN
Jan 83	646-76	A	F	Importer #2	74	—	M	LN

[a] A = adult
[b] S = single site.
[c] M = multiple site.
[d] LN = lymph node.

recognized. The majority of these cases, 19, have occurred in one group of wild-caught animals obtained from a single importer in 1976. Three were received from a second importer in 1975 and two were born at our facility. All wild-caught animals were mature on arrival. The average time spent in the colony was 44.8 months. A few animals were apparently quite aged at the time of death. The two colony-born monkeys were relatively young, only 20 and 31 months of age. The disease was seen in both sexes with a slightly higher incidence among males (15 males and 9 females).

In the summer and fall of 1980, in consideration of the high mortality rate in the colony, a strict procedure for identifying and treating sick animals was adopted.[16] Using weight loss as the single best indicator of a life threat to the animal,[14] each monkey was weighed monthly. When a loss in weight occurred, a rectal biopsy and culture were obtained and, depending on findings, the animal was treated by one of several regimens. The most effective treatment was found to be sulfasalazine (10 mg/kg) coupled with a synthetic liquid diet[16] (30 mℓ) administered by stomach tube three times daily for 6 weeks. This treatment resulted in remission of active colitis (Figures 1 and 3) and dramatic weight gain. Rectal biopsies established that in the four most recent cases of adenocarcinoma, colitis had preceded the diagnosis of cancer by 24 to 38 months (Figure 1). One tamarin (609-76) had severe colitis 28 months before death, but biopsies taken at 38 and 41 months prior to death had been normal. Rectal biopsy is adequate to diagnose colitis owing to the diffuse pattern, however, dysplasia and carcinoma are usually focal, hence they may be missed by this technique. Adenocarcinoma was diagnosed from a biopsy taken 22 months before death in one case (347-76) (Figure 6). At necropsy an invasive adenocarcinoma with extensive desmoplasia partially occluding the rectum was found. The colon was vastly dilated. The other three tamarins that died had large invasive adenocarcinomatous foci at the cecolic junction which had not been detected before death. These monkeys also had an extensive desmoplastic connective tissue response in the area of the tumor and in one there was perforation of the colon and peritonitis. All four of the animals that had histories of severe weight loss and diarrhea had been successfully treated with sulfasalazine and force fed a supplementary diet one or more times. This, no doubt, explains why they lived longer (over 70 months) and had more extensive invasion and metastases than those animals that died with colon cancer in previous years.

The incidence of colitis among infant and juvenile animals in our colony is not known. They are simply too small for adequate rectal biopsies and we are reluctant to disturb successful family groups and apparently healthy young. However, one infant with a history of poor growth and illness had severe colitis diagnosed from a biopsy taken at 10 months of age. Colitis has been found in a few juveniles at necropsy, but it is not known whether this is the same disease seen in adults.

V. ETIOLOGY

The etiologies of the colitis and/or colonic carcinoma are not known. The lesions are nonspecific and similar to those caused by various agents. Numerous attempts to isolate a causative virus have been unsuccessful. Bacterial cultures have resulted in the isolation of the usual gut flora, *E. coli, Klebsiella pneumoniae, Proteus* sp., and other presumably normal organisms. Pure cultures of *Klebsiella* have frequently been seen.[17] The only exception to these has been the finding of *Campylobacter fetus*, subsp. *jejuni*, in some animals. Statistical analysis of data correlating the presence of *Campylobacter* with the clinical observation of diarrhea and weight loss and histopathological findings of colitis in rectal biopsy on some 60 tamarins suggests that this organism has little significance. In a separate study rectal cultures were taken from animals five times over a 6-week period and the presence or absence of diarrhea was noted at the time of each culture. The results obtained seem to support the contention that no relationship exists between the presence of *Campylobacter* and the finding of diarrhea.

Various attempts have been made to transmit the disease to other species on the assumption that an infectious agent might be involved. Portions of tumor and colonic mucosa from tamarins that had histologically confirmed colitis and adenocarcinoma were macerated in normal saline. The suspension was given orally, rectally as an enema, and inoculated subcutaneously into three young guinea pigs, three young white mice, four young hamsters, and ten neonatal C57 black mice. Animals were sacrificed at various intervals up to 16 months for the hamsters and 22 months for the C57 black mice. There was no evidence of colitis in any of these animals.

Considering the morphological similarity between carrageenan-induced colitis in other laboratory animals and the chronic colitis in tamarins the possibility of some dietary ingredient or contaminant has been suggested as an etiological agent. Necessary studies on the relationship of diet composition to colitis are yet to be performed.

Similarities to human disease as described here and independently at Oak Ridge clearly establish the authenticity of carcinoma of the colon as an important disease of the cotton-top tamarin. It is intriguing that the disease has not been seen in closely related species housed at both facilities. That the cotton-top tamarin is an endangered species makes it imperative that every effort be made to better understand this disorder for the sake of preserving the species as well as possibly contributing to the understanding of the analogous human diseases.

REFERENCES

1. Lushbaugh, C. C., Humason, G. L., Swartzendruber, D. C., Richter, C. B., and Gengozian, N., Spontaneous colonic adenocarcinoma in marmosets, in *Primates in Medicine*, Goldsmith, E. I. and Moor-Jankowski, J., Eds., S. Karger, Basel, 1978, 119.
2. Chalifoux, L. V. and Bronson, R. T., Colonic adenocarcinoma associated with chronic colitis in cotton top marmosets, *Saguinus oedipus, Gastroenterology*, 80, 942, 1981.
3. Terrell, T. G., Gribble, D. H., and Osburn, B. I., Malignant lymphoma in macaques: a clinicopathologic study of 45 cases, *J. Natl. Cancer Inst.*, 64, 561, 1980.
4. Kirsner, J. B. and Shorter, R. G., Recent developments in "nonspecific" inflammatory bowel disease, I., *N. Engl. J. Med.*, 306, 775, 1982.
5. Kirsner, J. B. and Shorter, R. G., Recent developments in "nonspecific" inflammatory bowel disease. II., *N. Engl. J. Med.*, 306, 837, 1982.
6. Kennedy, P. C. and Cello, R. M., Colitis in boxer dogs, *Gastroenterology*, 51, 926, 1966.
7. Van Kruiningen, H. J., Granulomatous colitis of boxer dogs: comparative aspects, *Gastroenterology*, 53, 114, 1967.
8. Strandle, A., Sommers, S. C., and Petrak, M., Regional enterocolitis in cocker spaniel dogs, *Arch. Pathol.*, 57, 357, 1954.
9. Watt, J. and Marcus, R., Carrageenan-induced ulceration of the intestine in the guinea pig, *Gut*, 12, 164, 1971.
10. Anver, M. R. and Cohen, B. J., Animal model: ulcerative colitis induced in guinea pigs with degraded carrageenan, *Am. J. Pathol.*, 84, 431, 1976.
11. Boothe, A. D. and Cheville, N. F., The pathology of proliferative ileitis of the golden hamster, *Vet. Pathol.*, 4, 31, 1967.
12. Jonas, A. M., Tomita, Y., and Wyand, S., Enzootic intestinal adenocarcinoma in hamsters, *J. Am. Vet. Med. Assoc.*, 147, 1102, 1965.
13. Barthold, S. W., Coleman, G. L., Bhatt, P. N., Osbaldiston, G. W., and Jonas, A. M., The etiology of transmissible murine colonic hyperplasia, *Lab. Anim. Sci.*, 26, 889, 1976.
14. Chalifoux, L. V., Bronson, R. T., Escajadillo, A., and McKenna, S., An analysis of the association of gastroenteric lesions with chronic wasting syndrome of marmosets, *Vet. Pathol.*, 19(Suppl. 7), 141, 1982.

15. Escajadillo, A., Bronson, R. T., Sehgal, P., and Hayes, K. C., Nutritional evaluation in cotton-top tamarins *(Saguinus oedipus)*, *Lab. Anim. Sci.,* 31, 161, 1981.
16. Sehgal, P., Elliott, M. W., Chalifoux, L. V., Hayes, K. C., and Bronson, R. T., Efficacy of various therapeutic regimens in control of wasting and colonic disease in tamarins (abstract), presented at 32nd Annu. Session Am. Assoc. Lab. Anim. Sci., 1981.
17. Hajema, E. M., Unpublished observations, 1983.

Chapter 7

INTESTINAL TUMORS INDUCED IN THE RAT BY VARIOUS *N*-NITROSOUREAS

Toshiaki Ogiu, Akihiko Maekawa, and Tomio Narisawa

TABLE OF CONTENTS

I. INTRODUCTION

The incidence of human colonic or rectal carcinomas is high in North America, western Europe, and Australia and low in Asia and eastern Europe.[1] Efforts to induce intestinal tumors in animals as a model for human intestinal cancer have been made for a long time by many investigators and some effective ways are now available to induce tumors in various parts of the intestine in experimental animals.

A 500-ppm solution of *N*-ethyl-*N'*-nitro-*N*-nitrosoguanidine (ENNG) given continuously in the drinking water for 5 months induced a high incidence of duodenal adenocarcinomas in rats and mice.[2]

Ileal tumors were easily induced by bracken. About 20 to 34% of bracken in the basal diet of young rats for 4 months produced adenomas or adenocarcinomas in the small intestine, especially in the ileum, with very high frequency.[3,4]

In addition, two other distinct types of chemical carcinogens are now used to induce large-bowel tumors. The first type is *N,N'*-dimethylhydrazine (DMH) and its metabolites, such as azoxymethane (AOM), which act systematically. They are initially converted to a reactive intermediate, methylazoxymethanol (MAM), by enzymatic systems in the liver and subsequently produce tumors, primarily in the large bowel and occasionally in the small intestine, ear duct, and kidney.[5-7] The second type of carcinogen is represented by the *N*-alkyl-*N*-nitrosamides, such as *N*-methyl-*N*-nitrosourea (MNU),[8] *N*-methyl-*N*-nitro-*N*-nitrosoguanidine (MNNG),[9] and *N*-methyl-*N*-nitrosourethane (MNUT);[10] when given intrarectally these compounds can react directly without enzymatic activation and thus are topical, potent carcinogens that can cause tumor development in the large bowel.

On the other hand, there are many reports on the formation of N-nitrosamines from secondary amines and nitrite in vivo.[11-13] Nitrosoureas are probably important environmental carcinogens, not only in the digestive tract but also in various other organs, because some nitrosatable ureas formed in the environment, or some precursors of nitrosoureas, may also be nitrosated in vivo.[14-17] In this chapter, we review the development of intestinal tumors in rats given various nitrosoureas.

II. INDUCTION OF INTESTINAL TUMORS BY VARIOUS N-NITROSOUREAS

A. Oral Administration of *N*-Nitrosoureas

In our series of experiments, the carcinogenicities of various nitrosoureas in the intestine were compared in Donryu or F344 rats, in which spontaneous intestinal tumors are very rare.[18,19] In the first series, nitrosoureas in the drinking water were continuously administered to 11-week-old female Donryu rats (Table 1). Concentrations used in these experiments were 400, 200, and 100 ppm in distilled water for MNU, *N*-ethyl- (ENU), *N*-*n*-butyl- (BNU), *N*-*n*-amyl- (ANU), *N*-isobutyl- (IBNU), *N*-carboxymethyl- (CMNU), *N,N'*-dibutyl- (DBNU), and *N*-butyl-*N',N'*-dimethyl-*N*-nitrosourea (DmBNU) treatments, and 600, 300, and 150 ppm in distilled water for *N*-*n*-propyl-*N*-nitrosourea (PNU) treatment.

MNU induced no intestinal tumors except one hemangioma in the duodenum in the 100-ppm group, though forestomach papillomas were frequently induced in the highest-dose group (44%).[20]

ENU induced tumors predominantly in the forestomach.[21] Duodenal tumors were also induced though their incidence was low; 0, 9, and 6% in the 400-, 200-, and 100-ppm groups, respectively. Furthermore, one rat (3%) of the 100-ppm group had an ileal tumor and three rats (9%) of the 100 ppm group had colonic tumors. Almost all of the induced intestinal tumors were of the epithelial type.

Table 1
TUMORS INDUCED IN THE DIGESTIVE TRACT OF DONRYU RATS BY VARIOUS *N*-NITROSOUREAS IN DRINKING WATER

| Chemical | Conc. in drinking water (ppm) | No. of rats examined | Rats with digestive tract tumors | | No. of rats with tumors in | | | | | | | Ref. |
			No.	%	Oral cavity/ pharynx	Esophagus	Forestomach	Glandular stomach	Duodenum	Ileum/ jejunum	Colon/ rectum	
MNU	400	27	12	44	0	0	12	0	0	0	0	20
	200	33	1	3	0	0	0	1	0	0	0	
	100	36	2	6	0	0	0	1	1	0	0	
ENU	400	36	4	11	0	0	4	0	0	0	0	21
	200	35	7	20	0	0	5	1	3	0	0	
	100	33	8	24	0	0	4	2	2	1	3	
PNU	600	36	9	25	0	0	0	4	8	1	0	22
	300	35	14	40	0	0	1	4	11	3	1	
	150	38	8	21	0	0	0	5	5	0	1	
BNU	400	13	7	54	0	1	6	0	—	0	0	23
	200	21	17	81	0	2	14	0	—	1	0	
	100	20	20	100	0	5	16	0	—	0	0	
ANU	400	33	27	82	4	18	25	0	2	0	0	24
	200	33	27	82	7	15	27	2	1	0	0	
	100	35	24	69	4	20	21	0	0	0	0	
IBNU	400	28	25	89	0	0	4	5	21	6	0	25
	200	24	14	58	0	0	2	7	12	1	0	
	100	25	6	24	0	0	1	3	2	0	3	
CMNU	400	34	27	79	3	0	0	0	1	27	2	26
	200	38	19	50	1	0	0	0	0	19	0	
	100	40	6	15	1	0	0	0	0	5	0	
DBNU	400	28	0		0	0	0	0	0	0	0	27
	200	25	0		0	0	0	0	0	0	0	
	100	26	1	4	0	0	0	0	0	0	1	
DmBNU	400	33	4	12	0	0	3	0	—	1	0	28
	200	31	3	10	0	0	0	0	—	3	0	
	100	36	1	3	0	0	1	0	—	0	0	

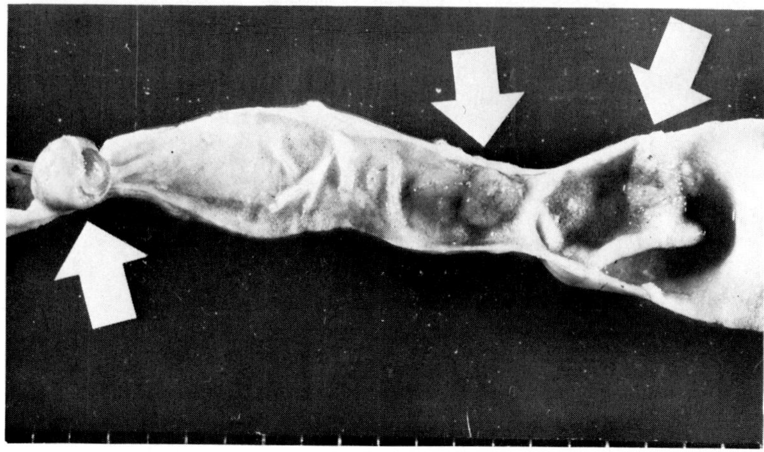

FIGURE 1.   Tumors induced in the ileum of a female Donryu rat given a 400-ppm
CMNU solution as the drinking water for 60 weeks prior to sacrifice.

PNU induced duodenal tumors in many rats.[22] The incidences of duodenal tumors
were 22, 31, and 13% in the 400-, 200-, and 100-ppm groups, respectively. In addition,
one tumor (3%) in the 400-ppm group and three tumors (9%) in the 200-ppm group
were seen in the jejunum/ileum and one large intestinal tumor (3%) was seen in both
the 200-ppm and the 100-ppm groups. About 40% were of the epithelial type.

Results of oral administration of BNU in the rat were first reported by Odashima.[23]
Although squamous cell carcinomas or papillomas were frequently induced in the
esophagus (15%) and forestomach (67%), intestinal tumors were not detected except
for one adenoma in the small intestine in the 200-ppm group.

ANU induced tumors predominantly in the digestive tract, although almost all tumors were present in the upper digestive tract.[24] Duodenal tumors were induced in two
rats in the 400-ppm group and one rat in the 200-ppm group, but not all of them were
epithelial tumors.

Oral administration of IBNU caused a high incidence of duodenal tumors, depending on the dose: 75% in the 400-ppm group, 50% in the 200-ppm group, and 8% in
the 100-ppm group.[25] Tumors of the jejunum/ileum were detected in six rats (21%) in
the 400-ppm group and one rat (4%) in the 200-ppm group, and tumors of the colon
were found in three rats (12%) of the 100-ppm group. Histologically, most of the
induced tumors were hemangiogenic.

CMNU possibly is a naturally occurring nitrosourea and this agent induced 1 adenoma of the duodenum, 20 adenomas (59%), 19 adenocarcinomas (56%) and 3 sarcomas (9%) of the jejunum/ileum, and 2 adenomas (6%) of the large intestine in the
400-ppm group; 15 adenomas (39%) and 9 adenocarcinomas (24%) of the jejunum/
ileum in the 200 ppm group; and 4 adenomas (10%) and 1 adenocarcinoma (3%) of
the jejunum/ileum in the 100-ppm group (Figure 1).[26]

DBNU induced colonic adenomas in only one rat (4%) of the 100-ppm group.[27]
DmBNU induced one adenoma and three mucinous carcinomas (6%) of the small intestine in the 400- and 200-ppm groups, and four forestomach papillomas (6%) in the
400- and 100-ppm groups.[28]

These results indicate that most nitrosoureas are not strong carcinogens for induction of intestinal tumors when they are administered orally to Donryu rats. Of nine
chemicals tested in our laboratory, the most effective carcinogen to induce intestinal
tumors was CMNU, which induced epithelial tumors in the jejunum/ileum. Although

oral administration of IBNU also frequently caused duodenal tumors, it is interesting that almost all of these tumors were hemangiogenic.

On the other hand, strain difference is a very important factor affecting the target organ for nitrosoureas in rats. A 400-ppm solution of three nitrosoureas was administered to both male and female F344 rats as their drinking water in our laboratory. Table 2 shows the incidence of digestive tract tumors in F344 rats.

Oral administration of ENU elicited a high yield of intestinal tumors, especially duodenal tumors.[29] The incidence of tumors found in the duodenum was 65 and 40%, that in the jejunum/ileum was 23 and 10%, and that in the colon was 23 and 1% in male and female rats, respectively. In other parts of the alimentary tract, glandular stomach tumors were detected in 18% of rats, followed by esophageal tumors (10%) and forestomach tumors (6%). All intestinal tumors were histologically of the epithelial type.

A 400-ppm PNU solution induced duodenal tumors in 83% of male rats and 72% of female rats.[30] The histologically predominant type was adenoma or adenocarcinoma; the nonepithelial type was scarce. In other parts of the small intestine, adenocarcinomas were found in three male rats (8%). Tumors of the glandular stomach, forestomach, and esophagus were also detected, though they were in the minority.

BNU induced predominantly upper digestive tract tumors.[31] The incidence of esophageal tumors was 54 and 56%, and that of forestomach tumor was 59 and 67% in male and female rats, respectively. In comparison with the incidence of upper digestive tract tumors, that of intestinal tumors was low. The incidence of duodenal tumors was 18 and 3% in male and female rats, respectively, that of jejunum/ileum tumors was 3% in male rats, and that of large bowel tumors was 8% in male rats and 5% in female rats. All digestive tract tumors induced by BNU were epithelial in nature.

These data show that ENU and PNU are potent carcinogens that induce epithelial tumors in the small intestine, especially in the duodenum, of F344 rats. However, the target organ for BNU is different from these two chemicals, more often affecting the upper digestive tract, especially the esophagus and forestomach.

In general, the duodenal epithelium of the F344 rat is more susceptible to nitrosoureas than that of the Donryu rats. When we consider the structure of these compounds, carcinogenicity of PNU in the intestine of Donryu rats is stronger than that of other nitrosoureas with linear alkyl group and is similar to ENU, and stronger than that of BNU in F344 rats when the compounds are administered continuously in the drinking water.

Results of continuous oral administration of various nitrosoureas in BD rats were reported by Druckrey and co-workers.[6,32] They examined the carcinogenicities of MNU, ENU, PNU, BNU, ANU, *N*-methyl-*N'*-acetyl-*N*-nitrosourea (AcMNU), and *N*-ethyl-*N'*-acetyl-*N*-nitrosourea (AcENU).[6,32] PNU was the most effective inducer of intestinal tumors in BD rats,[6] followed by AcENU,[6] but the others displayed very weak or no carcinogenicity in the intestines of this strain. On the other hand, MNU induced forestomach tumors,[32] AcMNU induced glandular stomach tumors,[6] and ANU induced upper digestive tract tumors.[6] These results in BD rats were very similar to the results found in Donryu rats. Pelfrene et al.[33] administered ENU in the drinking water continuously to MRC rats and induced large-bowel adenocarcinomas in 15% and sarcomas in 8% of treated rats.

Increasing molecular complexity seems to have no effect on the inducement of intestinal tumors. *N,N'*-Dimethyl- and *N,N',N'*-trimethyl-*N*-nitrosourea were given to rats in the drinking water by Druckrey et al.,[32] and *N,N',N'*-trimethyl-, *N*-methyl-*N',N'*-diethyl-, *N*-ethyl-*N',N'*-dimethyl-, and *N,N',N'*-triethyl-*N*-nitrosourea were administered in the drinking water by Lijinsky and Taylor.[34] However, long-term treatment with these chemicals did not cause neoplasms in the digestive tract of rats.

Table 2

TUMORS INDUCED IN THE DIGESTIVE TRACT OF F344 RATS GIVEN A 400-PPM SOLUTION OF VARIOUS *N*-NITROSOUREAS AS THE DRINKING WATER

Chemical	Sex	No. of rats examined	Rats with digestive tract tumors No.	%	No. of rats with tumors in Oral cavity/ pharynx	Esophagus	Forestomach	Glandular stomach	Duodenum	Ileum/ jejunum	Colon/ rectum	Ref.
ENU	M	40	32	80	1	2	2	7	26	9	9	29
	F	40	28	70	0	6	3	7	16	4	1	
PNU	M	36	32	89	0	1	3	2	30	3	0	30
	F	39	33	85	0	1	11	5	28	0	0	
BNU	M	39	36	92	11	21	23	0	7	1	3	31
	F	39	34	87	16	22	26	0	1	0	2	

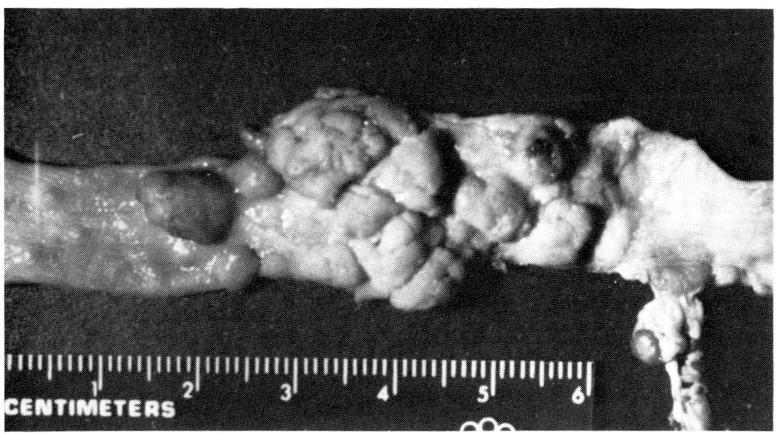

FIGURE 2. Multiple polyploid tumors induced in the large intestine of a male F344 rat given intrarectal administration of 2 mg of MNU three times per week for 5 weeks and sacrificed at the 35th experimental week.

A single, intragastric dose of MNU induced various digestive tract tumors in rats: 19% incidence in the small intestine, 52% incidence in the large bowel, and 29% incidence in the forestomach.[35] However, a single oral administration of ENU,[36] PNU,[37] or BNU[38] induced few or no intestinal tumors in rats.

B. Intrarectal Administration of *N*-Nitrosoureas

A high yield of large-bowel tumors in rats after the intrarectal instillation of aqueous solution of MNU or MNNG was first demonstrated by Narisawa et al.[8,9] Before then, various carcinogens, such as 20-methylcholanthrene[39,40] or benzo(*a*)pyrene,[41] were intrarectally administered by several investigators; however, they failed to induce large bowel tumors. On the other hand, 20-methylcholanthrene injected into the rectal wall of mice produced sarcomas originating in the wall.[42] The results of these experiments indicated that the mucosa of the large bowel is much more susceptible to the carcinogenic activity of MNU, and suggest that the direct-acting carcinogens, such as MNU or other *N*-alkyl-*N*-nitrosamides, which are absorbed into the large-bowel mucosa, especially via the large-bowel lumen, can readily cause tumor development. Thus, intrarectal administration of MNU may provide the simplest and most reliable model for the topical and selective production of multiple large-bowel tumors diffusely localized in the distal half of the large bowel of rats, mice,[8] and guinea pigs.[43,44]

A steep dose response of MNU given intrarectally, with respect to tumor development, was demonstrated in both rat and mouse experiments. In F344 rats, intrarectal doses of 2 mg, 1 mg, or 0.5 mg of MNU twice a week for 8 weeks induced large-bowel tumors with 95, 80, and 33% incidence, respectively, at weeks 22 to 26,[45] and 2 mg of MNU given three times a week for 1, 2, or 5 weeks produced large-bowel tumors with 22, 73, and 100% incidence, respectively, at week 50 (Figure 2). Tumor development is dependent upon the dose of MNU, exposure time to MNU, and the latent period after MNU treatment. In addition, the number of tumor nodules that develop seems to depend upon the dose of MNU and the latent period. An intrarectal dose of 2 mg of MNU 3 times a week for 5 weeks caused large-bowel tumors in ICR/Ha mice, with 49, 77, and 89% incidence at week 20, 25, and 30, respectively. Malignant thymic tumors and lung adenomas developed at high incidence concomitantly with large-bowel tumors.[8]

Since dialkyl- or other *N*-nitrosamines require enzymatic activation to be carcinogenic, failure of tumor induction in the large bowel after local or systemic administration of these carcinogens may be explained by a lack of necessary enzymes in this organ. Repeated intrarectal instillation of *N*-butyl-*N*-ethylnitrosamine to rats did not induce large-bowel tumors, but induced liver tumors.[46] Rice et al.[47,48] detected a high yield of large-bowel tumors in rats that were intraperitoneally administered a possible active metabolite of *N,N*-dimethylnitrosamine, *N*-acetoxymethyl-*N*-methylnitrosamine (AMMN). Subsequently, Habs et al.[49] demonstrated that AMMN, given intrarectally, selectively produced tumors in the descending colon and rectum.

The *N*-alkyl-*N*-nitrosamides, e.g., MNU and MNNG, are decomposed by hydrolysis under physiological conditions to form an intermediate, methyldiazohydroxide, which is probably an active form of these chemicals. Such a mechanism would explain the strong local action of these chemicals after intrarectal or other topical administration. Kamano et al.[50] demonstrated that the intrarectal injection of MNNG or ENNG produced large-bowel tumors in dogs. Therefore, these results suggest that the direct-acting carcinogen, MNU, and other carcinogenic *N*-alkyl-*N*-nitrosamides which are absorbed by the large-bowel mucosa, may cause large-bowel tumors in any animal species.

There have not been any reports on sex difference and age dependency in the development of large-bowel tumors after intrarectal administration of MNU, except one report by Balish et al.,[51] in which germ-free and conventional male rats were more susceptible to the carcinogen than female counterparts. The tumors induced in the large bowel of rats and mice by intrarectal doses of MNU, MNNG, or AMMN were polypoid or plaque-shaped and, histologically, most of them were well-differentiated adenocarcinomas though a few were signet-ring cell carcinomas and mucoid carcinomas. In contrast, tumors of guinea pigs were infiltrative or constrictive, and most of them were poorly differentiated adenocarcinomas.

C. Other Routes of Administration of *N*-Nitrosoureas

It is difficult to induce intestinal tumors by parenteral administration of *N*-nitrosoureas except by intravenous or intraperitoneal administration of MNU. Druckrey et al.[52,53] injected a single intravenous dose of MNU, at 70 to 100 mg/kg body weight, in BD rats and induced forestomach papillomas with 63% incidence and intestinal carcinomas with 25% incidence. Single intraperitoneal administrations of MNU at 50 mg/kg body weight to newborn or 5-week-old Wistar rats was examined by Terracini and Testa,[54] and incidences of intestinal adenocarcinomas were 16 and 10% in rats treated at birth and at 5 weeks of age, respectively.

Intravenous or subcutaneous injection of ENU[36] and subcutaneous administration of PNU[37] or BNU[32] did not cause digestive tract tumors in rats, although single intraperitoneal injections of BNU induced tumors at 100% incidence in the intestine, especially in the small intestine, in mice.[55]

III. PATHOLOGY OF INTESTINAL TUMORS INDUCED BY VARIOUS *N*-NITROSOUREAS

A. Sites and Macroscopic Findings of Intestinal Tumors

The sites and histological types of intestinal tumors induced in rats by various nitrosoureas seem to depend on the method or route of application of the chemicals, the strain of rats used, and the chemical structure of the nitrosourea. When nitrosoureas were administered orally, intestinal tumors developed most frequently in the small intestine (duodenum, jejunum, and ileum) and tumors of the large intestine were rare. On the other hand, when the chemicals were given intrarectally, tumors were localized only in the colon and/or rectum, and were especially restricted to the distal half, up to about 10 cm proximal to anus. In many cases, tumors were multiple in the intestine.

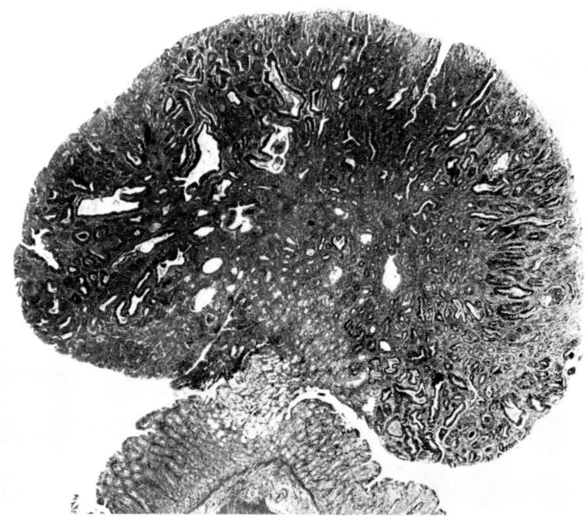

FIGURE 3.   Adenoma in the colon of a female Donryu rat given a 400-ppm CMNU solution as the drinking water for 60 weeks prior to sacrifice.

Macroscopically, these tumors were classified as polypoid, cauliflower-like, ulcerative, ulcerative-infiltrative, or plaque-shaped types. Histologically, most of these tumors were of epithelial origin. Intestinal invaginations due to induction of intestinal tumors were sometimes observed.

B. Histological Classification of Intestinal Tumors

1. Epithelial Tumors

a. Adenoma

Most of adenomas in the intestine are pedicular, and sessile tumors are very rare (Figure 3). Adenomas are composed of cylindrical or cuboidal cells with a few goblet cells. The structure of adenomas differs from that of the normal mucosa in the diversity of shape and size of the mucosal cells and number of mitotic figures. Nonetheless, cellular and structural atypia are slight and no invasion of tumor cells into the submucosa is observed. The stromata of adenomas are composed of loose connective tissue.

At the initial stage of carcinogenesis in the intestinal mucosa, foci of hyperplasia are detected as small swellings within the mucosa. Morphologically, they retain a mucous membrane with the normal glandular structure although there are some atypical histological findings, such as variations in the shape and size of glandular structure, in which mucosal cells are often basophilic with hyperchromatic nuclei and many mitotic figures (Figure 4). These foci eventually seem to progress to adenomas or adenocarcinomas at the final stage of carcinogenesis.

If there is severe distortion of cells and glandular structure in hyperplastic foci or adenomas without invasive growth of neoplastic cells, the diagnosis is "carcinoma *in situ*". However, histological differentiation between adenoma or adenocarcinoma *in situ* and adenocarcinoma is often very difficult.

b. Adenocarcinoma

Tubular adenocarcinomas are the most frequent type found in experimental animals,

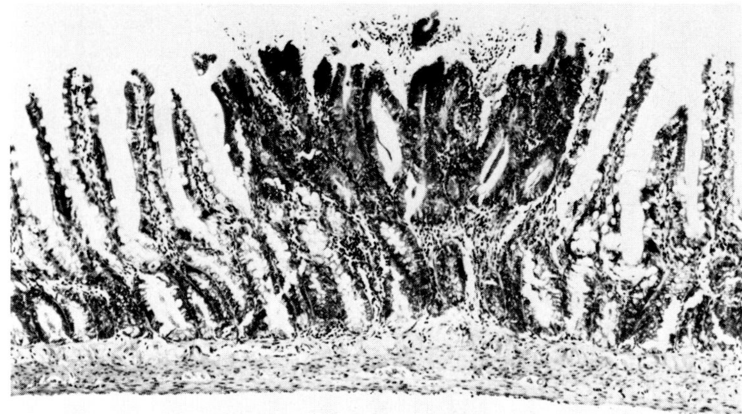

FIGURE 4.   Preneoplastic lesion in the mucosa of the small intestine in a female Donryu rat given a 400-ppm CMNU solution as the drinking water for 56 weeks prior to sacrifice.

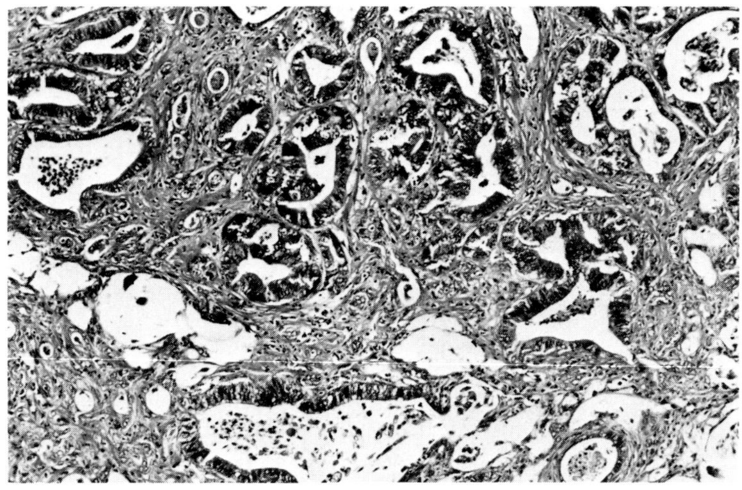

FIGURE 5.   Adenocarcinoma in the small intestine of a female Donryu rat given a 200-ppm CMNU solution as the drinking water for 67 weeks prior to sacrifice.

although a few are of the papillary type. They are composed of variable glandular structures, often with irregular arrangement, lined by one or more layers of high cylindrical cells with large, hyperchromatic and pleomorphic nuclei. The nucleus/cytoplasm ratio of tumor cells is increased considerably. Mitotic figures are frequently found and some of them are abnormal. The tumor cells often invade the submucosa, muscle layer, and serosa. Metastasis to remote organs or lymph nodes is observed in some cases (Figure 5).

Tumors are sometimes characterized by excess production of mucin; accordingly, the space between glandular structures is considerably expanded owing to mucin accumulation and the epithelial cells are distinctly flattened (Figure 6).

A few cases resemble human scirrhous carcinoma. Tumor cells tend to separate from each other and abundant connective tissues surround nests of tumor cells.

c. Mucinous Carcinoma and Signet-Ring Cell Carcinoma

Some of the mucin-secreting tumors are poorly differentiated or undifferentiated,

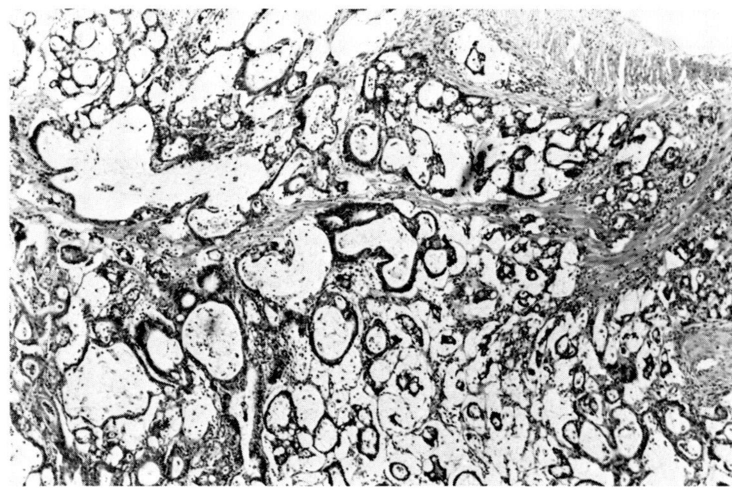

FIGURE 6. Mucinous adenocarcinoma in the small intestine of a female Donryu rat given a 400-ppm CMNU solution as the drinking water for 65 weeks prior to sacrifice.

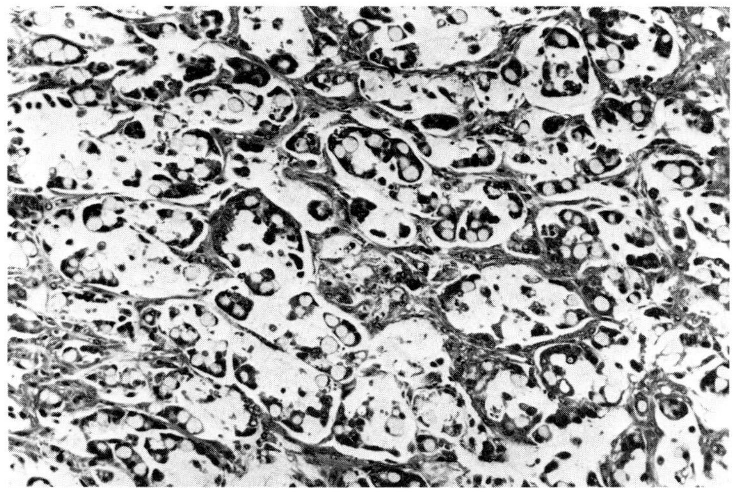

FIGURE 7. Signet-ring cell carcinoma in the duodenum of a female F344 rat given a 400-ppm ENU solution as the drinking water for 32 weeks prior to sacrifice.

without glandular formation, and are composed of highly pleomorphic and atypical tumor cells. In signet-ring cell carcinoma, intracellular accumulation of mucin is prominent and tumor cells appear characteristically like signet rings (Figure 7).

d. Squamous Cell Carcinoma

Squamous cell carcinoma is localized only in the rectum of rats given nitrosamides intrarectally and its incidence is very low. Histologically, tumor cells are markedly irregular in size and shape, and mitotic figures are frequent. Cancer pearls of concentrically arranged masses of keratin are generally formed in the central part of tumor clusters.

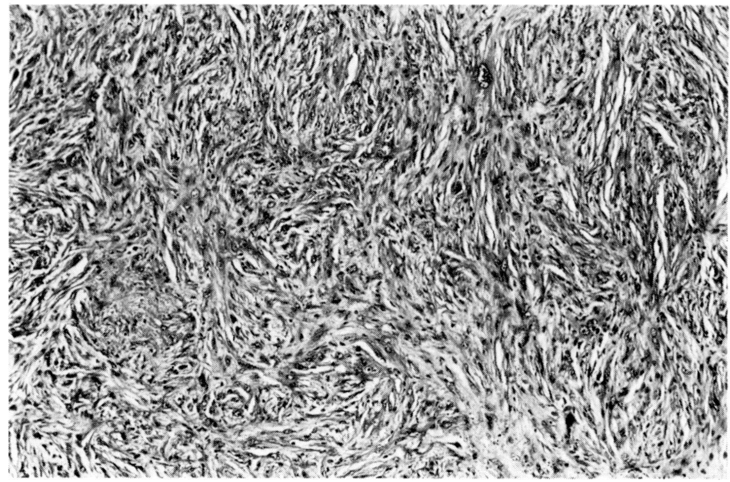

FIGURE 8.   Fibrosarcoma in the jejunum of a female Donryu rat given a 400-ppm CMNU solution for 67 weeks prior to sacrifice.

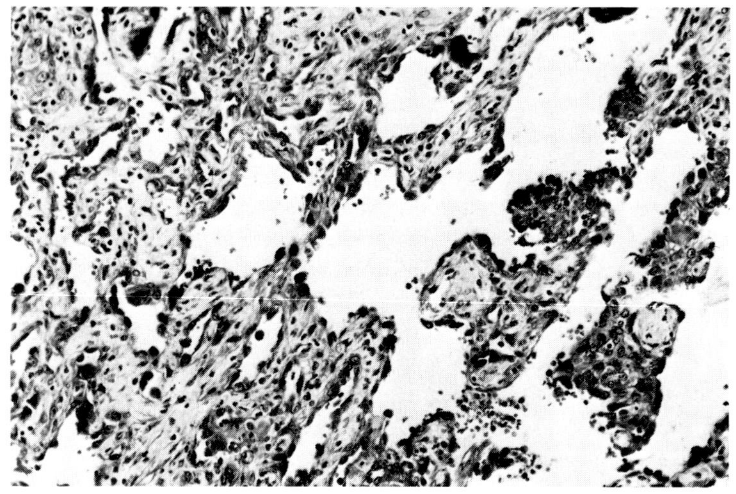

FIGURE 9.   Hemangioendothelioma in the duodenum of a female Donryu rat given a 400-ppm IBNU solution for 37 weeks prior to sacrifice.

2. Nonepithelial Tumors

As compared with epithelial tumors, nonepithelial tumors are rarely induced in the rat by nitrosoureas. Tumors are generally seen as nodules projecting from the serosal membrane and an ulcer is commonly found on the mucosal aspect of the nodules in malignant tumors.

Although the incidences are low, fibromas or leiomyomas are common in benign mesenchymal tumors. These tumors are often well circumscribed and capsulated with a fibrous membrane. In fibrosarcoma or leiomyosarcoma, spindle-shaped tumor cells proliferate and infiltrate the intestinal wall in all directions (Figure 8).

Angiogenic tumors, especially hemangioendotheliomas, are characteristically induced in Donryu rats by continuous oral administration of IBNU.[25] According to histological findings, hemangioendotheliomas can be subclassified into two types: benign and malignant. Benign hemangioendotheliomas consist of blood vessels lined by two

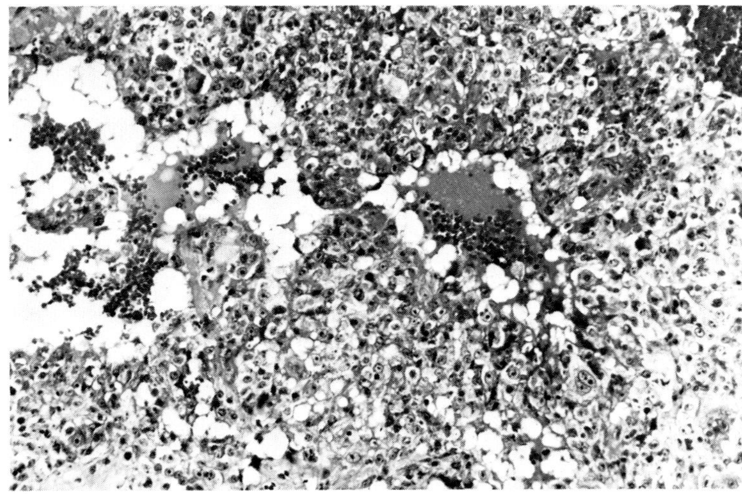

FIGURE 10. Malignant hemangioendothelioma in the duodenum of a female
Donryu rat given a 400-ppm IBNU solution for 40 weeks prior to sacrifice.

or more layers of endothelial cells. The lining cells are round rather than flat and are
mostly uniform in size and form. Mitotic figures are rarely seen. The blood spaces are
outlined by delicate collagen and lattice fibers which form a dense network throughout
the tumors (Figure 9).

In contrast, malignant hemangioendotheliomas consist of blood vessels lined by enlarged endothelial cells which are round or pleomorphic with numerous mitotic figures,
and giant cells are often seen (Figure 10). Occasionally, tumor cells completely occupy
the vesicular lumen and assume a lobular structure or a diffuse growth pattern, so that
it is difficult to discriminate these tumors from adenocarcinomas by hematoxylin-eosin
staining. However, there are no alcian blue-PAS or mucicarmine positive cells in these
tumors, and nests of tumor cells are surrounded irregularly by collagen and lattice
fibers.

In addition to these tumors, other angiogenic tumors such as hemangiomas and
hemangiopericytomas are rarely observed in the intestine.

Pozharisski[56] has described the pathology of intestinal tumors in rats. Histological
findings of intestinal tumors induced in rats by various nitrosoureas are similar to those
described by Pozharisski and also to those found in humans,[57] however the sites of rat
tumors are slightly different from those in the human.

IV. CARCINOGENESIS IN THE INTESTINE INDUCED BY PRECURSORS OF *N*-NITROSOUREAS

Bruce et al.[58] reported that mutagenic substances positive to the Ames test with and
without microsomal activation system were present in human feces. Moreover, it was
demonstrated that the feces of people residing in high-risk areas for large bowel cancer
were more mutagenic without microsomal activation than those of people from low-
risk areas.[59-61] It has been postulated that *N*-nitroso compounds can be formed in vivo
under some conditions, such as in the achlorhydric stomach, in the infected urinary
bladder, and in the large bowel whenever bacteria, nitrosatable amine, and nitrate or
nitrite coexist. Further, it was suggested by Kodama et al.[16] that alkylureas, which are
potential precursors of nitrosoureas, are formed from carbamyl amines or carbamyl
phosphate in our environment. Furthermore, it was surprisingly demonstrated that a

certain nitrosourea, CMNU, is formed from glycocyamine, which is a guanido compound present in foods, especially in meat products.[14,15] Another precursor component, nitrite, is formed from nitrate, the latter of which is widely distributed in our food.[62] Also, inhalation of nitrogen dioxide results in nitrite formation in vivo.[63,64]

Since Sander and Bürkle[65] first reported successful induction of malignant tumors in rats fed secondary amines and sodium nitrite, there have been many reports on induction of neoplasms in rats given alkylurea and sodium nitrite concurrently. Methylurea and sodium nitrite caused neurogenic, hematopoietic, and mammary tumors in Sprague-Dawley rats;[66] ethylurea and sodium nitrite induced neurogenic, mammary, and pituitary tumors in Sprague-Dawley rats[66] and neurogenic tumors in offspring of pregnant BD rats[67] and in E rats;[68] propylurea and sodium nitrite produced malignant reticulosis in E rats;[69] and butylurea and sodium nitrite caused malignant reticulosis in E rats[69] and neurogenic tumors in offspring of pregnant ACI rats.[70] In these experiments, parenteral tumors were induced in almost all rats examined. Further, Murthy et al.[71] fed butylurea and sodium nitrite in the diet in combination, and induced neoplasms of the lung, Zymbal's gland, forestomach, small intestine, and hematopoietic tissue in rats. The incidence of intestinal tumors in this experiment was 14% and was similar to that in F344 rats given 400 ppm BNU solution as the drinking water.[31] Therefore, it can be concluded that in vivo formation of nitrosourea caused the induction of various neoplasms, including intestinal tumors. However, multiple doses of intrarectal administration of methylurea concurrently with sodium nitrite failed to demonstrate carcinogenic activity in the large bowel of rats.[8]

Although it has been suggested that N-nitroso compounds are some of the most important carcinogens in our environment as inducers of not only intestinal tumors but also other tumors, it has not yet been demonstrated that human intestinal contents contain any form of *N*-nitroso compounds, including the direct-acting carcinogen *N*-alkyl-*N*-nitrosourea. Clearly, further investigations are needed to detect what specific kinds of mutagenic chemicals are contained in the human feces.

V. INDUCTION OF INTESTINAL TUMORS BY INTRARECTAL ADMINISTRATION OF MNU

Animal models for large-bowel carcinoma induced with intrarectal instillation of direct-acting carcinogens such as MNU, as well as parenteral administration of DMH and its metabolite AOM, are being used to study the multiple factors that are involved in the pathogenesis of human large-bowel cancer.

It has been demonstrated that induced large-bowel tumors only a few millimeters in diameter can be detected easily by endoscopic examination[72,73] or by X-ray examination with a barium enema[74,75] in surviving rats. The earliest lesions detected microscopically in grossly normal-appearing flat mucosa of the large bowel of MNU-treated rats are adenomatous lesions forming a single gland and found in the upper portion of the mucosa. However, Lev and Herp[76] reported that most invasive carcinomas of the large bowel of MNU-treated rats originated in the foci of epithelial atypia; a few carcinomas arose from adenomatous epithelia and subsequently grew into polypoid or plaque-shaped gross tumors. The histogenesis of large-bowel carcinomas in experimental animals is still controversial.

VI. ENVIRONMENTAL FACTORS AFFECTING DEVELOPMENT OF INTESTINAL TUMORS

Various environmental factors which affect induction of intestinal tumors have been well studied in rats treated with intrarectal administration of MNU. The possible role of dietary fat in the induction of human cancer of the large bowel was proposed from epidemiological studies[77] and, later, this proposal received support from experimental studies. A significantly higher incidence of large-bowel tumors was demonstrated in rats fed a high-fat diet (20% lard or 20% corn oil) than rats fed a 5% fat diet or standard laboratory chow after intrarectal administration of MNU.[78,79] A high-fat diet causes an increase in bile acid excretion into the bile and feces. These bile acids, especially secondary bile acids, may have a role in promoting activity (not initiation) on carcinogenesis in the large bowel.[80,81] This role has been postulated from the epidemiological studies.[82-84]

Cohen et al.[85] demonstrated that rats given an intrarectal dose of MNU and fed a diet containing 0.2% cholic acid, a primary bile acid, had more large-bowel tumors than rats fed a control diet. They also reported that a significant increase in fecal deoxycholic acid, a secondary bile acid, was detected in cholic acid-fed rats. However, a 0.2% cholesterol-supplemented diet significantly reduced the development of MNU-induced large-bowel tumors in rats when a twofold elevation of fecal cholesterol was detected.[86]

On the other hand, rats given an intrarectal instillation of MNU followed by long-term administration of the prostaglandin synthesis inhibitor, indomethacin, had significantly reduced development of large-bowel tumors.[87,88] Thus, indomethacin may suppress the promotional stage of MNU-initiated carcinogenesis in large-bowel mucosal epithelia, as demonstrated in benzo(a)pyrene-induced mouse skin carcinogenesis.[89,90] Furthermore, the development of large-bowel tumors induced by DMH or its metabolites was suppressed by the indomethacin treatment.[91,92]

It was demonstrated that the induction of large-bowel tumors in DMH-treated mice was inhibited by coadministration of various forms of antioxidants, such as disulfiram and butylated hydroxyanisole.[93]

Epidemiological[84,94,95] and also experimental studies[96] indicated that a diet rich in vegetables and fibers was associated with a low incidence of large-bowel cancer, though some kinds of fibers enhanced the development of MNU- or AOM-induced large-bowel tumors.[96,97] Raicht et al.[98] and Deschner et al.[99] reported that 0.2% dietary β-sitosterol, a plant sterol abundant in vegetables, decreased the incidence of large-bowel tumors of MNU-treated rats and lowered the proliferation rate of large-bowel epithelial cells.

Thus, large-bowel carcinogenesis is greatly influenced by multiple environmental factors, especially diet as described above, although vitamin A or C did not prevent the development of MNU-induced large-bowel tumors in rats.[100,101] Dietary factors influence the composition of intestinal microflora and the composition of the intestinal contents in which mutagenic activity is demonstrated, suggesting the presence of not only carcinogenic substances, but also cocarcinogenic or promoting factors such as certain bile acids. The luminal contents may also contain inhibiting factors such as dietary fibers or certain plant sterols. Thus, this animal model as well as other models with various chemical carcinogens such as DMH, is useful for elucidating large-bowel carcinogenesis, pathogenesis, tumor immunology, diagnosis, chemotherapy testing,[102-105] and prevention of human large-bowel cancers.

VII. CONCLUSIONS

Several effective methods are now available for inducing tumors in various parts of the intestines in rats. Currently, the most effective way to induce duodenal tumors is by continuous oral administration of ENNG in the drinking water; to induce ileal tumors is by oral administration of bracken in the diet; and to induce large bowel tumors is by the intragastric administration of DMH or AOM or intrarectal administration of nitrosamides.

The nitrosamides are important carcinogens in our natural environment. Various *N*-nitrosoureas were examined for their carcinogenicity in selected strains of rats with respect to target organs, and the continuous administration of these chemicals in the drinking water induced intestinal tumors with variable incidences. CMNU was most effective in inducing small-intestinal adenomas/adenocarcinomas in Donryu rats. IBNU also caused a high yield of duodenal tumors, though almost all intestinal tumors were hemangiogenic. ENU and PNU were potent inducers of duodenal tumors in F344 rats, and PNU and AcENU were effective inducers of duodenal tumors in BD rats. In addition, intrarectal administration of nitrosamides such as MNU, MNNG, or MNUT was a useful method for inducing large-bowel tumors. However, many parenteral treatments with nitrosoureas were less effective than oral or intrarectal treatment with nitrosoureas.

Histologically, many intestinal tumors induced by nitrosoureas were of the epithelial type: adenoma, adenocarcinoma, mucinous carcinoma, signet-ring cell carcinoma, and squamous cell carcinoma. A few were of the nonepithelial type: fibroma, leiomyoma, fibrosarcoma, leiomyosarcoma, and angiogenic tumors.

Nitrosoureas are formed in vivo from their precursors coexisting with nitrite. In some experiments using precursors of nitrosoureas, butylurea administered concurrently with sodium nitrite successfully induced intestinal tumors in rats and mice. Some nitrosatable precursors of nitrosoureas are present in our environment; therefore, nitrosoureas likely are important carcinogens for induction of human intestinal cancers. Mutagenic activity has actually been detected in human intestinal contents. Furthermore, dietary factors affect induction of intestinal tumors. Some act as cocarcinogenic or promoting factors and some act as inhibitory factors.

From a practical standpoint, intrarectal administration of nitrosamides is the most effective method to elicit a high yield of large-intestinal tumors in rats as a model for human intestinal cancer. This method provides a very useful model for further research on large-bowel carcinogenesis, pathogenesis, tumor immunology, diagnosis, chemotherapy testing, and prevention of intestinal cancer.

REFERENCES

1. International Agency for Research on Cancer, *Cancer Incidence in Five Continents*, Vol. 4, Waterhouse, J., Muir, C., Shanmugaratnam, K., and Powell, J., Eds., IARC, Lyon, 1982, 42.
2. Matsuyama, M., Nakamura, T., Suzuki, H., and Nagayo, T., Morphogenesis of duodenal adenocarcinomas induced by *N*-ethyl-*N*-nitro-*N*-nitrosoguanidine in mice and rats, *Gann Monogr.*, 17, 269, 1975.
3. Evans, I. A. and Mason, J., Carcinogenic activity of bracken, *Nature (London)*, 208, 913, 1965.
4. Hirono, I., Sasaoka, I., Shibuya, C., Shimizu, M., Fushimi, K., Mori, H., Kato, K., and Haga, M., Natural carcinogenic products of plant origin, *Gann Monogr.*, 17, 205, 1975.
5. Druckrey, H., Preussmann, R., Matzkies, F., and Ivankovic, S., Selektive Erzeugung von Darmkrebs bei Ratten durch 1,2-Dimethylhydrazin, *Naturwissenschaften*, 54, 285, 1967.
6. Druckrey, H., Organospecific carcinogenesis in the digestive tract, in *Proc. 2nd Int. Symp. Princess Takamatsu Cancer Res. Fund*, Nakahara, W., Takayama, S., Sugimura, T., and Odashima, S., Eds., University of Tokyo Press, Tokyo, 1972, 73.
7. Weisburger, J. H., Chemical carcinogens and their mode of action in colonic neoplasia, *Dis. Colon Rectum*, 16, 431, 1973.
8. Narisawa, T., Wong, C.-Q., Maronpot, R. R., and Weisburger, J. H., Large bowel carcinogenesis in mice and rats by several intrarectal doses of methylnitrosourea and negative effect of nitrite plus methylurea, *Cancer Res.*, 36, 505, 1976.

9. Narisawa, T., Sato, T., Hayakawa, M., Sakuma, A., and Nakano, H., Carcinoma of the colon and rectum of rats by rectal infusion of N-methyl-N'-nitro-N-nitrosoguanidine, *Gann*, 62, 231, 1971.
10. Corbett, T. H., Griswold, D. P., Jr., Roberts, B. J., Peckham, J. C., and Schabel, F. M., Jr., Tumor induction relationships in development of transplantable cancers of the colon in mice for chemotherapy assays, with a note on carcinogen structure, *Cancer Res.*, 35, 2434, 1975.
11. Archer, M. C., Lee, L., and Bruce, W. R., Analysis and formation of nitrosamines in the human intestine, *IARC Sci. Publ.*, 41, 357, 1982.
12. Fine, D., Ross, R., Rounbehler, D. P., Silvergleid, A., and Song, L., Formation *in vivo* of volatile N-nitrosamines in man after ingestion of cooked bacon and spinach, *Nature (London)*, 265, 753, 1977.
13. Tannenbaum, S. R., Young, V. R., Green, L., and Ruiz de Luzuriaga, K., Intestinal formation of nitrite and N-nitroso compounds, *IARC Sci. Publ.*, 31, 281, 1980.
14. Yamamoto, M., Yamada, T., and Tanimura, A., Studies on the formation of nitrosamines. III. The reaction products of glycocyamine and sodium nitrite, *J. Food Hyg. Soc. Jpn.*, 17, 176, 1976.
15. Yamada, T., Yamamoto, M., and Tanimura, A., Studies on the formation of nitrosamines. IV. Kinetical studies on the carboxymethylnitrosourea formation from glycocyamine and sodium nitrite, *J. Food Hyg. Soc. Jpn.*, 17, 182, 1976.
16. Kodama, M., Saito, H., and Yamaizumi, Z., Formation of alkylureas in the environment, *IARC Sci. Publ.*, 41, 131, 1982.
17. Mirvish, S. S. and Chu, C., Chemical determination of methylnitrosourea and ethylnitrosourea in stomach contents of rats, after intubation of the alkylureas plus sodium nitrite, *J. Natl. Cancer Inst.*, 50, 745, 1973.
18. Maekawa, A., Ogiu, T., and Odashima, S., Spontaneous tumors in Donryu rats (in Japanese), *Proc. Jpn. Cancer Assoc.*, 35, 36, 1976.
19. Maekawa, A., Kurokawa, Y., Takahashi, M., Kokubo, T., Ogiu, T., Onodera, H., Tanigawa, H., Ohno, Y., Furukawa, F., and Hayashi, Y., Spontaneous tumors in F-344/DuCrj rats, *Gann*, 74, 365, 1983.
20. Ogiu, T., Nakadate, M., Furuta, K., Maekawa, A., and Odashima, S., Induction of tumors of peripheral nervous system in female Donryu rats by continuous oral administration of 1-methyl-1-nitrosourea, *Gann*, 68, 491, 1977.
21. Ogiu, T., Nakadate, M., and Odashima, S., Rapid and selective induction of erythroleukemia in female Donryu rats by continuous oral administration of 1-ethyl-1-nitrosourea, *Cancer Res.*, 36, 3043, 1976.
22. Ogiu, T., Nakadate, M., and Odashima, S., Induction of leukemias and digestive tract tumors in Donryu rats by 1-propyl-1-nitrosourea, *J. Natl. Cancer Inst.*, 54, 887, 1975.
23. Odashima, S., Leukemogenesis of N-nitrosobutylurea in the rat. I. Effect of various concentrations in the drinking water to female Donryu rats, *Gann*, 61, 245, 1970.
24. Fujii, K., Nakadate M., Ogiu, T., and Odashima, S., Induction of digestive tract tumors and leukemias in Donryu rats by administration of 1-amyl-1-nitrosourea in drinking water, *Gann*, 71, 464, 1980.
25. Ogiu, T., Matsuoka, C., Furuta, K., Takeuchi, M., Maekawa, A., Nakadate, M., and Odashima, S., Induction of angiogenic tumors in the duodenum of female Donryu rats by continuous oral administration of N-isobutyl-N-nitrosourea, *Gann*, 74, 342, 1983.
26. Maekawa, A., Ogiu, T., Matsuoka, C., Onodera, H., Furuta, K., Tanigawa, H., and Odashima, S., Induction of tumors in the small intestine and mammary gland of female Donryu rats by continuous oral administration of N-carboxymethyl-N-nitrosourea, *J. Cancer Res. Clin. Oncol.*, 106, 12, 1983.
27. Ogiu, T., Kajiwara, T., Furuta, K., Takeuchi, M., Odashima, S., and Tada, K., Mammary tumorigenic effect of a new nitrosourea, 1,3-dibutyl-1-nitrosourea (B-BNU), in female Donryu rats, *J. Cancer Res. Clin. Oncol.*, 96, 35, 1980.
28. Takeuchi, M., Maekawa, A., Tada, K., and Odashima, S., Leukemias and vaginal tumors induced in female Donryu rats by continuous oral administration of 1-butyl-3,3-dimethyl-1-nitrosourea in the drinking water, *J. Natl. Cancer Inst.*, 56, 1177, 1976.
29. Takeuchi, M., Ogiu, T., Nakadate, M., and Odashima, S., Induction of duodenal tumors in F344 rats by continuous oral administration of N-ethyl-N-nitrosourea, *J. Natl. Cancer Inst.*, 64, 613, 1980.
30. Takeuchi, M., Ogiu, T., Nakadate, M., and Odashima, S., Induction of duodenal tumors and thymomas in Fischer rats by continuous oral administration of 1-propyl-1-nitrosourea, *Gann*, 71, 231, 1980.
31. Takeuchi, M., Ogiu, T., Matsuoka, C., Furuta, K., Maekawa, A., Nakadate, M., and Odashima, S., Induction of digestive tract tumors in Fischer rats by continuous oral administration of N-butyl-N-nitrosourea, *J. Cancer Res. Clin. Oncol.*, 107, 32, 1984.
32. Druckrey, H., Preussmann, R., Ivankovic, S., and Schmahl, D., Organotrope carcinogene Wirkungen bei 65 verschiedenen N-Nitroso-Verbindungen an BD-Ratten, *Z. Krebsforsch.*, 69, 103, 1967.

33. Pelfrene, A., Mirvish, S. S., and Garcia, H., Carcinogenic action of ethylnitroso cyanamide (ENC), 1-nitrosohydantoin (NH), and ethylnitrosourea (ENU) in the rat, *Proc. Am. Assoc. Cancer Res.,* 16, 117, 1975.
34. Lijinsky, W. and Taylor, H. W., Induction of neurogenic tumors by nitrosotrialkylureas in rats, *Z. Krebsforsch.,* 83, 315, 1975.
35. Leaver, D. D., Swann, P. F., and Magee, P. N., The induction of tumours in the rat by a single oral dose of *N*-nitrosomethyl-urea, *Br. J. Cancer,* 23, 177, 1969.
36. Druckrey, H., Schagen, B., and Ivankovic, S., Erzeugung neurogener Malignome durch einmalige Gabe von Athyl-nitrosoharnstoff (ANH) an neugeborene und junge BD IX-Ratten, *Z. Krebsforsch.,* 74, 141, 1970.
37. Ogiu, T., Nakadate, M., and Odashima, S., Induction of tumors in female Donryu rats by a single administration of 1-propyl-1-nitrosourea, *Gann,* 67, 121, 1976.
38. Odashima, S., Leukemogenic effects of *N*-butyl-*N*-nitrosourea in rats, *Gann Monogr.,* 12, 283, 1972.
39. Laurens, J. and Bacon, H. E., Studies of experimental carcinogenesis in the colon and rectum of the rat, *J. Natl. Cancer Inst.,* 12, 1237, 1952.
40. Rack, F. J., Kaufman, N., and Simeone, F. A., The effect of 20-methylcholanthrene applied directly to the colon in mice, *Cancer Res.,* 15, 722, 1955.
41. Toth, B., Tumorigenesis by benzo(*a*)pyrene administered intracolonically, *Oncology,* 37, 77, 1980.
42. Berenblum, I., Haran, N., and Rosin, A., The carcinogenic action in the mouse of 20-methylcholanthrene by rectal administration, *Am. J. Pathol.,* 32, 579, 1956.
43. Narisawa, T., Wong, C.-Q., and Weisburger, J. H., Induction of carcinoma of the large intestine in guinea pigs by intrarectal instillation of *N*-methyl-*N*-nitrosourea, *J. Natl. Cancer Inst.,* 54, 785, 1975.
44. O'Donnell, R. W. and Cockerell, G. L., Establishment and biological properties of a guinea pig colonic adenocarcinoma cell line induced by *N*-methyl-*N*-nitrosourea, *Cancer Res.,* 41, 2372, 1981.
45. Ward, J. M., Sporn, M. B., Wenk, M. L., Smith, J. M., Feeser, D., and Dean, R. J., Dose response to intrarectal administration of *N*-methyl-*N*-nitrosourea and histopathologic evaluation of the effect of two retinoids on colon lesions induced in rats, *J. Natl. Cancer Inst.,* 60, 1489, 1978.
46. Schmähl, D., Zur carcinogenen Wirkung von Butylathylnitrosamin bei rektaler Applikation an Ratten, *Z. Krebsforsch.,* 74, 110, 1970.
47. Rice, J. M., Joshi, S. R., Roller, P. P., and Wenk, M. L., Methyl(acetoxymethyl)nitrosamine: a new carcinogen highly specific for colon and small intestine, *Proc. Am. Assoc. Cancer Res.,* 16, 32, 1975.
48. Ward, J. M., Rice, J. M., Roller, P. P., and Wenk, M. L., Natural history of intestinal neoplasms induced in rats by a single injection of methyl(acetoxymethyl)nitrosamine, *Cancer Res.,* 37, 3046, 1977.
49. Habs, M., Schmähl, D., and Wiessler, M., Carcinogenicity of acetoxymethyl-methyl-nitrosamine after subcutaneous, intravenous and intrarectal applications in rats, *Z. Krebsforsch.,* 91, 217, 1978.
50. Kamano, T., Kurihara, M., Kishino, H., Mizukami, K., Azuma, N., Kidokoro, T., Izumi, T., Wakabayashi, K., Kuwabara N., and Kondo, S., Experimental colonic cancer in dogs (in Japanese), *Igaku-no-Ayumi,* 118, 255, 1981.
51. Balish, E., Shih, C. N., Croft, W. A., Pamukcu, A. M., Lower, G., Bryan, G. T., and Yale, C. E., Effect of age, sex, and intestinal flora on the induction of colon tumors in rats, *J. Natl. Cancer Inst.,* 58, 1103, 1977.
52. Druckrey, H., Steinhoff, D., Preussmann, R., and Ivankovic, S., Krebserzeugung durch einmalige Dosis von Methylnitrosoharnstoff und verschiedenen Dialkyl-nitrosaminen, *Naturwissenschaften,* 50, 735, 1963.
53. Druckrey, H., Steinhoff, D., Preussmann, R., and Ivankovic, S., Erzeugung von Krebs durch eine einmalige Dosis von Methylnitrosoharnstoff und verschiedenen Dialkylnitrosaminen an Ratten, *Z. Krebsforsch.,* 66, 1, 1964.
54. Terracini, B. and Testa, M. C., Carcinogenicity of a single administration of *N*-nitrosomethylurea: a comparison between newborn and 5-week-old mice and rats, *Br. J. Cancer,* 24, 588, 1970.
55. Ward, J. M. and Weisburger, E. K., Intestinal tumors in mice treated with a single injection of *N*-nitroso-*N*-butylurea, *Cancer Res.,* 35, 1938, 1975.
56. Pozharisski, K. M., Tumours of the intestines, *IARC Sci. Publ.,* 5, 119, 1973.
57. Horn, R. C., Jr. and Fine, G., Alimentary tract, in *Pathology,* 7th ed., Anderson, W. A. D. and Kissane, J. M., Eds., C. V. Mosby, St. Louis, Mo., 1977, 1277.
58. Bruce, W. R., Varghese, A. J., Furrer, R., and Land, P. C., A mutagen in the feces of normal humans, in *Origins of Human Cancer, Book C,* Hiatt, H. H., Watson, J. D., and Winsten, J. A., Eds., Cold Spring Harbor Laboratory, Cold Spring Harbor, N.Y., 1977, 1641.
59. Ehrich, M., Aswell, J. E., Van Tassell, R. L., Wilkins, T. D., Walker, A. R. P., and Richardson, N. J., Mutagens in the feces of 3 South-African populations at different levels of risk for colon cancer, *Mutat. Res.,* 64, 231, 1979.

60. Reddy, B. S., Sharma, C., Darby, L., Laakso, K., and Wynder, E. L., Metabolic epidemiology of large bowel cancer: fecal mutagens in high- and low-risk population for colon cancer, *Mutat. Res.,* 72, 511, 1980.
61. Mower, H. F., Ichinotsubo, D., Wang, L. W., Mandel, M., Stemmermann, G., Nomura, A., Heilbrun, L., Kamiyama, S., and Shimada, A., Fecal mutagens in two Japanese populations with different colon cancer risks, *Cancer Res.,* 42, 1164, 1982.
62. Ishidate, M., Tanimura, A., Ito, Y., Sakai, A., Sakuta, H., Kawamura, T., Sakai, K., Miyazawa, F., and Wada, H., Secondary amines, nitrites and nitrosamines in Japanese foods, in *Proc. 2nd Int. Symp. Princess Takamatsu Cancer Res. Fund,* Nakahara, W., Takayama, S., Sugimura, T., and Odashima, S., Eds., University of Tokyo Press, Tokyo, 1972, 313.
63. Saul, R. L. and Archer, M. C., Nitrate formation in rats exposed to nitrogen dioxide, *Toxicol. Appl. Pharmacol.,* 67, 284, 1983.
64. Van Stee, E. W., Sloane, R. A., Simmons, J. E., and Brunnemann, K. D., In vivo formation of N-nitrosomorpholine in CD-1 mice exposed by inhalation to nitrogen dioxide and by gavage to morpholine, *J. Natl. Cancer Inst.,* 70, 375, 1983.
65. Sander, J. and Bürkle, G., Induktion maligner Tumoren bei Ratten durch gleichzeitige Verfutterung von Nitrit und sekundaren Aminen, *Z. Krebsforsch.,* 73, 54, 1969.
66. Koestner, A., Denlinger, R. H., and Wechsler, W., Induction of neurogenic and lymphoid neoplasms by the feeding of threshold levels of methyl- and ethylnitrosourea precursors to adult rats, *Food Cosmet. Toxicol.,* 13, 605, 1975.
67. Ivankovic, S. and Preussmann, R., Transplazentare Erzeugung maligner Tumoren nach oraler Gabe von Äthylharnstoff und Nitrit an Ratten, *Naturwissenschaften,* 57, 460, 1970.
68. Osske, G., Warzok, R., and Schneider, J., Diaplazentare Tumorinduktion durch endogen gebildeten N-Äthyl-N-nitrosoharnstoff bei Ratten, *Arch. Geschwulstforsch.,* 40, 244, 1972.
69. Schneider, J., Bicker, U., Warzok, R., and Osske, G., Tumorenstehung durch endogen gebildete Kanzerogene nach Gabe von n-Propyl-, iso-Propyl- bzw. n-Butylharnstoff und Nitrit bei Ratten, *Arch. Geschwulstforsch.,* 44, 126, 1974.
70. Maekawa, A., Ishiwate, H., and Odashima, S., Transplacental carcinogensis and chemical determination of 1-butyl-1-nitrosourea in stomach content after simultaneous oral administration of 1-butylurea and sodium nitrite to ACI/N rats, *Gann,* 68, 81, 1977.
71. Murthy, A. S. K., Baker, J. R., Smith, E. R., and Zepp, E., Neoplasms in rats and mice fed butylurea and sodium nitrite separately and in combination, *Int. J. Cancer,* 23, 253, 1979.
72. Narisawa, T., Wong, G.-Q., and Weisburger, J. H., Evaluation of endoscopic examination of colon tumors in rats, *Dig. Dis.,* 20, 928, 1975.
73. Merz, R., Wagner, I., Habs, M., Schmähl, D., Amberger, A., and Bachmann, U., Endoscopic diagnosis of chemically induced autochthonous colonic tumors in rats, *Hepato-Gastroenterology,* 28, 53, 1981.
74. Rosengren, J. E. and Lindström, C. G., Experimental colonic tumors in the rat. II. Double contrast examination and microscopy, *Acta Radiol. Diagr.,* 19, 465, 1978.
75. Skucas, J., Gluckman, J. B., Fowler, E. H., Turner, M. D., and Narisawa, T., Radiological evaluation of rat colonic tumors, *Invest. Radiol.,* 13, 34, 1978.
76. Lev, R. and Herp, A., Pathogenesis of rat colon carcinomas induced by N-methyl-N-nitrosourea, *J. Natl. Cancer Inst.,* 61, 779, 1978.
77. Wynder, E. L., Kajitani, T., Ishikawa, S., Dodo, H., and Takano, A., Environmental factors of cancer of the colon and rectum. II. Japanese epidemiological data, *Cancer,* 23, 1210, 1969.
78. Reddy, B. S., Watanabe, K., and Weisburger, J. H., Effect of high-fat diet on colon carcinogenesis in F344 rats treated with 1,2-dimethylhydrazine, methylazoxymethanol acetate, or methylnitrosourea, *Cancer Res.,* 37, 4156, 1977.
79. Narisawa, T., Reddy, B. S., and Weisburger, J. H., Effect of bile acids and dietary fat on large bowel carcinogenesis in animal models, *Gastroenterol. Jpn.,* 13, 206, 1978.
80. Chonchai, C., Bhadrachari, N., and Nigro, N. D., The effect of bile on the induction of experimental intestinal tumors in rats, *Dis. Colon Rectum,* 17, 310, 1974.
81. Narisawa, T., Magadia, N. E., Weisburger, J. H., and Wynder, E. L., Promoting effect of bile acids on colon carcinogenesis after intrarectal instillation of N-methyl-N'-nitro-N-nitrosoguanidine in rats, *J. Natl. Cancer Inst.,* 53, 1093, 1974.
82. Hill, M. J., Crowther, J. S., Drasar, B. S., Hawksworth G., Aries, V., and Williams, R. E. O., Bacteria and etiology of cancer of large bowel, *Lancet,* 1, 95, 1971.
83. Reddy, B. S. and Wynder, E. L., Large-bowel carcinogenesis: fecal constituents of populations with diverse incidence rates of colon cancer, *J. Natl. Cancer Inst.,* 50, 1437, 1973.
84. Reddy, B. S., Hedges, A. K., Laakso, K., and Wynder, E. L., Metabolic epidemiology of large bowel cancer-fecal bulk and constituents of high-risk North American and low-risk Finnish populations, *Cancer,* 42, 2832, 1978.

85. Cohen, B. I., Raicht, R. F., Deschner, E. E., Takahashi, M., Sarwal, A. N., and Fazzini, E., Effect of cholic acid feeding on *N*-methyl-*N*-nitrosourea-induced colon tumors and cell kinetics in rats, *J. Natl. Cancer Inst.*, 64, 573, 1980.

86. Cohen, B. I., Raicht, R. F., and Fazzini, E., Reduction of *N*-methyl-*N*-nitrosourea-induced colon tumors in the rat by cholesterol, *Cancer Res.*, 42, 5050, 1982.

87. Narisawa, T., Sato, M., Tani, M., Kudo, T., Takahashi, T., and Goto, A., Inhibition of development of methylnitrosourea-induced rat colon tumors by indomethacin treatment, *Cancer Res.*, 41, 1954, 1981.

88. Narisawa, T., Sato, M., Sano, M., and Takahashi, T., Inhibition of development of methylnitrosourea-induced rat colonic tumors by peroral administration of indomethacin, *Gann*, 73, 377, 1982.

89. Fürstenberger, G. and Marks, F., Early prostaglandin E synthesis is an obligatory event in the induction of cell proliferation in mouse epidermis *in vivo* by the phorbol ester TPA, *Biochem. Biophys. Res. Commun.*, 92, 749, 1980.

90. Verma, A. K., Ashendel, C. L., and Boutwell, R. K., Inhibition by prostaglandin synthesis inhibitors of the induction of epidermal ornithine decarboxylase activity, the accumulation of prostaglandins, and tumor promotion caused by 12-O-tetradecanoylpholbol-13-acetate, *Cancer Res.*, 40, 308, 1980.

91. Kudo, T., Narisawa, T., and Abo, S., Antitumor activity of indomethacin on methylazoxymethanol-induced large bowel tumors in rats, *Gann*, 71, 260, 1980.

92. Pollard, M. and Luckert, P. H., Indomethacin treatment of rats with dimethylhydrazine-induced intestinal tumors, *Cancer Treat. Rep.*, 64, 1323, 1980.

93. Wattenberg, L. W., Inhibitors of chemical carcinogenesis, *Adv. Cancer Res.*, 26, 197, 1978.

94. Burkitt, D. P., Epidemiology of cancer of the colon and rectum, *Cancer*, 28, 3, 1971.

95. Hirayama, T., A large-scale cohort study on the relationship between diet and selected cancers of digestive organs, in *Gastrointestinal Cancer*, Banbury Report 7, Bruce, W. R., Correa, P., Lipkin, M., Tannenbaum, S. R., and Wilkins, T. D., Eds., Cold Spring Harbor Laboratory, Cold Spring Harbor, N.Y., 1981, 409.

96. Watanabe, K., Reddy, B. S., Weisburger, J. H., and Kritchevsky, D., Effect of dietary alfalfa, pectin, and wheat bran on azoxymethane- or methylnitrosourea-induced colon carcinogenesis in F344 rats, *J. Natl. Cancer Inst.*, 63, 141, 1979.

97. Watanabe, K., Reddy, B. S., Wong, C. Q., and Weisburger, J. H., Effect of dietary undegraded carrageenan on colon carcinogenesis in F344 rats treated with azoxymethane or methylnitrosourea, *Cancer Res.*, 38, 4427, 1978.

98. Raicht, R. F., Cohen, B. I., Fazzini, E. P., Sarwal, A. N., and Takahashi, M., Protective effect of plant sterols against chemically induced colon tumors in rats, *Cancer Res.*, 40, 403, 1980.

99. Deschner, E. E., Cohen, B. I., and Raicht, R. F., The kinetics of the protective effect of β-sitosterol against MNU-induced colonic neoplasia, *J. Cancer Res. Clin. Oncol.*, 103, 49, 1982.

100. Silverman, J., Katayama, S., Zelenakas, K., Lauber, J., Musser, T. K., Reddy, M., Levenstein, M. J., and Weisburger, J. H., Effect of retinoids on the induction of colon cancer in F344 rats by *N*-methyl-*N*-nitrosourea or by 1,2-dimethylhydrazine, *Carcinogenesis*, 2, 1167, 1981.

101. Reddy, B. S., Hirota, N., and Katayama, S., Effect of dietary sodium ascorbate on 1,2-dimethylhydrazine- or methylnitrosourea-induced colon carcinogenesis in rats, *Carcinogenesis*, 3, 1097, 1982.

102. Narisawa, T., Kono, K., Yamaguchi, T., and Takahashi, T., Cancer chemotherapy model using autochthonous large bowel cancer in rats, *Gann*, 69, 431, 1978.

103. Sych, F., Habs, M., and Schmähl, D., Chemotherapy studies in autochthonous rat tumors, intestinal cancer, *Z. Krebsforsch.*, 92, 105, 1978.

104. Narisawa, T., Kono, K., Yamaguchi, T., and Takahashi, T., Chemoprevention of development of colonic adenomatosis and carcinomatosis with intrarectal dose of 5-FU on animal model, *Cancer*, 45, 439, 1980.

105. Narisawa, T., Sato, M., Tani, M., and Takahashi, T., Chemoprevention of development of colonic adenomatosis and carcinomatosis with 5-fluorouracil and ftorafur on animal model, *J. Cancer Res. Clin. Oncol.*, 97, 223, 1980.

Chapter 8

MORPHOGENESIS OF EXPERIMENTAL COLONIC NEOPLASMS INDUCED BY DIMETHYLHYDRAZINE

Shinichi Nakamura and Isamu Kino

TABLE OF CONTENTS

I. INTRODUCTION

Adenomas are the most common type of neoplasms of the colon and it is known that larger adenomas often contain cancerous foci. Those investigators who have emphasized the coexistence of adenoma with cancer have hypothesized an adenoma-cancer sequence,[1-4] while other investigators have maintained that cancer appears *de novo* and does not pass through an adenoma stage.[5-7] There is still controversy over these two opinions.

It is also known that colonic cancers are frequently observed in young patients with familial adenomatosis coli, in which condition numerous adenomas develop in the colon. Thus, it is presumed that there is a close relationship between adenoma and cancer.[8] However, the exact early morphogenesis of adenoma still remains unknown. Following studies on human material, Dukes[9] and Lane and Lev[10] have proposed that adenomas originate from the deep part of the crypts, but many investigators have insisted that adenomas develop in the upper part of the crypt.[11-15]

Recently, there have been many studies with chemical carcinogens that induce colonic neoplasms in small experimental animals. One such chemical, dimethylhydrazine (DMH), is known to induce adenomas and carcinomas in the colon of rats, mice, and hamsters at high incidence.[16-27] These experimental systems are now widely used as models of human colonic neoplasms.

We have induced tumors in the colon of these animals by DMH in order to investigate the morphogenesis of adenoma and the cellular kinetics of the background mucosa. We report here the results of these experiments.

II. COLONIC NEOPLASMS INDUCED BY DMH IN RODENTS

A. Mice

ICR mice were obtained from the Shizuoka Agriculture Co-operative Association for Laboratory Animals. The animals were 9 weeks old and weighed 30 to 40 g at the start of DMH (*N,N*-dimethylhydrazine dihydrochloride, Tokyo Kasei, Tokyo) treatment. They were given a standard diet and water *ad libitum,* and injected subcutaneously with 20 mg/kg DMH once a week for up to 24 weeks. The 17 mice treated with DMH showed emaciation, ruffled hair, and tumor formation in the anal region between week 23 and 33.

These mice were sacrificed between 23 and 33 weeks after injection. Complete autopsies were performed, and the colon was sectioned longitudinally and examined macroscopically. After fixation in 10% phosphate-buffered formalin (pH 7.0), the colon was cut into 5-mm-long sections, which were embedded in paraffin. Thin sections were stained with hematoxylin and eosin (H.E.) for histologic examination.

The incidence and induction time of tumors in these 17 ICR mice are shown in Table 1. All 17 animals had multiple colonic adenomas of various sizes, which were usually hemispherical or sessile with no ulceration (Figure 1). Almost all the adenomas were located in the most distal 7 cm of the large intestine, which has longitudinal mucosal ridges. No adenomas were observed in the proximal colon which has distinct oblique mucosal ridges. Two adenomas were found in the cecum (Figure 2). In the only animal killed in week 33, an adenocarcinoma invading the muscularis was found in the distal colon, but no metastasis was present. Histologically, these lesions were tubular adenomas of the same histologic type as observed in the human colon (Figure 3). Besides the colonic adenomas, 11 circumanal gland tumors including squamous cell carcinomas, two hemangiomas of the liver, and a ceruminous gland tumor of the ear were also found in the animals treated with DMH (Table 1).

Table 1
INCIDENCE OF DMH-INDUCED TUMORS IN 17 ICR MICE

Organ	Histological type	No. of tumor-bearing mice	M/F	Induction time (weeks)
Large intestine	Adenoma	17	7/10	23—33
	Adenocarcinoma	1	0/1	33
Anal region	Squamous cell carcinoma	1	0/1	27
	Tumor of the circumanal gland	11	5/6	26—33
Liver	Hemangioma	2	1/1	27, 33
Ear	Tumor of the ceruminous gland	1	0/1	32

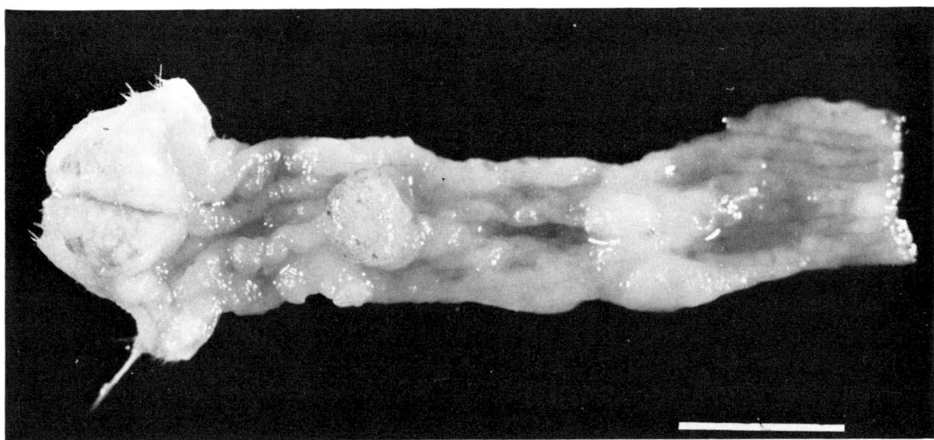

FIGURE 1. Multiple adenomas of the distal colon and a circumanal gland tumor in a DMH-treated mouse, sacrificed in week 27. Bar = 1 cm.

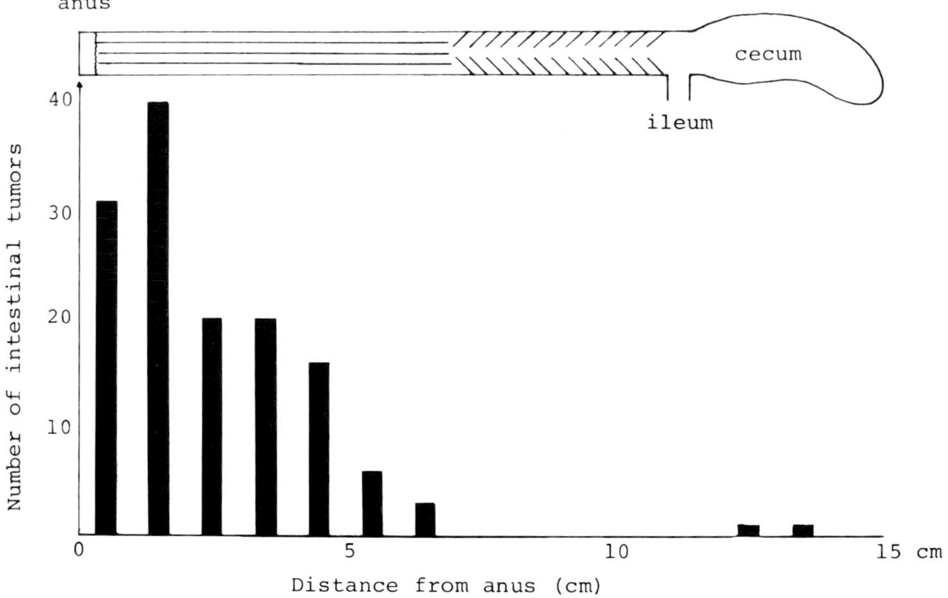

FIGURE 2. Distribution and number of adenomas in the large intestines of ICR mice treated with DMH (17 animals).

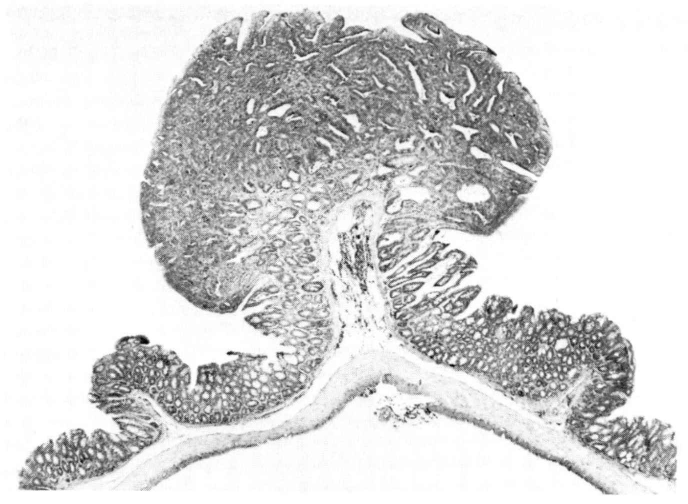

FIGURE 3.   A large hemispherical colonic adenoma in a mouse, sacrificed in week 33. (H.E.; magnification × 24.)

Table 2
INCIDENCE OF DMH-INDUCED TUMORS IN EIGHT SPRAGUE-DAWLEY RATS

Organ	Histology	No. of tumor-bearing rats	No. of rats with metastasis	Induction time (weeks)
Small intestine	Adenocarcinoma	3	2	24—33
Large intestine	Adenoma	5	0	25—33
	Adenocarcinoma	4	1	32—33
Ear	Squamous cell carcinoma	3	0	27—33
	Tumor of the ceruminous gland	3	0	32—33

B. Rats

Sprague-Dawley rats were 9 weeks old at the start of DMH treatment. A total of 15 animals were injected subcutaneously with 20 mg/kg DMH once a week for up to 24 weeks and 8 of the animals were killed between week 24 and 33. Three of the eight animals had signet-ring cell carcinomas of the small intestine, which had extensively metastasized to the peritoneum. Colonic adenomas and/or carcinomas were observed in all rats killed after 31 weeks (Table 2). Macroscopically, these tumors were of various shapes such as hemispherical, pedunculated, flatly protuberant, or ulcerated. Although these tumors were found in all parts of the colon, a majority were observed in the distal part (Figure 4).

Histologically, colonic tumors showed great diversity of cellular and structural atypism. Some were adenomas with mild atypia (Figure 5) and others were adenocarcinomas with severe atypia, invading the muscle and the subserosa (Figure 6). Signet-ring cell carcinomas were also observed. Besides the colonic tumors, squamous cell carcinomas of the ear and three ceruminous gland tumors were observed (Table 2).

C. Hamsters

Golden hamsters were 10 weeks old at the start of DMH treatment. A total of 30 animals were injected subcutaneously with 20 mg/kg DMH once a week for up 20 weeks and 27 of the animals died or were killed between week 10 and 25. The incidence of tumors in the 27 golden hamsters is shown in Table 3.

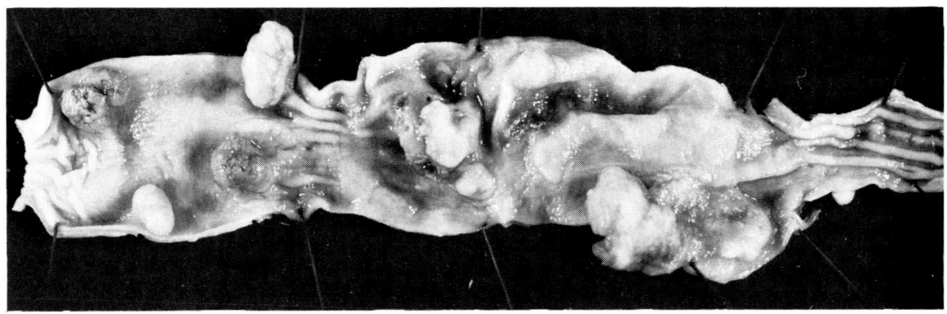

FIGURE 4. Multiple tumors of the distal colon in a DMH-treated rat, sacrificed in week 33.

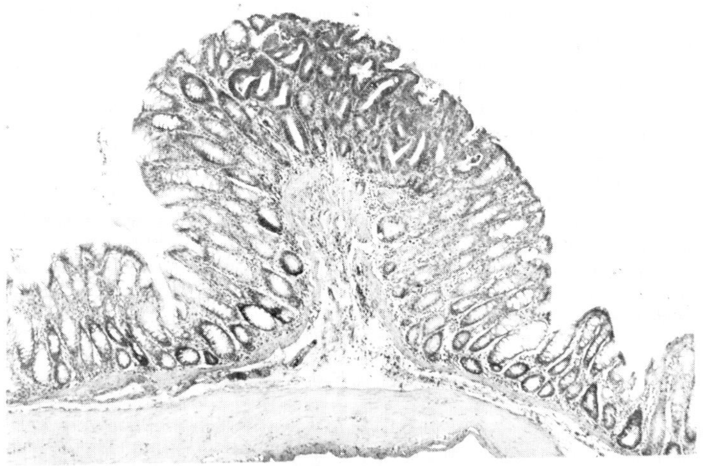

FIGURE 5. A small colonic adenoma with mild atypia in a rat treated with DMH. (H.E.; magnification × 45.)

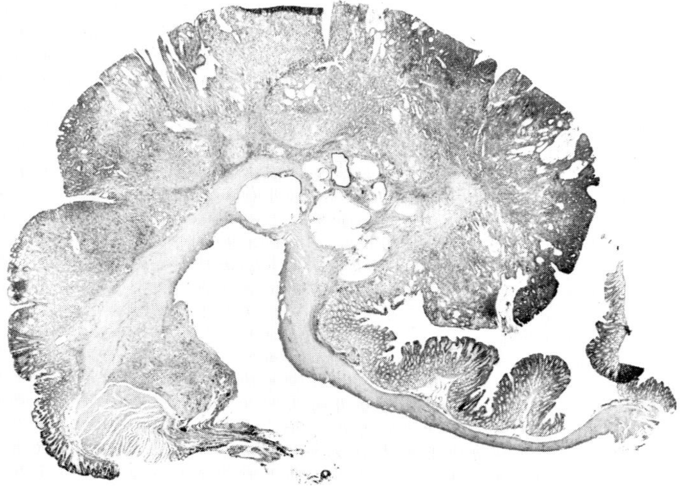

FIGURE 6. An advanced colonic adenocarcinoma in a rat with severe atypia. (H.E.; magnification × 30.)

Table 3
INCIDENCE OF DMH-INDUCED TUMORS IN 27 GOLDEN HAMSTERS

Organ	Histology	No. of tumor-bearing hamsters	Male/ female	Induction time (weeks)
Large intestine	Adenoma	27/27	14/13	10—25
	Adenocarcinoma	14/27	5/9	17—25
Liver	Proliferation of bile duct	18/27	6/12	16—25
	Cholangiocellular carcinoma	8/27	0/8	20—25
	Hepatocellular carcinoma	1/27	0/1	20

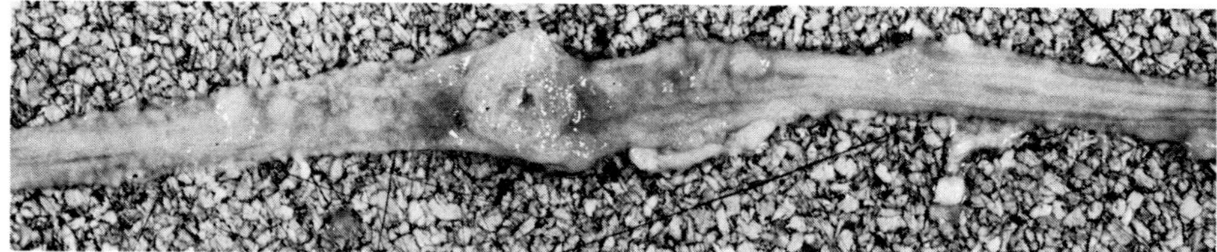

FIGURE 7.   Several colonic tumors in a hamster, sacrificed in week 22.

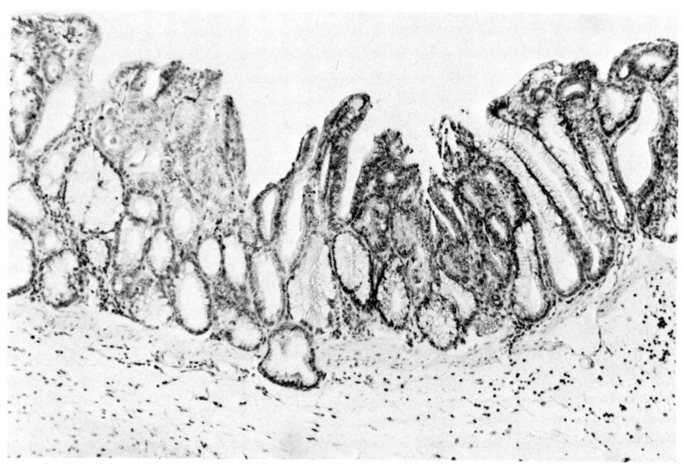

FIGURE 8.   A microscopic colonic adenoma in a hamster with mild atypia.
(H.E.; magnification × 80.)

Multiple tumors were observed in the colon at 4 to 18 cm from the anus (Figure 7). All of the 27 animals had multiple colonic adenomas (Figure 8). Adenocarcinoma was found in the colon of one animal killed in week 17 and 14 animals had colonic adenocarcinomas that invaded the muscle and subserosa, showing cystic dilatation, but which did not metastasize (Figure 9).

Adenocarcinomas showed mild cellular and structural atypism even at the point of invasion and there were no histologic differences between adenoma and adenocarcinoma except for invasion.

Besides the colonic tumors, liver lesions with proliferation of the bile ducts were found in 18 animals, 8 animals had cholangiocellular carcinomas, and a hepatocellular carcinoma was observed in 1 animal killed in week 20.

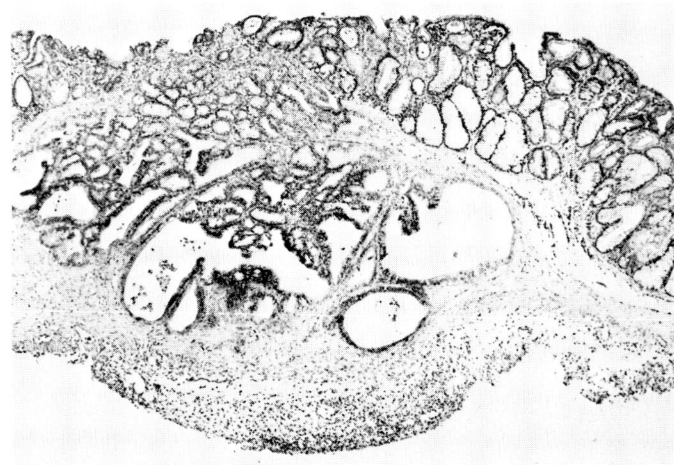

FIGURE 9. An advanced adenocarcinoma of the colon in the hamster. Submucosal growth and cyst formation are prominent. (H.E.; magnification × 45.)

D. Discussion

The metabolism and mode of action of the colonic carcinogen, DMH, is regarded to conform to the following steps: inoculated DMH is metabolized in the liver and the metabolite is excreted into the bile, transported to the colon, and ultimately broken down by intestinal bacteria to a carcinogen.[16,28,29] However, there are some reports that the carcinogenic metabolite of DMH enters directly into epithelial cells of the colon from the blood circulation.[18,30] In any case, there are no erosions or ulcers in the colons of animals treated with DMH except for tumor formations, so this experimental system is considered to be an excellent model to study the morphogenesis of human colonic tumors.[31]

Although in the present experiments highly susceptible ICR mice were used and a 100% incidence of adenoma in the distal colon was observed, it has been reported that some strains of mice show high incidence of DMH-induced tumors while others are completely resistant to DMH. This differential response to DMH-induced tumors is determined by the genotype of the mice.[32,33] Lobund Wistar rats were resistant to induction of colon tumors by DMH,[34] while Sprague-Dawley rats were very sensitive to DMH and showed a high incidence of colonic tumors in the present experiment.

We also confirmed the previous reports[25-27] that DMH treatment of golden hamsters induced colonic tumors. Emaciation became conspicuous in hamsters after about 10 weeks and extensive degeneration of the hepatocytes was observed at autopsy. Proliferation of the bile ducts and cholangiocellular and hepatocellular carcinomas were found in the livers of golden hamsters; this did not occur in mice or rats.

In regard to the distribution of colonic tumors, adenomas were confined to the distal parts of the colons of mice, but a considerable number of adenomas and carcinomas were observed in the proximal colons as well as the distal colons of rats and hamsters. Signet-ring cell carcinomas were observed in the small intestines of those rats that died from extensive peritoneal metastasis.

It has been reported that histologic structures and cell kinetics were different between the proximal vs. the distal colons of rats and mice.[35-38] There are no such differences in the human colon. Because the distal colon of the mouse is similar to that of man, this experimental model with mice seems to be suitable for analysis of human colonic tumors.

Almost all the colonic tumors of mice were adenomas and adenocarcinoma was found in only one case. The incidence of adenocarcinomas was much lower than those reported in previous studies,[22,24] probably owing to a shorter observation period[21] and differences in the strains tested.[32,33] A rather high incidence of adenocarcinomas was observed in rats treated with DMH and, histologically, many of these were poorly differentiated adenocarcinomas, including signet-ring cell carcinoma, which is rare in human colonic adenocarcinoma. DMH-induced adenocarcinoma in the colon of the hamster showed rather curious histologic features in which the carcinoma was initially a small lesion in the mucosa but developed to considerable size, with cystic glandular proliferation eventually invading the muscularis and subserosa. This histologic spectrum is rarely observed in man. There were no obvious differences in cell atypism between adenoma and carcinoma in the hamster, so the only distinction between adenoma and carcinoma was by the invasion of the tumor cells into the colonic wall.

From the present experiments, we stress that DMH-induced colonic adenoma of mice is a most excellent experimental model for study of the morphogenesis of human colonic adenoma for the following reasons: (1) DMH-induced tumors are found mainly in the colon; (2) distribution of the tumors is confined to the distal colon; (3) multiple tumors, including microscopic lesions, are induced; (4) most tumors are tubular adenomas; and (5) histologic appearance of adenomas is similar to that observed in man.

III. MORPHOGENESIS OF ADENOMA IN THE COLON OF MICE TREATED WITH DMH

Multiple adenomas induced in the colon of mice treated with DMH were investigated to reveal the mode of initiation and morphogenesis of adenomas. The mice were 9 weeks old, weighed 30 to 40 g, and were injected subcutaneously with 20 mg/kg DMH once a week for up to 20 weeks. Every 2 weeks, 2 or 3 DMH-treated mice and 2 control mice were sacrificed successively between week 2 and 20. The colon was cut into 5-mm lengths and examined by light microscopy. The 5-mm length of distal colon (0.5 mm to 1 cm proximal to the anus), where adenoma often develops, was examined by complete serial sectioning. More than 10,000 of these thin sections were stained and examined.

A. Sequential Observation

By week 4, hyperplastic glands were detected and these were usually observed in a scattered distribution until the end of the experiment. Microscopic adenomas, consisting of several atypical glands, were observed in the colons of animals sacrificed in week 10. Microscopic adenomas were always observed in the animals sacrificed after week 14. The number and the size of adenomas increased with longer periods of treatment (Table 4).

B. Morphogenesis Determined By Complete Serial Sectioning

Microadenomas that consisted of several atypical glands were easily found (Figure 10). This type of adenoma occupied the upper part of the colonic mucosa, and was slightly elevated from the surrounding normal mucosa. Smaller adenomas were the same height as the surrounding mucosa (Figure 11). In these adenomas the opening of the atypical gland was singular, as indicated by the arrow. Much smaller adenomas consisted of a single atypical gland (Figure 12). This single atypical gland was located in the upper half to upper two thirds of the mucosa and pushed aside the neighboring normal glands, thus showing endophytic growth. Adenomatous epithelia consisted of

Table 4
SEQUENTIAL OBSERVATION OF LARGE
INTESTINE OF ICR MICE TREATED WITH DMH

Time at sacrifice (weeks)	No. of animals	No. of animals with adenoma	No. of adenomas[a]
2	3	0	0
4	3	0	0
6	3	0	0
8	3	0	0
10	3	1	1
12	2	1	1
14	2	2	6
16	2	2	8
18	2	2	3
20	2	2	6

[a] Histological examination performed every 5 mm of the whole large intestine.

absorptive-type cells and a few goblet cells. This single atypical gland lesion was the smallest identifiable adenoma, and was designated as *single-gland adenoma*.[39]

Smaller single-gland adenomas located in the superficial part of the mucosa grew downward between adjacent normal glands, pushing them aside (Figure 13). This adenoma was the smallest one detected in the present study.

Complete serial sections also revealed the mode of development from single-gland adenomas to microscopic adenomas consisting of several atypical glands. One or more epithelial clusters appeared in the upper part of single-gland adenomas. These clusters then developed into small glands with narrow lumens, and branched out from the original single-gland adenoma, growing downward along the adenoma and pushing aside the adjacent normal crypts (Figure 14). These daughter glands shared their opening with the mother gland, so these microscopic adenomas initially had one opening. At the peripheral aspect of large adenomas, adenomatous epithelia often replaced the normal epithelia; this "branching" appeared to be the main way in which single-gland adenomas developed into microscopic adenomas, which consist of a central main gland surrounded by newly formed small glands. The initial mode of development of colonic adenomas induced by DMH is shown schematically in Figure 15.

C. Discussion

Complete serial sectioning allows the observation of the whole lesion from its beginning to its disappearance. Serial sectioning is especially important when the morphogenesis of adenomas is studied; minute lesions frequently cause interpretative problems because if the entire architecture of the adenomas is not assessed there is the possibility that the minute lesions represent only the peripheral part of a large adenoma.[39] It has already been reported that minute adenomas induced with DMH were observed in the upper part of the mucosa in the colons of rats and mice.[17,21-24] However, details of the early morphogenesis are not fully understood. The present complete serial sectioning reveals for the first time that adenomas originate from single-gland adenomas which are located in the upper part of the mucosa, through endophytic growth.

There are two opinions on the origin of human colonic adenomas. One is that adenomas originate from the deep part of glands[9,10] and the other opinion, based on cell kinetics studies using tritiated thymidine and measurements of mitotic indexes, is that adenomas develop in the upper part of the glands.[11-13] From cell kinetics studies of

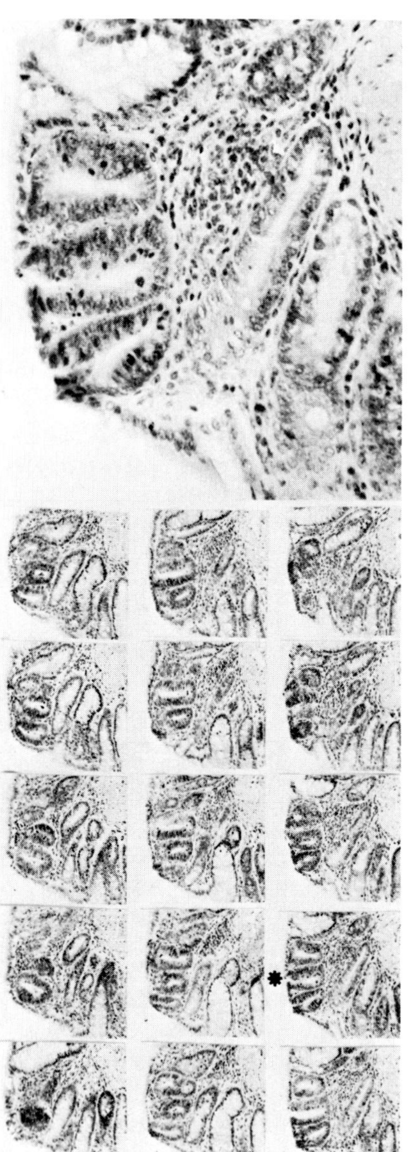

FIGURE 10.   A minute adenoma consisting of several atypical glands and occupying the upper part of the colonic mucosa. Right, higher magnification of one (*) of the sections. (H.E.; magnification × 95.)

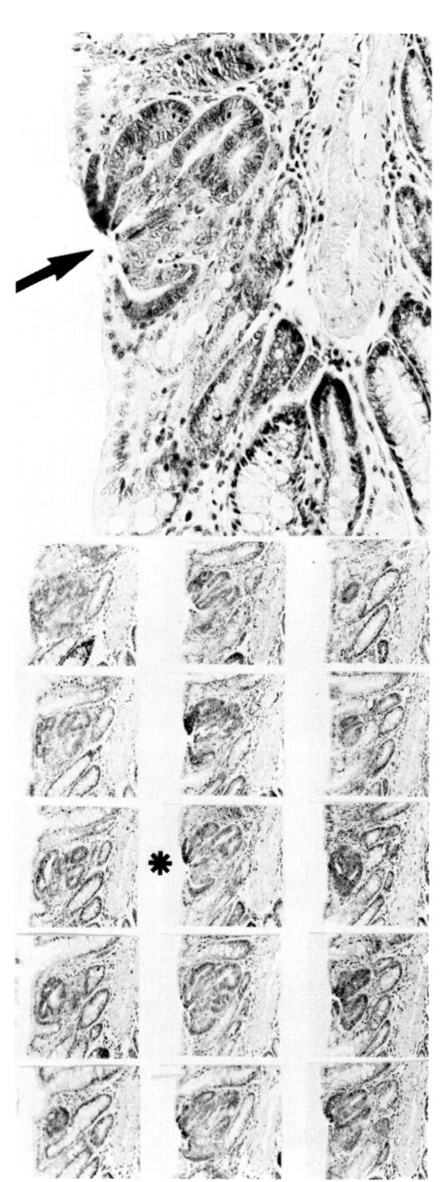

FIGURE 11.   Fifteen serial sections of a microscopic adenoma with a single crypt opening (left). (Right) Higher magnification of one (*) of the sections. The arrow shows the single crypt opening. (H.E.; magnification × 100.)

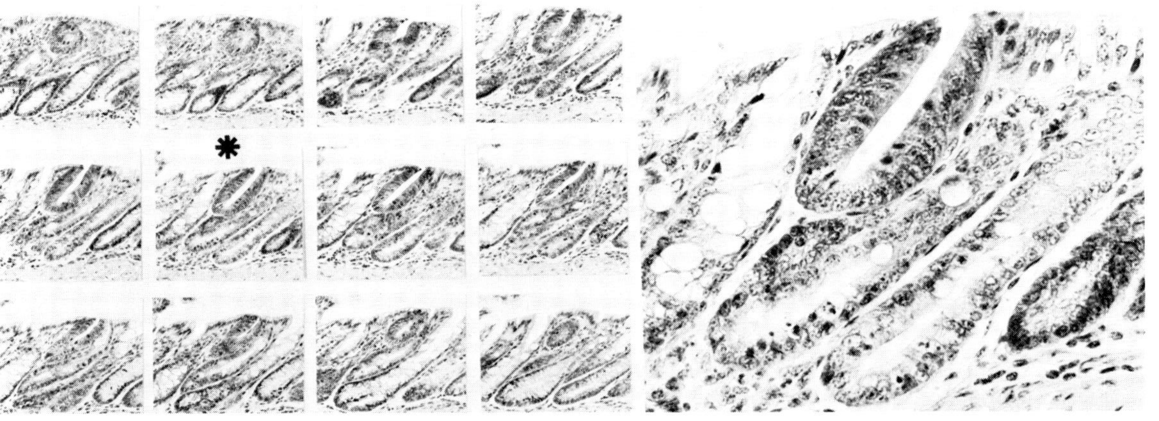

FIGURE 12. A single gland adenoma is located in the upper half of the mucosa with endophytic growth. (Right) Higher magnification of one (*) of the sections. (H.E.; magnification × 150.)

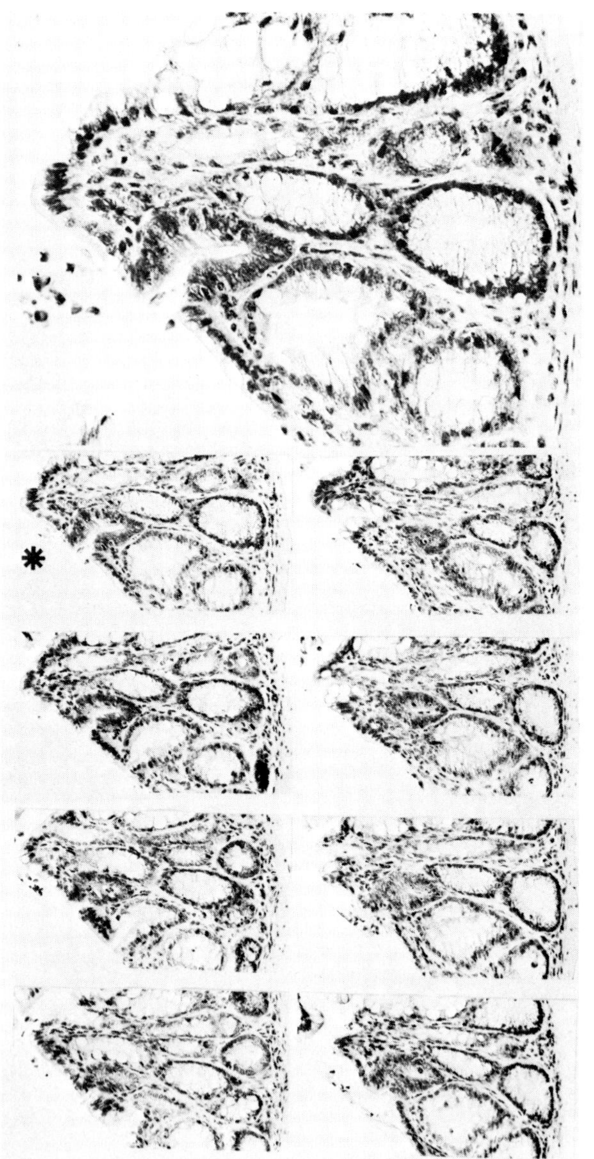

FIGURE 13. The smallest single-gland adenoma. The photograph on the right is a higher magnification of one (*) of the eight photographs on the left. (H.E.; magnification × 200.)

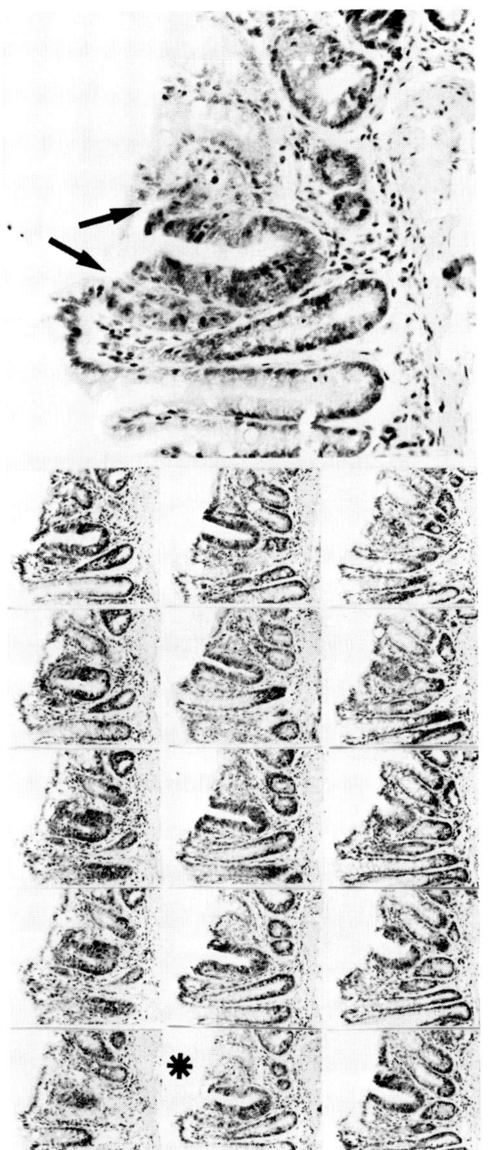

FIGURE 14. The photograph on the right shows an adenoma with a single gland with two little branches (arrows). (H.E.; magnification × 150.)

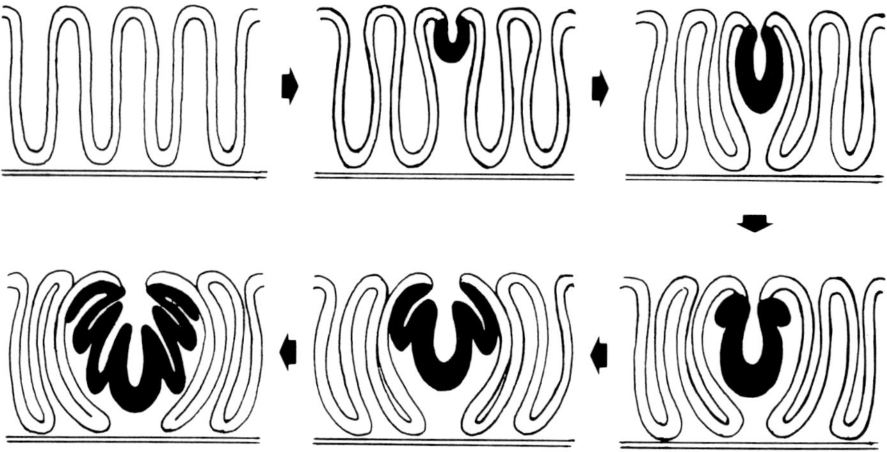

FIGURE 15.   Diagram of initial development of a colonic adenoma in an ICR mouse induced by DMH.

experimental animals, the expansion of the proliferative zone of colonic glands has been reported.[17,22-24,40-42]

The surface epithelium of the normal colonic mucosa of humans and mice has been shown to consist of many absorptive cells and a few goblet cells.[43,44] No immature cells with mitotic activity have been found in the surface epithelium. If a single-gland adenoma appears first from the superficial portion of the mucosa, there must be some proliferative cells in the upper part of the mucosa before the adenoma appears. If the background mucosa were investigated in detail, some precursor lesions of the adenoma may be detected. However, even though using complete serial sectioning, atypical cells or mitotic figures were not found in the upper part of the normal background mucosa of the colons of mice. Thus, we studied the cell kinetics of the mucosa of mice using tritiated thymidine (³H-TdR).

IV. CELL KINETICS OF COLONIC MUCOSA IN MICE TREATED WITH DMH

It had already been reported that different cell kinetics were observed in the background mucosa of the normal large intestine vs. that which has tumors.[13,42,45,46] In the present animal models with DMH-treated mice, we investigated the cell kinetics of background mucosa before and after development of an adenoma.

A. Sequential Observation of Cell Kinetics

The mice used were 14 weeks old, weighed 30 to 40 g, and were injected subcutaneously with 20 mg/kg DMH once a week for up to 20 weeks. Ten control animals were injected with phosphate-buffered saline (PBS). Two or three DMH-treated mice and one control animal were sacrificed successively every 2 weeks between week 2 and 20. Animals were given ³H-TdR (New England Nuclear, specific activity, 20 μCi/mmol) by intraperitoneal injection at a dosage of 0.5 μCi/g body weight. One hour after the injection the animals were sacrificed and their colons were fixed in PBS formalin. After fixation, the colon was cut into 5-mm-long sections which were embedded in paraffin and sectioned at 3 μm. Deparaffinized sections were dipped in Sakura NR-M2 emulsion (Konishiroku Photo Ind. Co.), stored at 4° for 6 weeks in a dark box, and stained with H.E. after development. Segments of 0.5 to 2 cm from the anus were examined mainly

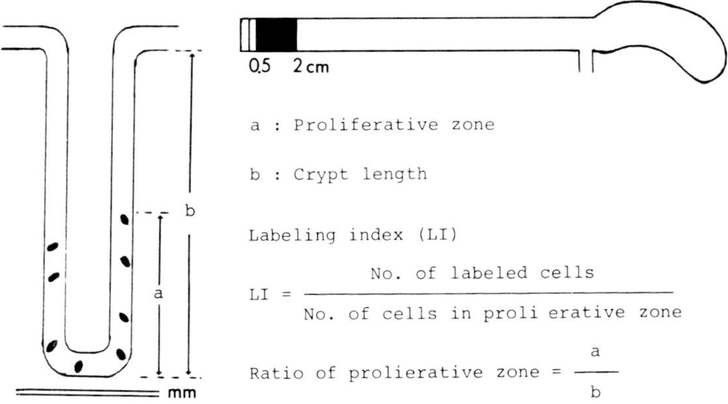

FIGURE 16. The method of observation on cell kinetics of the distal colonic mucosa (black area) in ICR mice treated with DMH.

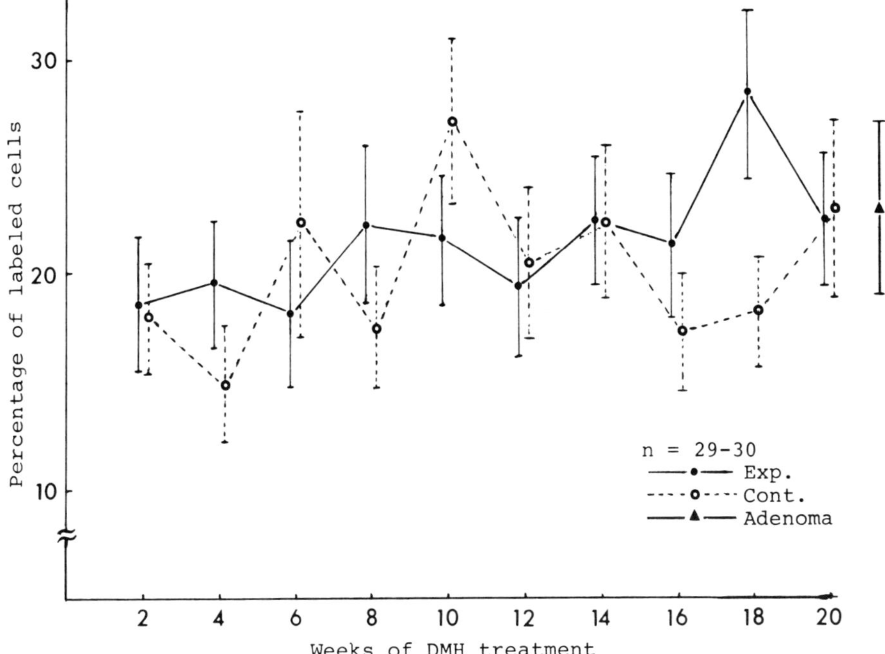

FIGURE 17. Labeling index of each group in each week. No significant difference was found in either experimental or control groups and labeling index of the adenoma was about 20%.

in the kinetics study because these segments of the distal colon were the most frequent sites of adenomas. Figure 16 shows the method of observation of cellular kinetics of the distal colonic mucosa. One side of the longitudinally sectioned crypts (crypt column) was analyzed. The proliferative zone (a) was tentatively defined to be between the uppermost-labeled cell and the base of the crypt. The length of the crypt column (b) was also recorded. The ratio of densely labeled cells to the total number of cells in the proliferative zone was expressed as the labeling index (LI). The ratio of the proliferative zone to the length of the crypt (a/b) was also calculated and was expressed as the proliferative zone rate.

Labeling index — Labeling indexes were about 20% in both the experimental and control groups, and there were no significant differences during each week (Figure 17). The labeling index of the adenomas observed in week 20 was also about 20%.

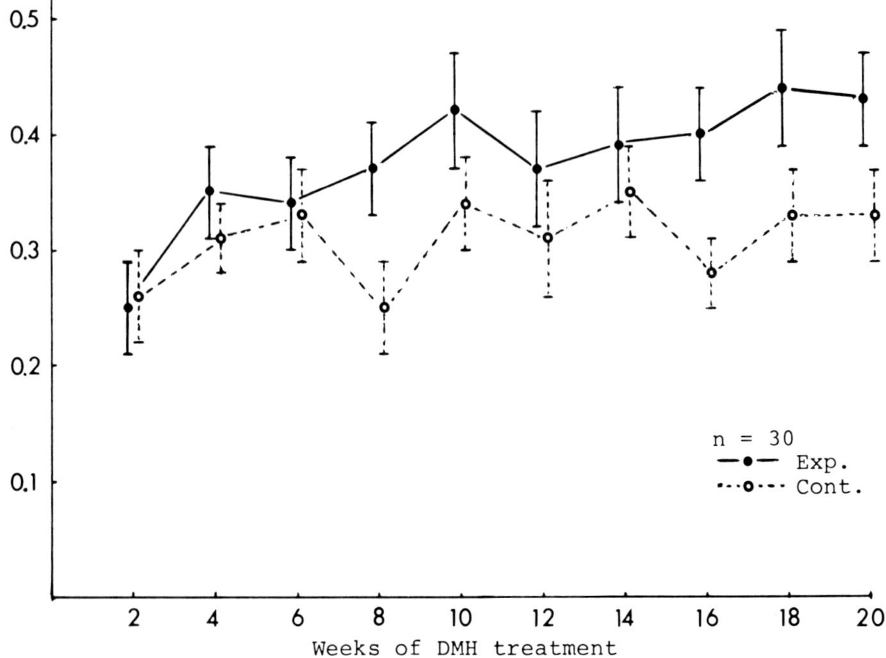

FIGURE 18.   The proliferative zone rates. After the week 16, the experimental group had a higher rate than the control group. However, the rate did not reach one half.

The proliferative zone rate — The rates for the experimental group were from 0.2 to 0.4, which were also observed for the control group, but after week 16 the experimental group had a higher rate than the control group. However, the rate did not increase even to one half (Figure 18).

Labeling index for segments along the crypt column — For study of the distribution of proliferating cells in the crypt, crypt columns were divided into ten equal segments and the labeling index was analyzed for each segment. Experimental and control animals killed in weeks 4, 12, and 18 were examined. A slight increase in the labeling index of the upper segments was observed in the animals killed in week 18, but no obvious cells or shift of main labeled segments from the lower region of the column to the upper part were found in the experimental animals (Figure 19). There was no significant difference between the control animals killed in weeks 4, 12, and 18 (Figure 20).

B. Cell Cycle Time of Colonic Epithelium in Mice By the Cumulative Labeling Method

The cell cycle time of the epithelium in the colons of experimental and control mice was investigated by the cumulative labeling method. We used 10 mice treated 20 times with DMH. They were given ^{3}H-TdR six times by intraperitoneal injection at a dosage of 0.5 μCi/g body weight every 5 hr for up to 25 hr. Two experimental animals and two control mice were sacrificed successively every 7 hr between the 1st and 28th hr, and labeling indexes were calculated (Figure 21). Each labeling index of 1, 7, 14, 21, and 28 hr, as shown in Figure 21, is aligned in a straight line. From this it is known that the S-phase (DNA synthetic phase) of both treated and control animals was 10 hr, and one cell cycle of the treated animals was 48 hr and of control mice was 54 hr. However, there was no significant difference between the two straight lines, nor significant difference in S-phase or cell cycle time between the DMH-treated and control animals.

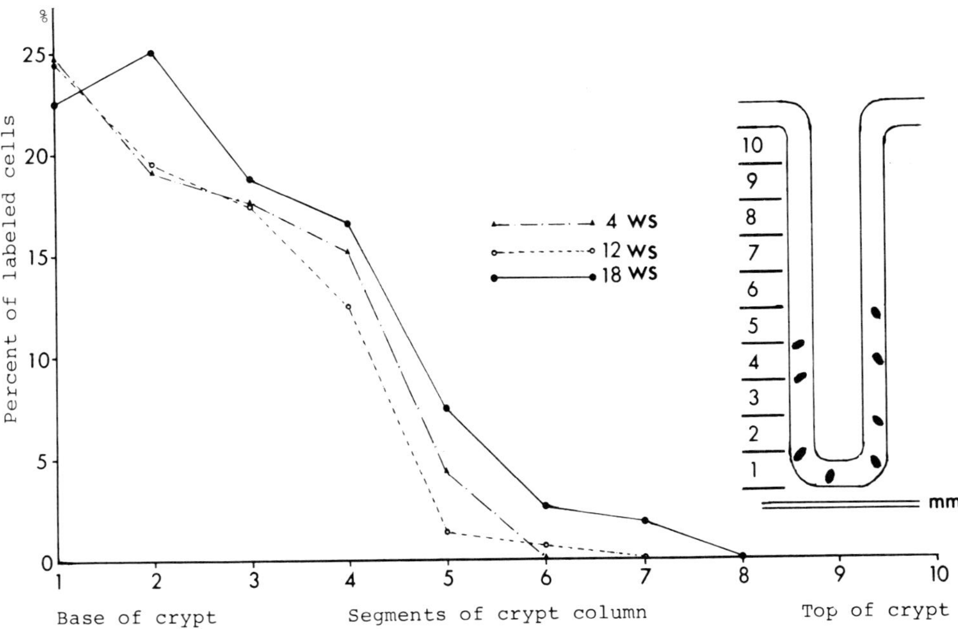

FIGURE 19.   Labeling index of each segment along the crypt column in the experimental animals. A slight increase in the labeling index of the upper segments was observed with an increase in DMH treatment. There was, however, no expansion or shift of the proliferative zone.

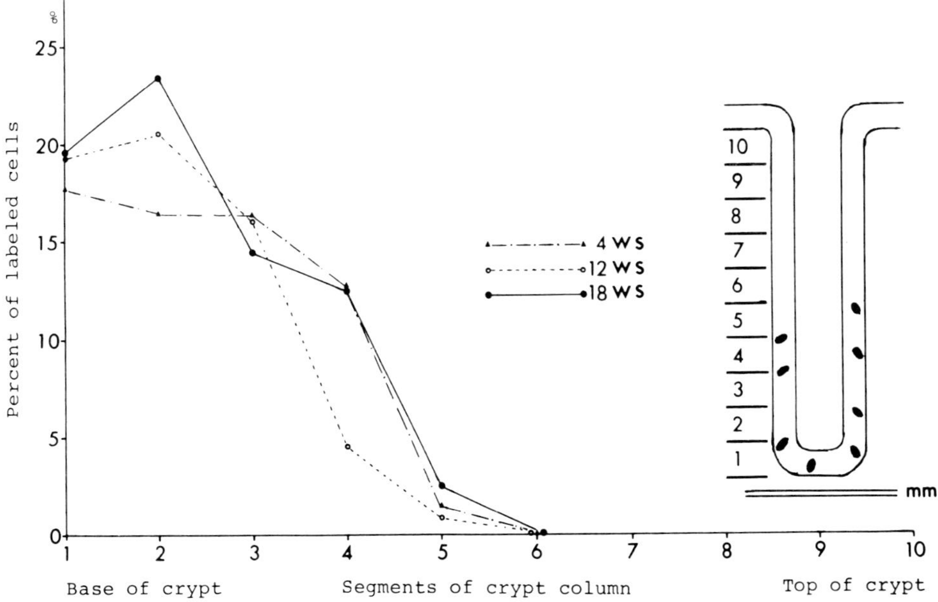

FIGURE 20.   Labeling index of each segment along the crypt column of the control animals. There was no difference between animals killed in weeks 4, 12, and 18.

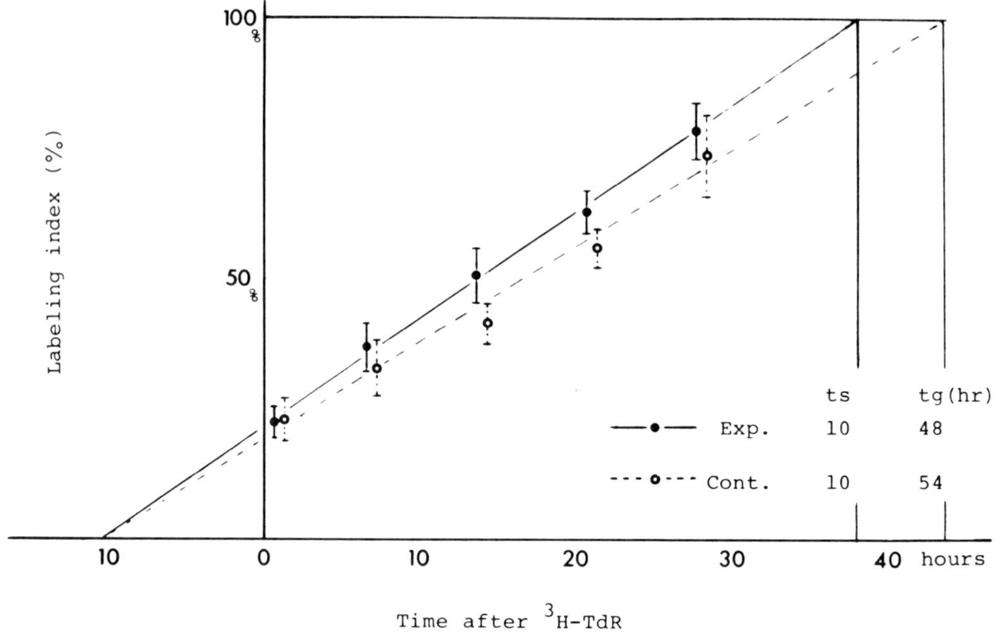

FIGURE 21.   The cell cycle time of the colonic epithelium of the mice by the cumulative labeling method. There were no significant differences between the two straight lines, one of which shows the experimental group and the other shows the control. It was calculated that the S-phase was 10 hr and one cell cycle was about 50 hr in each group.

C. Turnover Time of Colonic Epithelial Cells in Mice

The turnover time of the epithelial cells in the colons of DMH-treated and control mice was investigated. Eight experimental and four control animals were used in this experiment. After 16 DMH treatments, animals were injected with ³H-TdR intraperitoneally for flash labeling. The mice were sacrificed on days 8, 10, 15, and 20 after injection of ³H-TdR, and the turnover of labeled cells was observed. Labeled cells were observed both in experimental mice and control animals in the upper part of the mucosa on day 8, and also in superficial epithelium on day 10, but were rarely observed on day 15 (Figure 22). From this, the turnover time of colonic epithelial cells of mice was estimated to be about 10 days in both experimental and control groups.

D. Autoradiographs of Single Gland Adenoma

Mice with 20 DMH treatments were used in this experiment. Single-gland adenomas detected by complete serial sectioning were evaluated by microautoradiography. Figure 23 shows the autoradiograph of a single-gland adenoma in which labeled cells were diffusely distributed, while labeled cells were confined to the lower part of the surrounding normal glands.

E. Discussion

In our studies of cell kinetics, the proliferative zone rate (ratio of the proliferative zone to the length of the crypt column) was only slightly higher in DMH-treated mice than in control mice after week 16. The labeling index of each segment of the crypt column also showed no expansion or shift of the proliferation zone. Further, there were no differences in labeling indexes, cell cycle times, or turnover times of colonic epithelia between the experimental animals and control mice.

A shift or expansion of the proliferation zone from the base of the crypt toward the

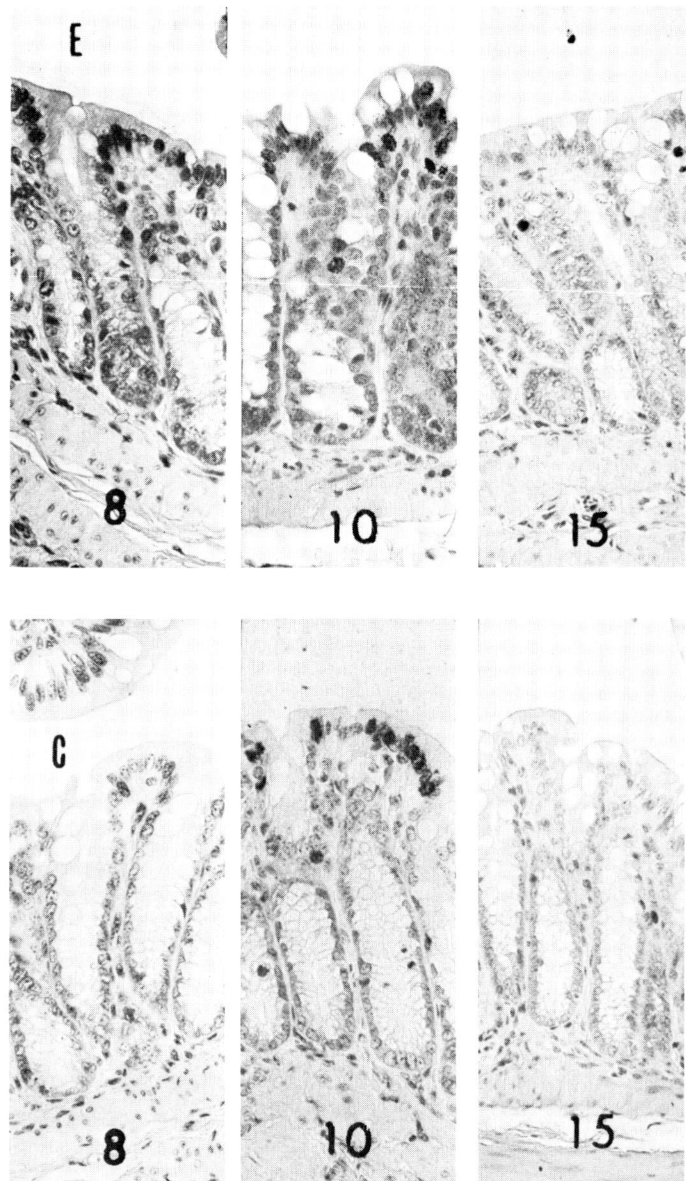

FIGURE 22. Autoradiographs of the mucosa of the colon of both experimental and control mice. Labeled cells were observed in both groups on day 8 and 10, but were rarely observed on day 15.

surface without any frank lesions has been described in colonic mucosa in patients with familial adenomatosis coli.[46,47] These findings were confirmed in the colonic mucosa of experimental animals treated with DMH.[17,22-24,40-42] A shift or expansion of the proliferation zone would logically explain why adenomas first appear in the upper part of the mucosa. As shown in the present studies, however, there was no expansion or shift of proliferation zone of the crypts during the process of development of adenomas in the mouse colon in animals treated with DMH. The effects of irradiation on changes in crypts of mouse colon during treatment with DMH were also studied by Richards and Tacha.[48] Although irradiated DMH groups had a markedly expanded

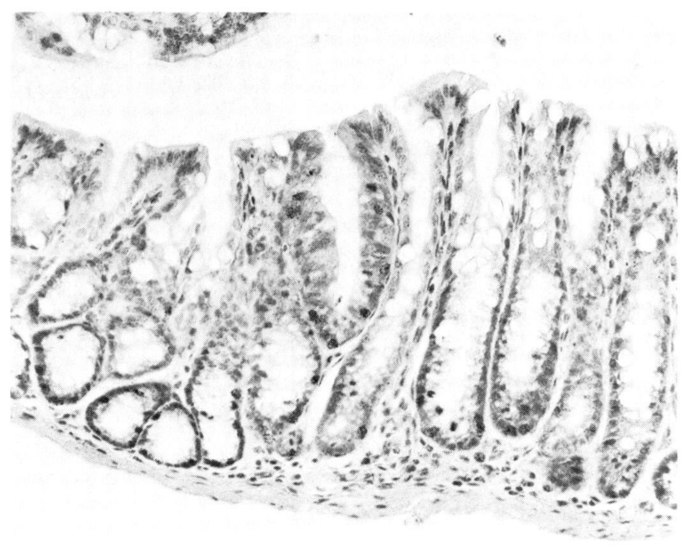

FIGURE 23.   The autoradiograph of a single-gland adenoma. Labeled nuclei were confined to the lower two third thirds of the mucosa, while they were diffusely scattered in a single-gland adenoma. (H.E.; magnification × 150.)

proliferation zone, the group treated with DMH only showed almost the same distribution of labeled cells as the control group. Five cases of surgically resected colon (one case of familial adenomatosis coli and four cases of ordinary colonic carcinoma) were treated by ex vivo autoradiography in cell kinetics studies. Results showed no significant difference between the labeled figures in normal colonic mucosa of cases of familial adenomatosis or in ordinary colonic cancer. Also, no significant expansion or shift of the proliferation zone of the crypts in the case of adenomatosis coli was observed.[49]

Detailed observation of the cell kinetics of normal epithelial cells in the colon of the mouse has been previously reported.[43,50] The replacement time of the colonic epithelial cell was about 10 days,[50] similar to our observation.

It has been presumed that if there were no derangement in the proliferation zone, an adenoma would not develop because of the rapid turnover time of epithelial cells within 10 days. Even if neoplastic cells appeared in the proliferation zone of the lower part of the crypt, they would soon migrate out of the crypt to the surface epithelium and desquamate before they proliferated and stabilized as neoplastic tissue. The rapid turnover time of epithelial cells in the small intestine has been suggested as a partial explanation why epithelial neoplasms are rare in the small intestine.[51]

It is of interest, however, that in a study of the morphogenesis of chemically induced duodenal adenocarcinomas in rodents by Matsuyama et al.,[52] the earliest carcinoma was found in an atypical gland located in the intravillous stroma. It was hypothesized that this lesion escaped the rapid turnover of epithelial cells of the duodenal mucosa, and subsequently developed into a macroscopic adenocarcinoma. If a similar change were to occur in the development of adenoma of the colon, derangement of the proliferative zone would not be required for adenoma development.

Chang[53] studied carcinogenesis in mice treated with DMH and reported that colonic neoplasms originated at the crypt base, or occurred as an outpocketing pouch in the proliferative zone of the crypt. It is interesting that this outpocketing pouch found in mice treated with DMH was similar to the adenoma bud which the present authors previously observed in the development of adenoma of the colon in patients with familial adenomatosis coli.[54] The pouch or bud could easily succeed in developing to an adenoma without extrusion with migrating normal, colonic epithelial cells.

V. SUMMARY

When the morphogenesis of colonic adenoma is investigated, there is an important interpretative problem as to whether a very small lesion, such as a single gland adenoma, might be regarded as an antecedent lesion of adenoma. If any ulcers or erosions were observed in the colon of the mice treated with DMH, the regenerative processes must be considered and this would complicate the study of early morphogenesis of adenomas. Fortunately, however, ulcers or erosions were not observed in the background mucosa of the colon of mice treated with DMH in our experiments.

Evaluation of the antecedent lesion is also difficult when adenomas and cancers are induced by DMH in the colon of rats and hamsters. Almost all DMH-induced colon tumors of mice are adenomas. Therefore, this mouse tumor model may be equivalent to the familial adenomatosis coli of man.

One problem is the acute cytotoxic effect of DMH, with resultant reparative hyperplasia.[55-57] In the present study mucosal hyperplasia was first observed in the colon of mice killed in week 4. This mucosal hyperplasia with mild atypia adds to the difficulty in investigating very small lesions. Lesions smaller than single-gland adenomas were still obscure in the present study, even after complete serial sectioning.

Richards[57] studied whether the hyperplasia of the colonic mucosa of mice, as induced by DMH, was reversible or not. The relationship between number of DMH treatments and periods of recovery after termination of treatment was analyzed, and it was revealed that reduction of mucosal hyperplasia occurred 9 weeks after termination of less than 12 treatments.[57] It might be desirable, after termination of several treatments with DMH, to allow for a period of recovery in which the acute hyperplastic effect of DMH is reduced, prior to observation of the morphogenesis of the adenomas. We plan to investigate the morphogenesis of adenomas in this modified model with mice.

It has been revealed that branching seems to be the main way in which single-gland adenomas develop into microscopic adenomas. This consists of a central mother gland surrounded by newly formed daughter glands.

There was no significant difference in cell kinetics in the background mucosa between the experimental animals and controls before or after development of adenomas. It may be considered that a derangement in cell kinetics, such as a shift or expansion of the proliferation zone did not influence the development of adenoma, but that other mechanisms were operative.

Lesions smaller than single-gland adenomas were detected in the investigation on the early morphogenesis of colonic adenomas of patients with familial adenomatosis. These smaller lesions (buds of single-gland adenomas) originated in the proliferation zone of the normal crypts.[54] Chang[53] also found the evaginating pouch in the proliferation zone of the crypt in the colon of the mice treated with DMH. It will be important to probe the bud of the adenoma by complete serial sectioning in this mouse tumor model.

REFERENCES

1. Lane, N., The precursor tissue of ordinary large bowel cancer, *Cancer Res.*, 36, 2669, 1976.
2. Muto, T., Bussey, H. J. R., and Morson, B. C., The evolution of cancer of the colon and rectum, *Cancer*, 36, 2251, 1975.
3. Morson, B. C. and Dawson, I. M. P., Adenomas and the adenoma-carcinoma sequence, in *Gastrointestinal Pathology*, 2nd ed., Morson, B. C. and Dawson, I. M. P., Eds., Blackwell Scientific, Oxford, 1979, chap. 38.
4. Rickert, R. R., Auerbach, O., Garfinkel, L., Hammond, E. C., and Frasca, J. M., Adenomatous lesions of the large bowel. An autopsy survey, *Cancer*, 43, 1847, 1979.
5. Castleman, B. and Krickstein, H., Do adenomatous polyps of the colon become malignant? *N. Engl. J. Med.*, 267, 469, 1962.
6. Kino, I. and Nakamura, S., Pathological characteristics of colonic early cancers — from the viewpoint of histogenesis (in Japanese), *Stomach Intestine*, 15, 357, 1980.
7. Spratt, J. S., Jr. and Ackerman, L. V., Small primary adenocarcinomas of the colon and rectum, *JAMA*, 179, 337, 1962.
8. Bussey, H. J. R., Polyposis syndromes, in *The Pathogenesis of Colorectal Cancer*, Morson, B. C., Ed., W.B. Saunders, Philadelphia, 1978, chap. 8.
9. Dukes, C. E., An explanation of the difference between a papilloma and an adenoma of the rectum, *Proc. R. Soc. Med.*, 11, 829, 1947.
10. Lane, N. and Lev, R., Observations on the origin of adenomatous epithelium of the colon. Serial section studies of minute polyps in familial polyposis, *Cancer*, 16, 751, 1963.
11. Cole, J. W. and McKalen, A., Studies on the morphogenesis of adenomatous polyps in the human colon, *Cancer*, 16, 998, 1963.
12. Wiebecke, B., Brandts, A., and Eder, M., Epithelial proliferation and morphogenesis of hyperplastic adenomatous and villous polyps of the human colon, *Virchows Arch. A. Pathol. Anat. Histol.*, 364, 35, 1974.
13. Lipkin, M., Phase 1 and phase 2 proliferative lesions of colonic epithelial cells in diseases leading to colonic cancer, *Cancer*, 34, 878, 1974.
14. Maskens, A. P., Histogenesis of adenomatous polyps in the human large intestine, *Gastroenterology*, 77, 1245, 1979.
15. Hashimoto, D., Observations on the origin of adenomatous epithelium of the colon — three-dimensional analysis of the unicryptal adenoma in familial polyposis (in Japanese), *J. Jpn. Surg. Soc.*, 83, 308, 1982.
16. Druckrey, H., Production of colonic carcinomas by 1,2-dialkylhydrazines and azoxyalkanes, in *Carcinoma of the Colon and Antecedent Epithelium*, Burdette, W. J., Ed., Charles C Thomas, Springfield, Ill., 1970, 267.
17. Pozharisski, K. M., Morphology and morphogenesis of experimental epithelial tumors of the intestine, *J. Natl. Cancer Inst.*, 54, 1115, 1975.
18. Pozharisski, K. M., Kapustin, Y. M., Likhachev, A. J., and Shaposhnikov, J. D., The mechanism of carcinogenic action of 1,2-dimethylhydrazine (SDMH) in rats, *Int. J. Cancer*, 15, 673, 1975.
19. Fisher, E. R. and Paulson, J. D., Genesis of 1,2-dimethylhydrazine-induced colon cancer. A light and electron microscopic study, *Arch. Pathol. Lab. Med.*, 105, 29, 1981.
20. Wiebecke, B., Lohrs, U., Gimmy, J., and Eder, M., Production of tumors in the intestines of mice by 1,2-dimethylhydrazine, *Z. Ges. Exp. Med.*, 149, 277, 1969.
21. Haase, P., Cowen, D. M., Knowles, J. C., and Cooper, E. H., Evaluation of dimethylhydrazine induced tumors in mice as a model system for colorectal cancer, *Br. J. Cancer*, 28, 530, 1973.
22. Thurnherr, N., Deschner, E. E., Stonehill, E. H., and Lipkin, M., Induction of adenocarcinomas of the colon in mice by weekly injections of 1,2-dimethylhydrazine, *Cancer Res.*, 33, 940, 1973.
23. Deschner, E. E., Experimentally induced cancer of the colon, *Cancer*, 34, 824, 1974.
24. Chang, W. W. L., Histogenesis of symmetrical 1,2-dimethylhydrazine-induced neoplasms of the colon in the mouse, *J. Natl. Cancer Inst.*, 60, 1405, 1978.
25. Osswald, H. and Krüger, F. W., Die cancerogene Wirkung von 1,2-Dimethylhydrazine beim Goldhamster, *Arzneim. Forsch.*, 19, 1891, 1969.
26. Toth, B., Tumorigenesis studies with 1,2-dimethylhydrazine dihydrochloride, hydrazine sulfate, and isonicotinic acid in golden hamsters, *Cancer Res.*, 32, 804, 1972.
27. Winneker, R. C., Tompkins, M., Westenberger, P., and Harris, J., Morphological studies of chemically induced colon tumors in hamsters, *Exp. Mol. Pathol.*, 27, 19, 1977.
28. Fiala, E. S., Investigations into the metabolism and mode of action of the colon carcinogen 1,2-dimethylhydrazine, *Cancer*, 36, 2407, 1975.
29. Fiala, E. S., Kulakis, C., Bobotas, G., and Weisburger, J. H., Detection and estimation of azomethane in expired air of 1,2-dimethylhydrazine-treated rats, *J. Natl. Cancer Inst.*, 56, 1271, 1976.

30. Zedeck, M. S., Grab, D. J., and Sternberg, S. S., Differences in the acute response of the various segments of rat intestine to treatment with the intestinal carcinogen, methylazoxymethanol acetate, *Cancer Res.*, 37, 32, 1977.
31. LaMont, J. T. and O'Gorman, T. A., Experimental colon cancer, *Gastroenterology*, 75, 1157, 1978.
32. Evans, J. T., Shows, T. B., Sproul, E. E., Paolini, N. S., Mittelman, A., and Hauschka, T. S., Genetics of colon carcinogenesis in mice treated with 1,2-dimethylhydrazine, *Cancer Res.*, 37, 134, 1977.
33. Diwan, B. A., Meier, H., and Blackman, K. E., Genetic differences in the induction of colorectal tumors by 1,2-dimethylhydrazine in inbred mice, *J. Natl. Cancer Inst.*, 59, 455, 1977.
34. Pollard M. and Zedeck, M. S., Induction of colon tumors in 1,2-dimethylhydrazine-resistant Lobund Wistar rats by methylazoxymethanol acetate, *J. Natl. Cancer Inst.*, 61, 493, 1978.
35. Martin, B. F., The goblet cell pattern in the large intestine, *Anat. Rec.*, 140, 1, 1961.
36. Sunter, J. P., Wright, N. A., and Appleton, D. R., Cell population kinetics in the epithelium of the colon of the male rat, *Virchows Arch. B.*, 26, 275, 1978.
37. Sunter, J. P., Watson, A. J., Wright, N. A., and Appleton, D. R., Cell proliferation at different sites along the length of the rat colon, *Virchows Arch. B.*, 32, 75, 1979.
38. Sunter, J. P., Appleton, D. R., De Rodriguez, M. S. B., Wright, N. A., and Watson, A. J., A comparison of cell proliferation at different sites within the large bowel of the mouse, *J. Anat.*, 129, 833, 1979.
39. Nakamura, S. and Kino, I., Morphogenesis of colonic adenomas in mice treated with N,N'-dimethylhydrazine dihydrochloride, *Acta Pathol. Jpn.*, 32, 473, 1982.
40. Barthold, S. W., Autoradiographic cytokinetics of colonic mucosal hyperplasia in mice, *Cancer Res.*, 39, 24, 1979.
41. Barthold, S. W., Relationship of colonic mucosal background to neoplastic proliferative activity in dimethylhydrazine-treated mice, *Cancer Res.*, 41, 2616, 1981.
42. Deschner, E. E. and Maskens, A. P., Significance of the labeling index and labeling distribution as kinetic parameters in colorectal mucosa of cancer patients and DMH treated animals, *Cancer*, 50, 1136, 1982.
43. Chang, W. W. L. and Leblond, C. P., Renewal of the various types of epithelial cells in the descending colon in the mouse, in *Carcinoma of the Colon and Antecedent Epithelium*, Burdette, W. J., Ed., Charles C Thomas, Springfield, Ill., 1970, 197.
44. Kaye, G. I., Fenoglio, C. M., Pascal, R. R., and Lane, N., Comparative electron microscopic features of normal, hyperplastic, and adenomatous human colonic epithelium. Variations in cellular structure relative to the process of epithelial differentiation, *Gastroenterology*, 64, 926, 1973.
45. Maskens, A. P. and Deschner, E. E., Tritiated thymidine incorporation into epithelial cells of normal-appearing colorectal mucosa of cancer patients, *J. Natl. Cancer Inst.*, 58, 1221, 1977.
46. Frommer, D., Logue, T., and Moore, F., Mitosis in rectal epithelial surface cells in controls and in patients with colorectal tumors, in *Colonic Carcinogenesis*, Malt, R. A. and Williamson, R. C. N., Eds., MTP Press, Lancaster, England, 1981, 145.
47. Iwama, T., Utzunomiya, J., and Sasaki, J., Epithelial cell kinetics in the crypts of familial polyposis of the colon, *Jpn. J. Surg.*, 7, 230, 1977.
48. Richards, T. C. and Tacha, D. E., Effects of sublethal irradiation on changes in crypts of the mouse colon during treatment with 1,2-dimethylhydrazine, *J. Natl. Cancer Inst.*, 69, 693, 1982.
49. Nakamura, S., Kino, I., and Baba, S., *Ex vivo* autoradiography of the human gastrointestinal tract: a new approach to cell kinetic studies of surgically removed tumor-bearing organs, *Gann*, 74, 116, 1983.
50. Tsubouchi, S., Kinetic analysis of epithelial cell migration in the mouse descending colon, *Am. J. Anat.*, 161, 239, 1981.
51. Rijke, R. P. C., Some speculations on control mechanisms of cell proliferation in intestinal epithelium, in *Cell Proliferation in the Gastrointestinal Tract*, Appleton, D. R., Sunter, J. P., and Watson, A. J., Eds., Pitman Medical, Kent, England, 1980, 57.
52. Matsuyama, M., Nakamura, T., Suzuki, H., and Nagayo, T., Morphogenesis of duodenal adenocarcinomas induced by *N*-ethyl-*N*-nitro-*N*-nitroso-guanidine in mice and rats, *Gann Monogr. Cancer Res.*, 17, 269, 1975.
53. Chang, W. W. L., Morphological basis of multistep process in experimental colonic carcinogenesis, *Virchows Arch. B.*, 41, 17, 1982.
54. Nakamura, S. and Kino, I., Morphogenesis of minute adenomas in familial polyposis coli, *J. Natl. Cancer Inst.*, 93, 41, 1984.
55. Barthold, S. W. and Jonas, A. M., Morphogenesis of early 1,2-dimethylhydrazine-induced lesions and latent period reduction of colonic carcinogenesis in mice by a variant of *Citrobacter freundii*, *Cancer Res.*, 37, 4352, 1977.

56. Barthold, S. W. and Beck, D., Modification or early dimethylhydrazine carcinogenesis by colonic mucosal hyperplasia, *Cancer Res.*, 40, 4451, 1980.
57. Richards, T. C., Changes in crypt cell populations of mouse colon during recovery from treatment with 1,2-dimethylhydrazine, *J. Natl. Cancer Inst.*, 66, 907, 1981.

Chapter 9

ANTIBIOTIC-INDUCED ENTEROCOLITIS IN ANIMALS

Gary D. Rifkin and F. Robert Fekety, Jr.

TABLE OF CONTENTS

I. INTRODUCTION

Pseudomembranous colitis, first described in association with abdominal surgery by Finney in 1893[1] and recently recognized as a complication of antibiotic usage,[2,3] is the result of toxin production in the large bowel by *Clostridium difficile*.[4] While the disease has been noted as an infrequent complication of surgery, bowel obstruction, vascular insufficiency, uremia, and the use of various antibiotics, its etiology remains unclear.[6] Theories proposed include changes in intestinal microbial flora, direct toxic effects of antibiotics or their metabolites on intestinal mucosa, hypersensitivity reactions, and production of toxic substances by intestinal flora.[7] An increase in the number of cases following the use of the lincosamides in the early 1970s prompted studies of the pathogenesis of pseudomembranous colitis and a search for an animal model. Adverse effects of antibiotics on the gastrointestinal tract of rodents were well recognized. Guinea pigs given penicillin, chlortetracycline, bacitracin, or erythromycin developed lethal diarrhea and pathologic findings of acute hemorrhagic colitis.[8,9] Similar findings were noted with subcutaneous injection and oral administration of lincomycin to hamsters.[10] With renewed interest in antimicrobial-induced enterocolitis (AIC) in the 1970s, investigations began using the hamster as a model of colitis.

There were early reservations regarding the applicability of the hamster as a model for AIC.[11] In contrast to the disease in humans, AIC in hamsters involves the ileocecal rather than the distal colonic area, pseudomembranes are not as well developed, and lethality is quite common.[12] However, reliable induction of colitis with antimicrobials known to produce human pseudomembranous colitis, compatibility of the histological lesions with those in man, and the availability and ease in working with the animal fit well with criteria for a good research animal[13] and encouraged the development of the hamster model.

Although other animals are susceptible to AIC, investigations by several groups using the hamster have (1) characterized the model,[12,14] (2) documented pathologic changes,[15-17] (3) compared effects of various antibiotics,[4,18] (4) performed bacteriologic studies of fecal and cecal flora,[19,20] (5) documented and characterized the presence of fecal toxins,[7,21-27] (6) outlined therapeutic and preventive measures,[4,28-31] and (7) provided insight into the epidemiology of the disease.[32,33]

This work has established toxin-producing *Clostridium difficile* as the causative agent of AIC in both hamsters and humans, led to the development of a fast, reliable cell culture cytotoxicity assay for diagnosis, established oral vancomycin as effective first line treatment for the disease, and brought forth recommendations regarding possible prevention of transmission of the pathogen in epidemic settings.

II. ANTIBIOTIC-INDUCED ENTEROCOLITIS IN THE HAMSTER

A. The Model

As the impetus to develop the hamster model derived from an increasing number of cases of pseudomembranous colitis after the introduction of lincomycin and clindamycin, the latter was used in initial studies to induce the disease. Hamsters given small doses (1 mg/kg) of clindamycin by orogastric, intraperitoneal, intramuscular, intravenous, or percutaneous routes, developed a characteristic "wet-tail" syndrome that culminated in death within 7 days.[12,14] Food and water intake fell off within 24 to 48 hr. Watery, brown diarrhea ensued with staining of the paws and tail, animals became lethargic, their fur ruffled, and they huddled in the corners of their cages. When prompted to move, they often were noted to be ataxic. Death followed shortly thereafter in nearly 100% of animals.

The pathologic findings on gross examination of the cecum and distal ileum[12,15] were most striking. In normal animals the intestinal contents of the cecum had a pasty green quality and there were fecal pellets in the large bowel, while in clindamycin-treated animals the cecum and distal ileum were hemorrhagic, congested, and distended with fluid. No fecal pellets were found in the large bowel.

Histologically there was mucosal and submucosal congestion, leukocytic infiltration in the lamina propria and submucosa, and degenerative changes in surface enterocytes.[12,15,16] Foci of mucosal erosions were seen and patches of cellular debris and mucopurulent exudate formed microscopic pseudomembranes resembling that seen in human cases of pseudomembranous colitis.[15] Similar histologic inflammatory changes were found in the distal ileum and colon.

On scanning electron microscopy, the normal smooth mucosal surface was disrupted, crypts were distorted and dilated, sloughing of surface epithelial cells was seen, and spirilliform bacteria, normally present, were no longer evident.[12] Transmission electron microscopy revealed microvilli that were distorted, twisted, or totally lost.[12,16] Intracellular edema led to cell surface bulging and, in some instances, displacement of the microvillous border.

The "wet-tail" syndrome could be induced with many other antibiotics including all penicillins, cephalosporins, cephamycins, erythromycin, gentamicin, tobramycin, trimethoprim-sulfamethoxazole, thienamycin, and vancomycin.[4,12,18,34] While administration of chloramphenicol, metronidazole, and tetracyclines led to disease, the route of administration and dosage used was more critical.[4,35] Rifampin also caused enterocolitis, but only when resistant isolates of *C. difficile* were present. Antineoplastic agents such as methotrexate and 5-fluorouracil also produced an entercolitis.[36,37] Occasionally, the disease occurred in one or more animals spontaneously or after physical injury.

Although the hamster's response to all of the agents was similar and predictable, the time of onset varied with the specific agent, dosage, route of administration, and exposure to other animals. For example, while clindamycin doses of 100 mg/kg produced the typical picture and mortality rate, the onset of disease was delayed as compared with doses of 1 or 5 mg/kg.[12] The reason for the delayed response remains unclear, but investigators have speculated on longer suppression of the organism in the bowel before regrowth and toxin production or a direct effect of the antibiotics on toxin production. With vancomycin, hamsters remained well until the drug was stopped — then the typical picture occurred — most likely because of regrowth of susceptible toxigenic *C. difficile* that had been suppressed or reaquisition from the environment.[28-30]

While attack rates of 80 to 100% were expected with usual doses of clindamycin, environmental factors influenced the model. To reproduce the disease reliably, in addition to a susceptible hamster one needed the presence of toxigenic *C. difficile* and one of the inducing agents listed above. Most experiments were carried out with hamsters housed in small groups of five to ten per cage. Once *C. difficile* was present in one or more animals, the coprophagic and cannibalistic nature of the hamster ensured the passage of the organism to all cage mates. Animals housed separately in plastic isolators or in laminar air flow racks did not reliably develop disease.[35] Environmental surfaces have been documented to be colonized with *C. difficile,* but the role of surface colonization or spread by personnel, formites, or airborne routes remains unclear.[32,33,38]

Hamsters given a large number of toxigenic *C. difficile* via the orogastric route remained in good health.[39] If given antibiotics either before the administration of the organism or at the same time, typical enterocolitis occurred. This suggested that normal stool flora played a role in resisting colonization with *C. difficile* or in suppressing its overgrowth and toxin production. Changes in this flora as a result of antimicrobial administration allowed for colonization by as few as two *C. difficile* per milliliter, its growth and toxin production, and eventual fatal enterocolitis.[39]

Attempts at replacement of the normal flora after administration of antibiotics but before colonization with *C. difficile,* in order to protect animals from colitis, has had mixed results.[32,40]

B. The Role of *Clostridium difficile* and Its Toxins

Once the hamster was established as a reliable model for AIC, investigators concentrated on the cecal contents of hamsters dying with clindamycin-induced enterocolitis for clues to the etiology of the disease. Serial passage of the cecal contents or sterile filtrates prepared from these contents were found to produce the disease in normal hamsters.[7,22] Further, intraperitoneal injection of as little as 100 $\mu\ell$ of sterile filtrate produced intestinal, omental, and mesenteric fat hemorrhages, exudative peritonitis, pleural effusions, and death within 24 hr.[7] Smaller doses produced a more prolonged syndrome, with diarrhea and hemorrhagic cecitis 3 to 4 days after challenge. Attempts to reproduce the same results by the administration of clindamycin intraperitoneally were unsuccessful.[7] In other experiments, removing clindamycin from cecal contents by dialysis indicated that clindamycin was not the factor responsible for the toxicity.[3]

As the results seen with intraperitoneal injection of infiltrates were reminiscent of effects produced by clostridial enterotoxins,[41] neutralization of the toxic moiety by polyvalent clostridial antitoxin was attempted and successfully demonstrated.[7,14] Further, monovalent *C. sordellii* antitoxin was identified as the active constituent in polyvalent antitoxin.[23]

At the same time, *C. difficile* was consistently isolated from stool cultures of hamsters and humans developing clindamycin-enterocolitis.[5,22] Administration of this organism to hamsters challenged with antibiotics produced an identical enterocolitis.[39] Intraperitoneal injection of sterile culture filtrates of *C. difficile* led to disease identical to that induced by cecal filtrates from hamsters dying of enterocolitis.[23] In addition, toxic filtrates from *C. difficile* were neutralized by *C. sordellii* antitoxin. Except for the S-4 strain used to produce the initial U.S. Standard *C. sordellii* antitoxin, attempts at reproducing the disease with *C. sordellii* isolates or toxin were unsuccessful. With this strain, death occurred after injection of the toxin, but the pathologic findings differed from that produced by *C. difficile* or cecal filtrates.[23] Thus toxigenic *C. difficile* appeared to be the agent responsible for AIC.

Attempts at culturing *C. difficile* from the intestines of healthy hamsters revealed only a 3 to 5% isolation rate.[33] Current culture methods, however, will not detect concentrations of organisms below 100 colony-forming units per milliliter. It would appear that antibiotics either disturb the equilibrium of intestinal flora so that the initially very low numbers of organisms proliferate or they set up conditions allowing for the acquisition and growth of the organism from environmental sources. Even in the face of disease, *C. difficile* only makes up a minor component of hamster or human fecal flora, with concentrations in the range of less than 10^8 colony-forming units per gram wet weight cecal contents.[5]

Of interest has been the known susceptibility of *C. difficile* to many of the agents causing AIC.[4] The production of disease in hamsters and humans does not appear to be due solely to the overgrowth of resistant organisms, but the factors responsible for the organism's growth, toxin production, and release have not yet been clearly defined.

While identification of a toxic substance in the fecal contents of hamsters with clindamycin enterocolitis led to the identification of *C. difficile* as the causative agent for the disease, investigation into the properties and action of the toxin was also undertaken. Initial experiments demonstrated the toxic agent to be nondialyzable, acid and alkaline labile, and instantaneously but reversibly bound to *C. sordellii* antitoxin.[14,42,43] Further, as a stool extract from a patient with clindamycin-associated colitis had recently been demonstrated to be toxic for WI-38 cell fibroblasts,[21] filtrates of cecal contents from hamsters with clindamycin enterocolitis were tested in similar systems. Both cecal filtrates and sterile broth filtrates of *C. difficile* produced in vitro cytotoxicity for most cell lines.[14,23] Cells were damaged within 20 to 30 min and surface changes were detectable within 1 hr. Actinomorphic changes manifested by radiation of cell processes in various directions were followed by cellular rounding within 4 hr. These changes appeared to result from irreversible disruption of actin microfilament bundles.[44] Uncoupling of oxidative phosphorylation in mitochondrial respiration prevented toxicity. Cytotoxic effects were specifically neutralized by *C. sordellii* antitoxin.[14,23] This assay of cell cytotoxicity and neutralization has subsequently become the simplest test for the presence of toxigenic *C. difficile* colitis in patients.[45,46]

The effect of the toxin on cell cultures in vitro was paralleled by its effect on hamster epithelium in vivo. Within 4 hr, surface epithelial cells were distorted, ballooned, and they began to desquamate into the lumen.[17] The lamina propria became congested and there was increasing purulent inflammation such that by 8 hr a severe enterocolitis with inflammatory pseudomembranes could be seen.

Recent work has demonstrated the existence of two immunologically separate *C. difficile* toxins.[25,47] Both toxins, A and B, caused rounding of cells, but toxin B was uniformly more active. Each was neutralized by homologous but not heterologous antiserum. Toxin A elicited a positive hemorrhagic fluid response in rabbit ileal loops more characteristic of that produced by *Shigella* enterotoxin than by enterotoxins of *E. coli* (LT) or *V. cholera*.[27] Injection of toxin A into hamster ceca was lethal, causing severe hemorrhage, villous disruption, and cecal edema. Toxin B caused some focal hemorrhage but was not lethal.[25] Both toxins appeared important in causing the enterocolitis, as hamsters immunized against either toxin alone were not protected from enterocolitis after clindamycin challenge while immunization against both toxins was protective.[25] The relative roles of these toxins in the production of disease have not been established in the hamster model or human cases of AIC.

C. Therapy and Prevention

The hamster has also proven to be an excellent model for assessing the role of therapeutic agents in the treatment of *C. difficile* colitis. Nonspecific agents such as methylprednisolone, atropine-diphenoxylate, cholestyramine, and parenteral fluids as well as immunization and multiple antibiotics have been evaluated for prevention and treatment.

Most *C. difficile* species are inhibited by low concentrations of vancomycin, metronidazole, rifampin, and ampicillin.[4] Inhibition of the organism, however, is not enough to prevent the onset of clindamycin-induced *C. difficile* enterocolitis as agents such as ampicillin, which are effective against *C. difficile* in vitro, readily induce the disease in vivo. Recent work suggested that administration of ampicillin suppressed growth of *C. difficile*, but also induced β-lactamase production by other gut flora.[49] This destroyed ampicillin activity, allowed regrowth of *C. difficile*, toxin production, and resulted in colitis. Animals given a β-lactamase inhibitor as well as ampicillin remained in good health. As ampicillin is a major cause of human *C. difficile* colitis,[2,4,20] its usage for treatment is unlikely.

Daily oral vancomycin in doses comparable to those used in humans prevented the development of clindamycin-induced enterocolitis in hamsters as long as it was continued.[28,29] Once stopped, animals died with typical enterocolitis even if the sole clindamycin challenge had been as long as 3 months earlier. Recent experiments have shown that enterocolitis and death in the vancomycin-treated animals were due to environmental acquisition of *C. difficile,* as animals receiving the same treatment, but kept environmentally isolated, all survived.[32,33] In fact, treatment of isolated hamsters with vancomycin for 3 weeks before challenge with clindamycin effectively prevented clindamycin-induced enterocolitis, suggesting that vancomycin eradicated toxigenic *C. difficile* from hamster intestines and reinfection did not occur in the isolated setting.[24,32]

There is evidence to suggest that vancomycin itself may kill or inhibit intestinal organisms that prevent acquisition of *C. difficile*. Administration of *C. difficile* suspension to animals not previously given antibiotics did not produce enterocolitis.[24] Prior treatment with vancomycin, however, produced changes in bowel flora such that as few as two *C. difficile* organisms could produce an infection and culminate in a fatal enterocolitis.[39] Intestinal concentrations of vancomycin were inhibitory for many facultative anaerobic as well as aerobic intestinal microorganisms that may have competed with or been antagonistic to *C. difficile* within the bowel. Which organisms may have been responsible for the colonization resistance remains unknown.[50]

Orogastric metronidazole also protected hamsters from lethal clindamycin-induced enterocolitis when given daily.[4,18] Like vancomycin, once metronidazole was discontinued the animals acquired *C. difficile* and died. Protection with metronidazole was less predictable than with vancomycin, but similar mechanisms are likely.

Bacitracin has been used successfully for therapy of a few cases of human *C. difficile* colitis,[51] but supportive hamster experiments are scarce.[30] In vitro tests suggest that most *C. difficile* are sensitive to bacitracin, but isolates resistant to the drug do occur.[76]

Anion exchange resins, cholestyramine, and colestipol are felt to bind *C. difficile* toxins within the gut.[52] They have had little effect on survival in the hamster model,[19,29] but there have been several reports of their effectiveness in man.[53] Nonspecific therapy with methylprednisolone, maintenance of hydration, and atropine-diphenoxylate also have failed to decrease mortality or shorten the duration of disease in the hamster.[19,29] It has been suggested that the latter agent may, in fact, be deleterious by causing retentin of toxins within the bowel.[54]

The possible role of immunotherapy in treatment or prevention of *C. difficile* colitis remains unclear. Administration of *C. sordellii* antitoxin to hamsters was associated with significant protection from colitis and death after challenge with clindamycin.[31] Further, these animals remained healthy for more than 3 months after challenge, in spite of likely colonization with *C. difficile*. Recent studies of actively immunized hamsters, using toxoids to both *C. difficile* toxin A and toxin B, have also demonstrated protection from clindamycin challenge.[25] As most cases of *C. difficile* colitis occur sporadically, the role of immunization in the future prevention of AIC in man is doubtful, but a vaccine might prove useful in certain hospitals where the endemic rate is high.[38]

III. OTHER ANIMAL MODELS OF ANTIBIOTIC-INDUCED COLITIS

A. Rabbits

Although recognized as a cause of rabbit deaths in conventional colonies since the 1920s, spontaneous enteritis emerged as a significant problem in the mid-1950s.[55,56] Variable rates of isolation of *E. coli* and *Clostridium perfringens* were demonstrated, but the etiology of the enteritis remained unclear.[56] Tetracycline prevented the disease.

Rabbits given either oral lincomycin or clindamycin died within 3 days of a lethal enterocolitis affecting mainly the cecum and large bowel and resembling the findings of spontaneous enteritis.[57] Gentamicin and vancomycin were protective. Cecal filtrates from dying animals were toxic when injected intraperitoneally or into rabbit intestinal loops.[58] Further work demonstrated that the toxic activity was neutralized by antiserum to *C. perfringens* type E iota toxin, but not by other specific monovalent or polyvalent clostridial antitoxins.[59,60] Recently, helically coiled *C. spiroforme*, capable of producing iota-like toxin neutralized by antitoxin to *C. perfringens* type E iota toxin, was isolated from rabbits with both spontaneous enteritis and AIC.[61] This organism was found in diseased animals, but rarely in healthy ones, and must be strongly implicated as the major etiology of antibiotic-induced and spontaneous colitis in rabbits. Whether this organism is a cause of antibiotic diarrhea in man remains unknown.

C. difficile in concentrations of greater than 10^8 g wet weight of fresh feces has also been demonstrated to cause hemorrhagic colitis in rabbits.[62] Other clostridial species such as *C. perfringens* and *C. tertium* may, by unknown mechanisms, increase the growth of *C. difficile* in vivo and potentiate its toxicity. While probably not the major cause of colitis in rabbits, *C. difficile* colitis has been reported to occur.[63]

B. Guinea Pigs

Conventional but not axenic guinea pigs given small doses of penicillin, lincomycin, or clindamycin also developed enterocolits.[64-67] The course of the disease, pathologic changes, and protection experiments paralleled that demonstrated in the hamster, but lethality was not as reproducible. Pseudomembranous plaques similar to those found in human pseudomembranous enterocolitis have occasionally been noted.[65] Recent investigations have documented the presence of cecal toxins neutralizable by *C. sordellii* and *C. difficile* antitoxins, as well as cultures positive for *C. difficile* in many of the animals.[68,69] Further, rabbits immunized with toxic guinea pig cecal extracts produced antibodies neutralizing the cytotoxicity of human stool filtrates from patients with *C. difficile* colitis and filtrates of *C. difficile* cultures.[69] Other isolated reports of clindamycin-induced enterocolitis due to toxigenic *Bacillus pumilus*,[70] or associated with the production of a toxin neutralized by antitoxin to *C. histolyticum*,[66] have not as yet been confirmed by other investigators and have not been associated with human cases of antibiotic-associated diarrhea.

Of interest, guinea pigs given lincomycin were also noted to develop distended, hyperemic gall bladders with purulent nodules resembling pseudomembranes.[71,72] Cell proliferation and increased production of mucus was followed by inflammatory infiltration and ulceration. Bile cultures remained sterile. Animals surviving the challenge developed pigment stones similar to that seen in humans with gall bladder disease. These studies raised the intriguing possibility of clostridial toxin absorbed from the gut leading to gall bladder injury. As of this time, there is no known association of *C. difficile* colitis with acute cholecystitis or subsequent gallstone formation in humans.

C. Mice and Rats

Gnotobiotic mice have been used to study the effects of *C. difficile* in an animal without interference from other bacteria. Although *C. difficile* toxin can be demonstrated at 10^{-6} dilution, these animals developed inflammation in the lamina propria of the cecum and mild diarrhea without weight loss. Lethality was rare.[73] Treatment with vancomycin decreased viable cell density, increased spore formation, and decreased toxin to undetectable levels within 24 hr. When vancomycin was discontinued, all parameters returned to the pretreatment levels and symptomatic diarrhea resumed. Vancomycin induction of *C. difficile* spore formation and subsequent regrowth of the organism as seen here may explain the 10% relapse rate after treatment in human cases. Clindamycin did not change *C. difficile* counts or cytotoxin production. Despite the use of a clindamycin-sensitive strain, resistant *C. difficile* emerged suggesting either induction of resistance, or growth of a previously low number of resistant organisms.

When germ-free rats were monoassociated with a toxigenic strain of *C. difficile,* 17% of the animals died with enterocolitis, hepatitis, and interstitial pneumonia. The organism was cultured not only from bowel, but also from spleen, kidney, and liver.

Cecal filtrates were positive for *C. difficile* toxin. Rats monoassociated with a poorly toxigenic strain of *C. difficile* were colonized, but did not develop disease.[74]

While conventional rats were also resistant to the lethal effects of clindamycin, they have been used to investigate the etiology of watery diarrhea without colitis that occurs in 10 to 15% of patients receiving clindamycin.[74] Perfusion of the rat intestine with clindamycin at levels readily achievable after oral ingestion in man had no significant effect on morphology but decreased water and sodium absorption, particularly in the ileum. The cause of the defect is unknown but it was not associated with cyclic AMP or cyclic GMP systems, glucose transplant, or disturbance of villous absorptive cells. Further work on the etiology of antibiotic-induced watery diarrhea without colitis is needed.

IV. CONCLUSIONS AND FUTURE INVESTIGATIONS

The development of the hamster model for antibiotic-induced colitis has resulted in the recognition of toxigenic *C. difficile* as the responsible pathogen, led to the development of a rapid, sensitive test for the disease, and allowed for testing of effective treatment regimens. The role of *C. difficile* as part of the intestinal microflora, its interaction with other bacteria, and the mechanisms and site of action of its toxins remain to be elucidated. The humoral immune response of the hamster and man to the organism and toxins has not been adequately addressed. Further, investigation into the mechanism(s) of antibiotic-induced diarrhea without colitis, one of the most common side effects limiting antibiotic usage in man and animals, may be undertaken using the models and approaches enumerated here.

REFERENCES

1. Finney, J. M. T., Gastroenterostomy for cicatrizing ulcer of the pylorus, *Bull. Johns Hopkins Hosp.,* 4, 53, 1893.
2. Mogg, G. A. G., Keighley, M. R. B., Burdon, D. W., Alexander-Williams, J., Youngs, D., Johnson, M., Bently, S., and George, R. H., Antibiotic-associated colitis — a review of 66 cases, *Br. J. Surg.,* 66, 738, 1979.
3. Bartlett, J. G., Antibiotic-associated pseudomembranous colitis, *Rev. Infect. Dis.,* 1, 530, 1979.
4. Fekety, R., Silva, J., Toshniwal, R., Allow, M., Armstrong, J., Browne, R., Ebright, J., and Rifkin, G., Antibiotic-associated colitis: effects of antibiotics on *Clostridium difficile* and the disease in hamsters, *Rev. Infect. Dis.,* 1, 386, 1979.
5. Bartlett, J. G., Chang, T. W., Taylor, N. S., and Onderdonk, A. B., Colitis induced by *Clostridium difficile, Rev. Infect. Dis.,* 1, 370, 1979.
6. Price, A. B. and Davies, D. R., Pseudomembranous colitis, *J. Clin. Pathol.,* 30, 1, 1977.
7. Rifkin, G. D., Silva, J., Jr., and Fekety, R., Gastrointestinal and systemic toxicity of fecal extracts from hamsters with clindamycin-induced colitis, *Gastroenterology,* 74, 52, 1978.
8. Hamre, D. M., Rake, G., McKee, C. M., and MacPhillamy, H. B., Toxicity of penicillin as prepared for clinical use, *Am. J. Med. Sci.,* 206, 642, 1943.
9. Silva, J., Jr., Animal models of antibiotic-induced colitis, *Microbiology,* 258, 1979.
10. Small, J. D., Fatal enterocolitis in hamsters given lincomycin hydrochloride, *Lab. Anim. Care,* 18, 411, 1968.
11. Bartlett, J. G. and Grbach, S. C., Pseudomembranous enterocolitis (antibiotic related colitis), *Adv. Intern. Med.,* 22, 455, 1977.
12. Lusk, R. H., Fekety, R., Silva, J., Browne, R. A., Ringler, D. H., and Abrams, G. D., Clindamycin-induced enterocolitis in hamsters, *J. Infect. Dis.,* 137, 464, 1978.
13. Hughes, H. C., Jr. and Lang, C. M., Basic principles in selecting animal species for research projects, *Clin. Toxicol.,* 13, 611, 1978.

14. Chang, T. W., Bartlett, J. G., Gorbach, S. L., and Onderdonk, A. B., Clindamycin-induced enterocolitis in hamsters as a model of pseudomembranous colitis in patients, *Infect. Immunol.*, 20, 526, 1978.
15. Price, A. B., Larson, H. E., and Crow, J., Morphology of experimental antibiotic-associated enterocolitis in the hamster: a model for human pseudomembranous colitis and antibiotic-associated diarrhoea, *Gut*, 20, 467, 1979.
16. Humphrey, C. D., Lushbaugh, W. B., Condon, C. W., Pittman, J. C., and Pittman, F. E., Light and electron microscopic studies of antibiotic associated colitis in the hamster, *Gut*, 20, 6, 1979.
17. Abrams, G. D., Allo, M., Rifkin, G. D., Fekety, R., and Silva, J., Jr., Mucosal damage mediated by clostridial toxin in experimental clindamycin-associated colitis, *Gut*, 21, 493, 1980.
18. Bartlett, J. G., Chang, T. W., Moon, N., and Onderdonk, A. B., Antibiotic-induced lethal enterocolitis in hamsters: studies with eleven agents and evidence to support the pathogenic role of toxin-producing clostridia, *Am. J. Vet. Res.*, 39, 1525, 1978.
19. Fekety, R., Silva, J., Browne, R. A., Rifkin, G. D., and Ebright, J. R., Clindamycin-induced colitis, *Am. J. Clin. Nutr.*, 32, 244, 1979.
20. Bartlett, J. G., Taylor, N. S., Chang, T. W., and Dzink, J., Clinical and laboratory observation in *Clostridium difficile* colitis, *Am. J. Clin. Nutr.*, 33, 2521, 1980.
21. Larson, H. E., Parry, J. V., Price, A. B., Davies, D. R., Dolby, J., and Tyrrell, D. A. J., Undescribed toxin in pseudomembranous colitis, *Br. Med. J.*, 1, 1246, 1977.
22. Bartlett, J. G., Onderdonk, A. B., Cisneros, R. L., and Kasper, D. L., Clindamycin-associated colitis due to a toxin-producing species of clostridium in hamsters, *J. Infect. Dis.*, 136, 701, 1977.
23. Rifkin, G. D., Fekety, R., and Silva, J., Neutralization by *Clostridium sordelli* antitoxin of toxins implicated in clindamycin-induced cecitis in the hamster, *Gastroenterology*, 75, 422, 1978.
24. Larson, H. E., The experimental pathogenesis of antibiotic related colitis, *Scand. J. Infect. Dis.*, 22(Suppl.), 7, 1980.
25. Libby, J. M., Jortner, B. S., and Wilkins, T. D., Effects of the two toxins of *Clostridium difficile* in antibiotic-associated cecitis in hamsters, *Infect. Immunol.*, 36, 822, 1982.
26. Sullivan, N. M., Pellett, S., and Wilkins, T. D., Purification and characterization of toxins A and B of *Clostridium difficile*, *Infect. Immunol.*, 35, 1032, 1982.
27. Lyerly, D. M., Lockwood, D. E., Richardson, S. H., and Wilkins, T. D., Biological activities of toxins A and B of *Clostridium difficile*, *Infect. Immunol.*, 35, 1147, 1982.
28. Browne, R. A., Fekety, R., Jr., Silva, J., Jr., Boyd, D. I., Work, C. O., and Abrams, G. D., The protective effect of vancomycin on clindamycin-induced colitis in hamsters, *Johns Hopkins Med. J.*, 141, 183, 1977.
29. Bartlett, J. G., Chang, T. W., and Onderdonk, A. B., Comparison of five regimens for treatment of experimental clindamycin-associated colitis, *J. Infect. Dis.*, 138, 81, 1978.
30. Bartlett, J. G., Onderdonk, A. B., and Cisneros, R. L., Clindamycin-associated colitis in hamsters: protection in vancomycin, *Gastroenterology*, 73, 722, 1977.
31. Allo, M., Silva, J., Jr., Fekety, R., Rifkin, G., and Waskin, H., Prevention of clindamycin-induced colitis in hamsters by *Clostridium sordellii* antitoxin, *Gastroenterology*, 76, 351, 1979.
32. Larson, H. E., Price, A. B., and Borriello, S. P., Epidemiology of experimental enterocecitis due to *Clostridium difficile*, *J. Infect. Dis.*, 142, 408, 1980.
33. Fekety, R., Kyung-Hee, K., Batts, D. H., Browne, R. A., Cudmore, M. A., Silva, J., Jr., Toshniwal, R., and Wilson, K. H., Studies on the epidemiology of antibiotic-associated *Clostridium difficile* colitis, *Am. J. Clin. Nutr.*, 33, 2527, 1980.
34. Ebright, J. R., Fekety, R., Silva, J., and Wilson, K. W., Evaluation of eight cephalosporins in hamster colitis model, *Antimicrob. Agents Chemother.*, 19, 980, 1981.
35. Toshniwal, R., Fekety, R., and Silva, J., Jr., Etiology of tetracycline-associated pseudomembranous colitis in hamsters, *Antimicrob. Agents Chemother.*, 16, 167, 1979.
36. Syrjamaki, C. E., Silva, J., Rifkin, G. D., and Fekety, R., Effects of methotrexate in a hamster model of enterocolitis, *Clin. Res.*, 26, 742A, 1978.
37. Cudmore, M. A., Silva, J., and Fekety, R., Clostridial enterocolitis produced by antineoplastic agents in hamsters and humans, *Current Chemotherapy in Infant Diseases*, American Society for Microbiology, Washington, D.C., 1980, 1460.
38. Burdon, D. W., *Clostridium difficile*: the epidemiology and prevention of hospital-acquired infection, *Infection*, 10, 203, 1982.
39. Larson, H. E., Price, A. B., Honour, P., and Borriello, S. P., *Clostridium difficile* and the oetiology of pseudomembranous colitis, *Lancet*, 1063, 1978.
40. Wilson, K. H., Silva, J., and Fekety, F. R., Suppression of *Clostridium difficile* by normal hamster cecal flora and prevention of antibiotic-associated cecitis, *Infect. Immunol.*, 34, 626, 1981.
41. MacLennan, J. D., The histotoxic clostridial infections of man, *Bacteriol. Rev.*, 26, 177, 1962.

42. Rifkin, G. D., Fekety, F. R., Silva, J., Jr., and Sack, R. B., Antibiotic-induced colitis implication of a toxin neutralized by *Clostridium sordellii* antitoxin, *Lancet*, 1103, 1977.
43. Bartlett, J. G., Experimental studies of antibiotic associated colitis, *Scand. J. Infect. Dis.*, 22(Suppl.), 11, 1980.
44. Thelestam, M. and Bronnegard, M., Interaction of cytopathogenic toxin from *Clostridium difficile* with cells in tissue culture, *Scand. J. Infect. Dis.*, 22(Suppl.), 16, 1980.
45. Silva, J., Jr. and Fekety, R., Clostridia and antimicrobial enterocolitis, *Ann. Rev. Med.*, 32, 327, 1981.
46. Tedesco, F. J., Antibiotic associated pseudomembranous colitis with negative proctosigmoidoscopy examination, *Gastroenterology*, 77, 295, 1979.
47. Taylor, N. S. and Bartlett, J. G., Partial purification and characterization of a cytotoxin from *Clostridium difficile*, *Rev. Infect. Dis.*, 1, 379, 1979.
48. Donta, S. T., Sullivan, N., and Wilkins, T. D., Differential effects of *Clostridium difficile* toxins on tissue-cultured cells, *J. Clin. Microbiol.*, 15, 1157, 1982.
49. Rolfe, R. D. and Finegold, S. M., Intestinal B-lactamase activity in ampicillin-induced *Clostridium difficile*-associated ileocecitis, *J. Infect. Dis.*, 147, 227, 1983.
50. Rolfe, R. D. and Finegold, S. M., Inhibitory interactions between normal fecal flora and *Clostridium difficile*, *Am. J. Clin. Nutr.*, 33, 2539, 1980.
51. Tedesco, F. J., Bacitracin therapy in antibiotic-associated pseudomembranous colitis, *Dig. Dis. Sci.*, 25, 783, 1980.
52. Taylor, N. S. and Bartlett, J. G., Binding of *Clostridium difficile* cytotoxin and vancomycin by anion-exchange resins, *J. Infect. Dis.*, 141, 92, 1980.
53. Kreutzer, E. W. and Milligan, F. D., Treatment of antibiotic-associated pseudomembranous colitis with cholestyramine resin, *Johns Hopkins Med. J.*, 143, 67, 1978.
54. Novak, E., Lee, J. G., Seckman, E., Phillips, J. P., and Disanto, A. R., Unfavorable effect of atropinediphenoxylate (Lomotil) therapy in lincomycin-caused diarrhea, *JAMA*, 235, 1451, 1976.
55. Whitney, J. C., A review of non-specific enteritis in the rabbit, *Lab. Anim.*, 10, 209, 1976.
56. Kruijt, B. C., Enteritis in conventional rabbit colony, *Lab. Anim.*, 10, 189, 1976.
57. Fesce, A., Ceccarelli, A., Fesce, E., and Balsari, A., Ecophylaxis: preventive treatment with gentamicin of rabbit lincomycin-associated diarrhea, *Folia Vet. Lat.*, 7, 225, 1977.
58. Katz, L., LaMont, J. T., Trier, J. S., Sonnenblick, E. B., Rothman, S. W., Broitman, S. A., and Riet, S., Experimental clindamycin-associated colitis in rabbits, *Gastroenterology*, 74, 246, 1978.
59. LaMont, J. T., Sonnenblick, E. B., and Rothman, S., Role of clostridial toxin in the pathogenesis of clindamycin colitis in rabbits, *Gastroenterology*, 76, 356, 1979.
60. Rehg, J. E. and Pakes, S. P., Implication of *Clostridium difficile* and *Clostridium perfringens* iota toxins in experimental lincomycin-associated colitis of rabbits, *Lab. Anim. Sci.*, 32, 253, 1982.
61. Borriello, S. P. and Carman, R. J., Association of iota-like toxin and *Clostridium spiroforme* with both spontaneous and antibiotic-associated diarrhea and colitis in rabbits, *J. Clin. Microbiol.*, 17, 414, 1983.
62. Dabard, J., Dubos, F., Martinet, L., and Ducluzeau, R., Experimental reproduction of neonatal diarrhea in young gnotobiotic hares simultaneously associated with *Clostridium difficile* and other clostridium strains, *Infect. Immunol.*, 24, 7, 1979.
63. Rehg, J. E. and Lu, Y. S., *Clostridium difficile* colitis in a rabbit following antibiotic therapy for pasteurellosis, *J. Am. Vet. Med. Assoc.*, 179, 1296, 1981.
64. Formal, S. B., Abrams, G. D., Schneider, H., and Laundy, R., Penicillin in germ-free guinea pigs, *Nature (London)*, 198, 712, 1963.
65. Lee, S. P. and Thomsen, L. L., Toxin-induced cell membrane injury in guinea pigs given lincomycin, *Pathology*, 14, 317, 1982.
66. Knoop, F. C., Clindamycin-associated enterocolitis in guinea pigs: evidence for a bacterial toxin, *Infect. Immunol.*, 23, 31, 1979.
67. Rehg, J. E., Yarbrough, B. A., and Pakes, S. P., Toxicity of cecal filtrates from guinea pigs with penicillin-associated colitis, *Lab. Anim. Sci.*, 30, 524, 1980.
68. Rehg, J. E., Cecal toxin(s) from guinea pigs with clindamycin-associated colitis, neutralized by *Clostridium sordellii* antitoxin, *Infect. Immunol.*, 27, 387, 1980.
69. Rothman, S. W., Presence of *Clostridium difficile* toxin in guinea pigs with penicillin-associated colitis, *Med. Microbiol. Immunol.*, 169, 187, 1981.
70. Brophy, P. F. and Knoop, F. C., *Bacillus pumilus* in the induction of clindamycin-associated enterocolitis in guinea pigs, *Infect. Immunol.*, 35, 289, 1982.
71. Scott, A. J., Lincomycin-induced cholecystitis and gallstones in guinea pigs, *Gastroenterology*, 71, 814, 1976.
72. Lee, S. P. and Scott, A. J., Further observations in lincomycin-induced cholelithiasis in guinea pigs, *J. Pathol.*, 131, 117, 1980.

73. Onderdonk, A. B., Cisneros, R. L., and Bartlett, J. G., *Clostridium difficile* in gnotobiotic mice, *Infect. Immunol.*, 28, 277, 1980.
74. Czuprynski, C. J., Johnson, W. J., Balish, E., and Wilkins, T., Pseudomembranous colitis in *Clostridium difficile*-monoassociated rats, *Infect. Immunol.*, 39, 1368, 1983.
75. Giannella, R. A., Serumaga, J., Walls, D., and Drake, K. W., Effect of clindamycin on intestinal water and glucose transport in the rat, *Gastroenterology*, 80, 907, 1981.
76. Rifkin, G. D. and Fekety, F. R., Jr., Unpublished observations.

Chapter 10

EQUINE GRANULOMATOUS ENTERITIS

Ronnie E. Cimprich

TABLE OF CONTENTS

I. INTRODUCTION

Crohn's disease (regional enteritis) is a disease not only in search of an etiology, but also of an animal model. This chapter describes what the author sees as the spontaneous animal model that most closely approximates the disease in man — granulomatous enteritis in the horse. Inconveniently, as models go, the disease in horses is also in search of an etiology and case material is not readily available. However, equine granulomatous enteritis is well-defined clinically and, as a result of networking of researchers in the field, when a case does present there is a wealth of material available for study. To date, cases have been reported in the U.S.,[1-3] Australia,[4-6] and South Africa.[7] This chapter will also discuss other spontaneous and induced animal models of granulomatous enteritis.

II. GRANULOMATOUS ENTERITIS OF HORSES

A. Clinical Presentation

Horses present with a history of chronic weight loss of several months duration in spite of normal appetite. One series of 22 horses included thoroughbreds, standardbreds, and crossbreeds varying in age from 1 to 13 years.[8] There was either no history of diarrhea or one of intermittent diarrhea with semiformed feces constantly present. Dermatitis, arthritis, spondylitis, and vulva linear erosion were sometimes present. The horses were uniformly hypoalbuminemic with varying gamma globulin levels. ^{51}Cr-albumin clearances performed in several animals were elevated when compared to controls, indicating intestinal protein loss. Xylose absorption tests performed in several horses showed almost flat curves, with absorption of only 5 mg/dℓ at 60 min compared to a peak of 20 mg/dℓ in normal horses. Peritoneal fluid obtained by paracentesis showed a marked reduction in phagocytic material within peritoneal mesothelial cells when compared to normal controls. When lymphocyte transformation tests were performed, there was a marked reduction in response to phytohematagglutinin and pokeweed antigen. When compared to controls, cultures of staphlycocci grown with polymorphonuclear leukocytes showed decreased kill rates when induced with serum of affected horses. Other serum and urine parameters, including hematology, were generally within normal limits.

Multiple, firm nodules or masses were consistently palpable at the root of the mesentery on rectal examination. Ileal biopsies obtained by standing left flank laparotomy were diagnostic of the disease.[2]

B. Post-Mortem Examination
1. Gross Findings

The horses were thin or emaciated. The peritoneal cavity in some animals contained 500 mℓ to 15 ℓ of turbid yellow or serosanguinous fluid. Prominent gross changes were most common in the ileum, and consisted of firm nodules or annular or raised plaques (Figure 1). The nodules and plaques were either restricted to the serosa or extended to the mucosa. In other areas, the serosal surface had a diffuse, raised, fine, granular appearance. The gross mucosal changes varied greatly from animal to animal but were present most often in the ileum. The following changes were seen: a finely granular appearance and thickening (Figure 2), corrugated mucosa in annular or raised patches (Figure 3), and depressed foci 5 to 10 mm in diameter or depressed red streaks (fissures) 3- to 4-cm long. The duodenal and jejunal mucosae were usually not remarkable grossly.

The colonic mucosa was usually normal grossly, but numerous linear erosions 2- to 3-mm wide and 40-mm long were present in some animals (Figure 4). Swollen, wet

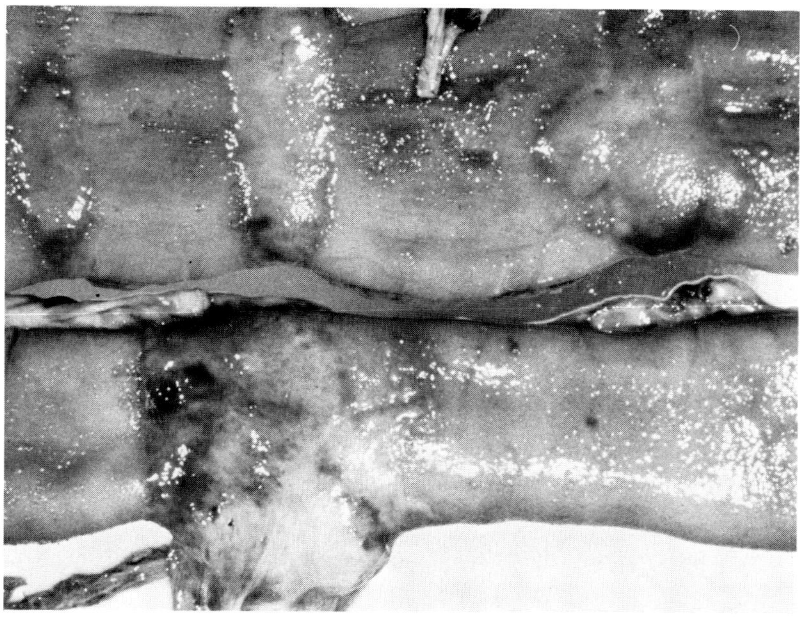

FIGURE 1.   Nodules and plaques on the serosal surface of the ileum.

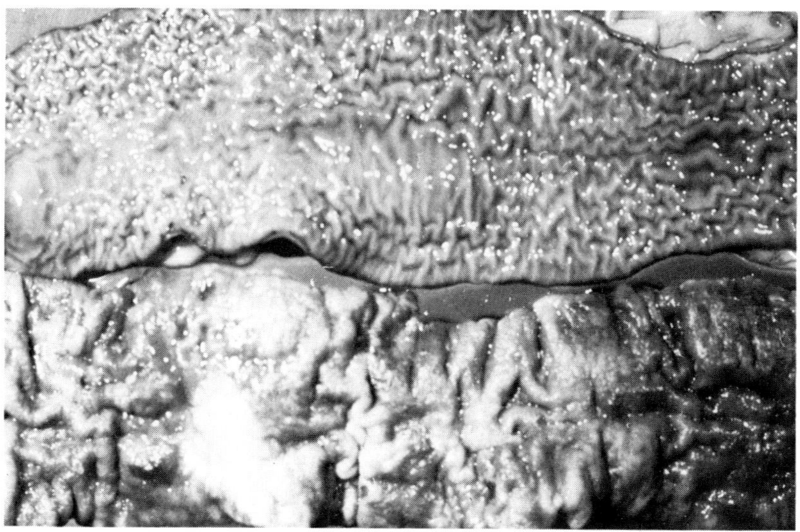

FIGURE 2.   Normal mucosa above and thickened mucosa below. From the ileum of an affected horse.

mucosa covered with irregular red patches 3- to 10-mm wide and 1-mm deep were present in some horses. The latter were often opposite areas of serosal adhesions.

Masses as large as 20-cm long and 5-cm thick encircling the small bowel and adherent to other abdominal viscera were sometimes present. Adhesions of gut to gut, or gut to omentum, mesentery, or abdominal wall were a common feature.

The lymph nodes were normal except for the mesenteric nodes which were enlarged (3 to 6 cm in diameter), often wet, firm, and mottled gray-white (Figure 5). The surfaces had irregularly shaped, firm to hard white nodules 3 to 5 mm in diameter. On

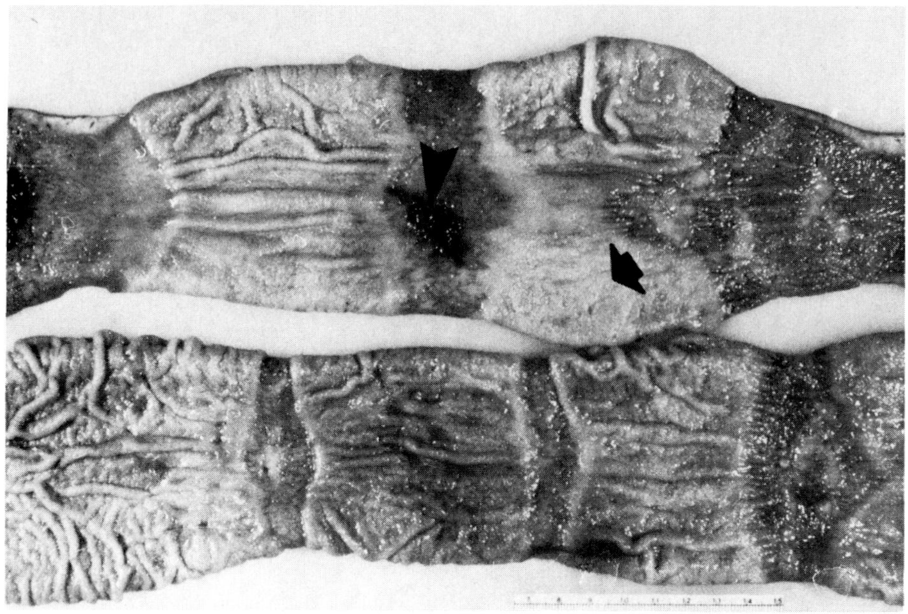

FIGURE 3.   Annular areas of abnormal mucosa with adjacent raised thickened foci (arrow). Ulcerated foci were sometimes present (arrowhead).

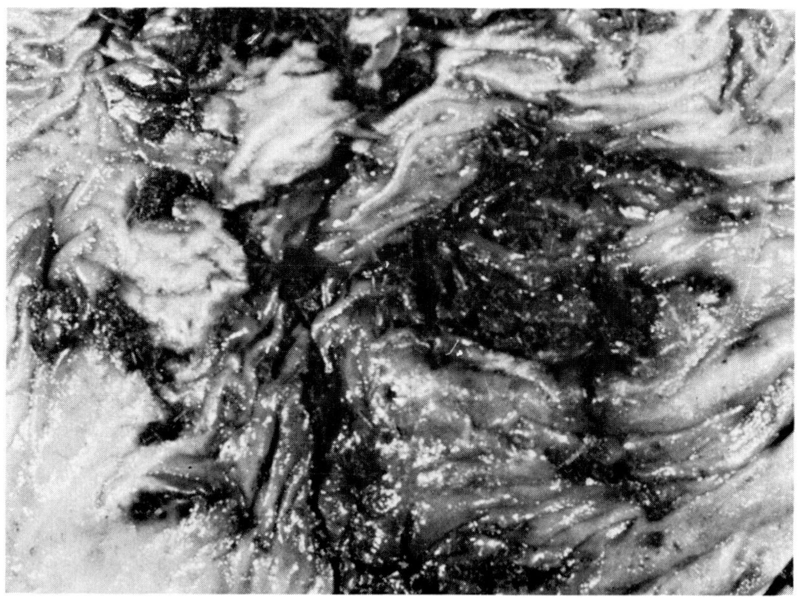

FIGURE 4.   Colonic mucosa with linear erosions.

cut surfaces, the normal architecture was often obliterated by homogeneous wet gray firm tissue or multiple firm white nodules.

In occasional animals, the gastric mucosa was also thickened and cobblestone in appearance. Some animals also had firm livers with either dilated bile ducts or firm 1 to 2 mm gritty yellow or white nodules. The remaining viscera in the abdominal and thoracic cavities were generally normal.

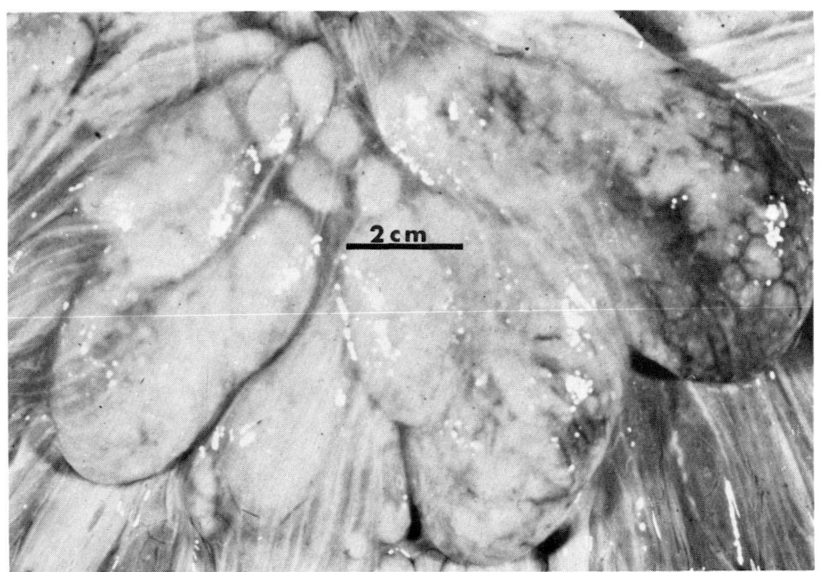

FIGURE 5.   Enlarged, edematous mesenteric lymph nodes.

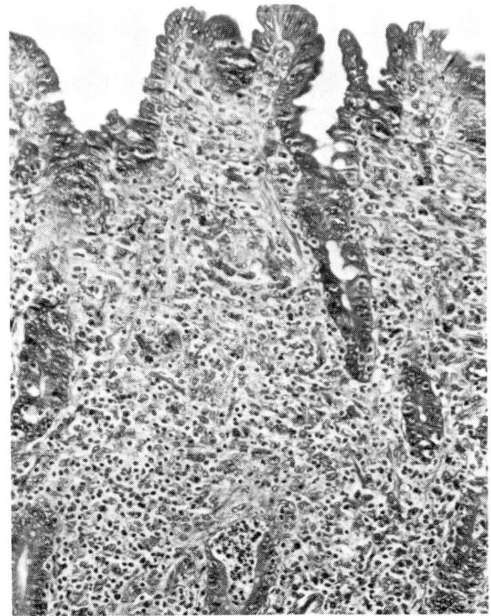

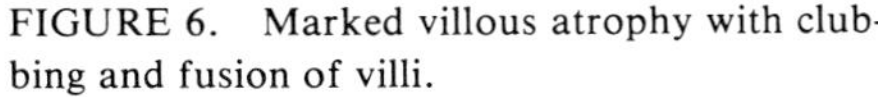

FIGURE 6.   Marked villous atrophy with clubbing and fusion of villi.

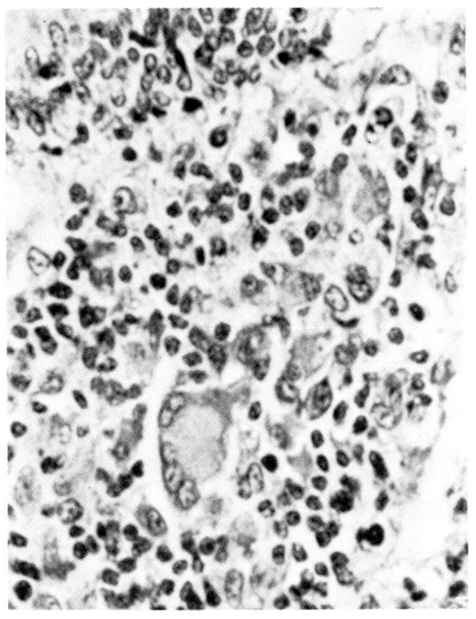

FIGURE 7.   Higher-power photomicrograph of
mixed mononuclear cell infiltrates and giant
cells.

2. Microscopic Pathology

Although the bowel was usually grossly abnormal only segmentally, histologically
the entire bowel was involved. In general, the ileum was most severely affected; other
parts of the small intestine were also affected, and the large intestine least affected.
Marked villous atrophy with clubbing and fusion of villi was present throughout the
entire length of the small intestine (Figure 6). Mixed populations of lymphocytes and
epitheloid cells with sparse scatterings of plasma cells diffusely infiltrated the lamina
propria (Figure 7) and submucosa with transmural extension to the serosa present in

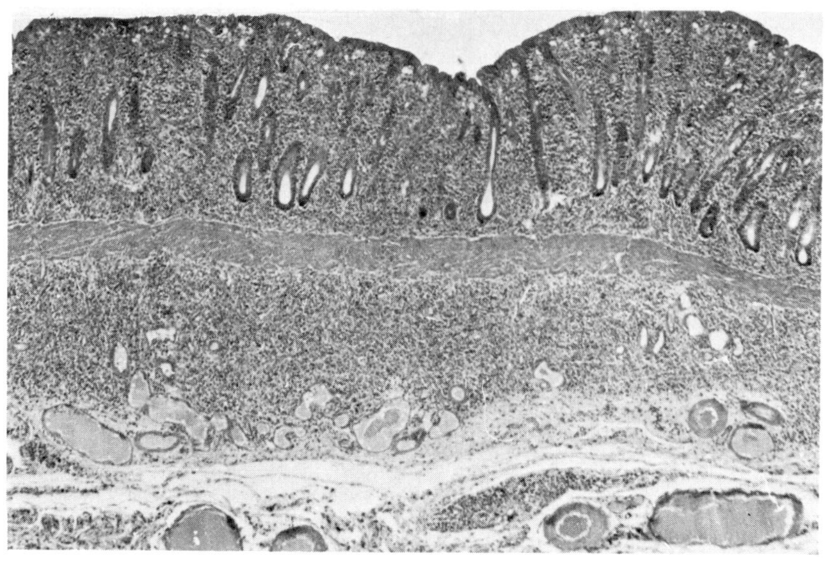

FIGURE 8.   Transmural inflammatory cell infiltration and villous atrophy in the small intestine.

some segments (Figure 8). Many foci in the small intestine had flat cuboidal epithelium, squamous metaplasia, or necrosis of cells of the tips of small intestinal villi. Occasional well-defined granulomas were present in the small intestine. Vasculitis of medium-sized vessels was sometimes present. Edema of the lamina propria and submucosa of the small intestine was a common feature, but varied in degree and distribution. Dilation of submucosal lymphatics was an inconsistent feature. Serosal thickening due to proliferation of fibrous tissues, small vessels, and mesothelial cell hyperplasia was a common feature. In general, the cellular infiltrate in the large intestine was restricted to the lamina propria and submucosa, and was less severe than that described in the small bowel.

The reaction in mesenteric lymph nodes varied from diffuse lymphoid hyperplasia to a focal or diffuse infiltration of mixed mononuclear cells. Fibrous tissue proliferation with extension of the mononuclear cell infiltrate into and through the capsule was common (Figure 9). Histologic changes in the stomach, when present, were similar to that described for the bowel. Minimal to moderate portal fibrosis with a mixed mononuclear cell infiltrate was a consistent finding. The amount of infiltrate did not distort the normal architecture of the hepatic parenchyma, which was otherwise not remarkable. Bacterial, fungal, and acid-fast stains on multiple sections of gut and lymph node were negative.[1]

C. Transmission Studies

Only one transmission study has been attempted. Following the method of Cave et al.,[9] homogenized and centrifuged ileum from a diseased horse was filtered through a 0.2-cm Nalgene filter and 0.1 mℓ aliquots were injected into 10 to 12 subserosal sites in the ileum of each of four rabbits. The same procedure was repeated in four control rabbits using ileum from a normal horse. After 4 months the animals were killed and examined grossly and histologically. There was no evidence of granulomatous inflammation in any of the animals.[10]

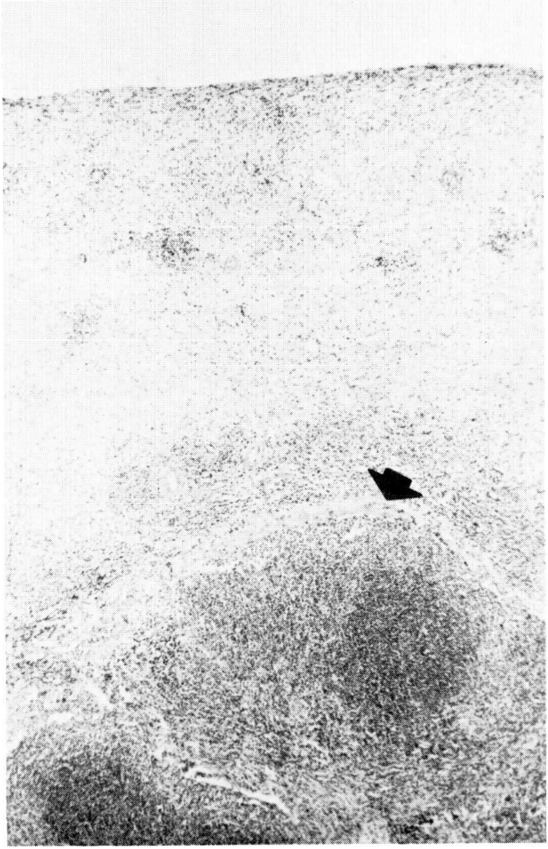

FIGURE 9.   Thickened capsule of a mesenteric lymph node.
Arrow shows edge of node.

III. OTHER SPONTANEOUS ANIMAL MODELS

A. Dogs

In 1954, Strand et al.[11] described a regional enteritis in cocker spaniels that grossly and histologically had features in common with Crohn's disease. Although the syndrome appeared to be a good animal model for Crohn's disease, it has not been described in the breed since the initial report.

Individual cases in dogs have been reported by both Van Kruiningen[12] and DiBartola et al.[13] When examined as a group, these dogs provide good material for an animal model. There was, however, considerable variability between the cases represented, and any one animal had only a few characteristics of regional enteritis. The diversity of clinical presentation and pathologic findings limits their potential for a consistent spontaneous animal model.

B. Cattle

Johne's disease of cattle, caused by *Mycobacterium paratubulerculosis* (johnei), presented clinically with chronic weight loss and diarrhea in spite of good appetite. Grossly, the mucosa of the terminal ileum and ileocecal valve was rugous or cobblestone in appearance. Histologically, mucosal granulomatous inflammation, typically characterized by large foamy epitheloid cells containing large numbers of myobacteria, predominated. The submucosa was occasionally involved, but the muscularis and serosa were not affected. Mesenteric lymph nodes contained similar epithelioid infiltrates.

Although presented as a model,[14] this disease has limited applicability as the gross appearance, inflammatory infiltrates, and etiology make it distinct from Crohn's disease.

C. Swine

Regional or terminal ileitis has also been proposed as an animal model.[15] Lesions were most prominent in the ileum and were characterized by mucosal hyperplasia and muscular hypertrophy. Granulomatous inflammation was not a histologic feature. The disease is caused by a vibrio-like bacterium, *Campylobacter sputorum* subsp. *mucosalis.*[16]

D. Miscellaneous

Recently, Mayberry et al.[17] have reviewed enteric infectious diseases of animals including hamsters, mice, rats, primates, and sheep and their relevance to Crohn's disease. Although interesting, parallels between most of the diseases described and Crohn's disease were limited.

IV. INDUCED ANIMAL MODELS

A. Immunologic Model of Inflammatory Bowel Disease Induced by Dinitrochlorobenzene (DNCB)

This model was produced by initially sensitizing animals (rabbits or guinea pigs) to DNCB by skin painting, with an anomestic response induced by colonic instillation. These cell-mediated lesions induced colonic lesions comparable with inflammatory bowel disease although, morphologically, more compatible with ulcerative colitis. After repeated application of DNCB, delayed hypersensitivity skin tests became positive when challenged by colonic antigen. The model shows that exogenous antigens may initiate a cellular immune response to endogenous antigens, and that an immune response may be responsible for the pathogenesis of the disease in some patients.[18]

B. Experimental Regional Enteritis in Pigs

Kalima and colleagues[19] obstructed mesenteric lymphatics to the terminal ileum by injecting formalin into regional lymph nodes. Grossly mucosal ulcers, reddening edema, and eventually fistula formation were present. Histologically, submucosal edema with lymphoid hyperplasia and round and giant cell infiltrates were present, especially in the subserosa. The authors hypothesized that destruction of lymphatic function with resulting inhibition of absorption of large particles led to chronic irritation and edema. The compromised edematous tissue might be more easily infected by intestinal microbes. The authors felt the model closely simulates Crohn's disease in both its acute and chronic phase.

C. Mouse

Ginsburg et al.[20] proposed a new animal model in mice: studying the effect of thymus-derived (T) cell regulation of antigen-specific, T cell-dependent granuloma formation. This was done by priming A/J (H-2^a lgh-1^e) mice by subcutaneous injection of azobenzenarsonate (ABA) coupled with spleen cells. Primed animals were challenged by insertion of ABA-coupled polyacrylamide beads into the intestinal wall. Histologic examination done 24 and 32 hr after insertion showed granuloma formation.

D. Dog

Intravenous injection of cinchophen in the dog[21] induced ulcers in the stomach and small intestine. Ulcers in the small bowel always lay over lymphoid follicles with granuloma formation present in follicles adjacent to the ulcer. Early lesions showed crypt abscesses as well as dilatation of lymphatics in the lamina propria. Suppression of H[3]-thymidine in lymphocytes and impaired phytohematagglutinin was present after injection. The authors felt the model mimicked many of the early features of Crohn's disease.

V. ANIMAL MODELS INDUCED BY CROHN'S DISEASE TISSUE

A. Mice

Crohn's disease tissue homogenates were injected into CBA and C5FB10 mice. Although no overt disease developed in the animals, their splenic cells showed indirect immunofluorescence when Crohn's disease sera and goat anti-human IGM sera were applied. Complete blocking of fluorescence with unlabeled goat anti-human serum was obtained. Pooled homogenized spleens with antigen-positive cells injected into neonatal mice caused failure to thrive, diarrhea, rectal bleeding, perianal ulceration, and colitis within 6 weeks. Antigen was once again detected in the spleens of these animals.[22]

Normal and immunodeficient CBA and A_2G strain mice were injected in the footpad with both crude and cell-free (0.2 mℓ) Crohn's disease filtrates. Histologic examination between 9 and 27 months showed progression of granulomas in the footpad and systemically with both the crude and cell-free filtrates in normal and immunodeficient mice. The authors felt that the induction of granulomas by the granuloma-inciting agent was not strain- or species-specific and was independent of the immune status in CBA mice.[23]

Kiran[24] and colleagues, although not creating a model, have studied the etiology of Crohn's disease using athymic nude mice. When homogenates of Crohn's disease from either the ileum or lymph node were injected into T-cell-deficient nude mice (nu/nu), the mice developed either lymphoid hyperplasia or lymphomas. Indirect immunofluorescence, using sera from Crohn's disease patients, stained hyperplastic nodes and lymphoma tissues from affected mice, thus indicating that these tissues contained an antigen recognized by Crohn's disease sera.

B. Rabbits

New Zealand white rabbits were inoculated intramurally in the intestine with 0.2 mℓ of the filtrates of homogenates of ileum or colon from Crohn's disease patients. Animals necropsied at a mean of 42.8 weeks (range 12 to 150 weeks) showed positive gross and histologic findings. Gross changes included ileal thickening and crypt abscess formation. Histologically, granulomatous infiltrates or granulomas comprised of epithelioid cells were considered positive findings. The authors felt that these data further substantiated the presence of a transmissible agent or agents in Crohn's disease tissue.[9]

VI. CONCLUSION

Granulomatous enteritis in the horse shares many features in common with chronic Crohn's disease of man. Like Crohn's disease, it is a granulomatous enteritis of unknown etiology. Gross lesions predominate in the ileum and often are segmental. The mucosa may be cobblestoned, thickened, or edematous with linear fissures or ulcerations. Loops of bowel often adhere to each other or to the abdominal wall. The mesenteric nodes are enlarged and firm.

Histologically, all layers of the bowel wall may be infiltrated with a mixed mononuclear cellular infiltrate including giant cells. In man, 50% of patients present with typical granulomas, 25% with diffuse granulomatous inflammation, and 25% with transmural inflammation.[15] All the horses have diffuse granulomatous infiltrates with occasional discrete granulomas and giant cells. In both man and the horse, granulomas and/or granulomatous inflammation may be present in regional lymph nodes and adjacent organs such as the liver and stomach. In both, the liver often shows a mild pericholangitis which is sometimes granulomatous.

Although the disease in horses is different from that in man in that the entire small intestine and, to a lesser degree, the large intestine is involved histologically, recent histologic studies via gastric biopsy show gastroduodenal involvement in as high as 24% of Crohn's disease patients.[26] Recent studies have shown that even histologic sections from a "normal" bowel in these patients may show significant reductions in disaccharidase, a brush border enzyme, again indicating a much more diffuse disease process than originally thought.[27]

As in man, the immune status of the horses seems to be altered, but whether this is a consequence of, or precedes the disease is unknown.

The lack of transmissibility in the horse/rabbit experiment may be questioned in that the rabbits were examined only 16 weeks after inoculation while the range in time for development of lesions in rabbits injected with Crohn's disease filtrates was 12 to 105 weeks.[9]

REFERENCES

1. Cimprich, R. E., Equine granulomatous enteritis, *Vet. Pathol.*, 11, 535, 1974.
2. Merritt, A. M., Cimprich, R. E., and Beech, J., Granulomatous enteritis in nine horses, *J. Am. Vet. Med. Assoc.*, 169, 603, 1976.
3. Meuten, D. J., Butler, D. G., Thompson, G. W., and Lumsden, J. H., Chronic enteritis associated with malabsorption and protein-losing enteropathy in the horse, *J. Am. Vet. Med. Assoc.*, 172, 326, 1978.
4. Hodgson, D. R. and Allen, J. R., Granulomatous enteritis in a thoroughbred horse, *N. Z. Vet. J.*, 30, 180, 1982.
5. Pass, D. A. and Bolton, J. R., Granulomatous enteritis in horses in western Australia, *Aust. Adv. Vet Sci.*, 218, 1981.
6. Roberts, M. C. and Norman, P., A re-evaluation of the D(+) xylose absorption test in the horse, *Equine Vet. J.*, 11, 239, 1979.
7. Bester, R. C. and Coetzer, J. A. W., A wasting syndrome in a horse associated with granulomatous enteritis, *J. S. Afr. Vet. Assoc.*, 49, 351, 1978.
8. Pathology records, New Bolton Center School of Veterinary Medicine, University of Pennsylvania, Philadelphia, 1972—1983.
9. Cave, D. R., Mitchell, M. D., and Brooke, B. N., Experimental animal studies of the etiology and pathogenesis of Crohn's disease, *Gastroenterology*, 69, 618, 1975.
10. Merritt, A. M., Cimprich, R. E., and Beech, J., Granulomatus enteritis in horses — clinical and transmission studies, *Am. J. Dig. Dis.*, 22, 570, 1977.
11. Strand, A., Semmers, S. C., and Petrac, M., Regional enterocolitis in Cocker Spaniel dogs, *AMA Arch. Pathol.*, 57, 357, 1954.
12. Van Kruiningen, H. J., Canine colitis comparable to regional enteritis and mucosal colitis in man, *Gastroenterology*, 62, 1128, 1972.
13. DiBartola, S. P., Rogers, W. A., Boyce, J. T., and Grimm, J. P., Regional enteritis in two dogs, *J. Am. Vet. Med. Assoc.*, 181, 94, 1982.
14. Patterson, D. S. P. and Allen, W. M., Chronic mycobacterial enteritis in ruminents as a model of Crohn's disease, *Proc. R. Soc. Med.*, 65, 998, 1972.
15. Embso, P., Terminal or regional enteritis in swine, *Nord. Vet. Med.*, 3, 1, 1951.
16. Rowland, A. C. and Lawson, G. H. K., Porcine intestinal adenomatosis: a possible relationship with necrotic enteritis, regional ileitis, and proliferative hemorrhagic enteropathy, *Vet. Rec.*, 97, 178, 1975.
17. Mayberry, J. F., Rhodes, J., and Heatly, R. V., Infections which cause ileocolic disease in animals: are they relevant to Crohn's disease? *Gastroenterology*, 78, 1080, 1980.

18. Rabin, B. S., Immunologic model of inflammatory bowel disease, *Am. J. Pathol.,* 99, 253, 1980.
19. Kalima, T. V., Saloniemi, H., and Rahko, T., Experimental regional enteritis in pigs, *Scand. J. Gastroenterol.,* 11, 353, 1976.
20. Ginsburg, C. H., Falchuk, Z. M., Benaccerrat, B., and Green, M. I., Regulation of granuloma formation in the mouse intestine: a new model for Crohn's disease, *Gastroenterology,* 80, 1157, 1981.
21. Stewart, T. H. M., Heteny, C., Rowsell, H., and Orizaga, M., The induction of acute ulcerative enteritis in the dog, *Clin. Res.,* 20, 928, 1972.
22. Cave, D. R., Riddel, R. H., Ford, H., and Kirsner, J. B., An antigen, antibody and animal model from Crohn's disease tissues, *Clin. Res.,* 28, 763, 1980.
23. Cave, D. R., Mitchell, D. N., and Brooke, M. D., Induction of granulomas in mice by Crohn's disease tissue, *Gastroenterology,* 75, 632, 1978.
24. Kiran, M. D., Valenzuela, I., Williams, S. E., and Soeiro, R., Studies of the etiology of Crohn's disease using athymic nude mice, *Gastroenterology,* 84, 364, 1983.
25. Donaldson, R. M., Regional enteritis, in *Gastrointestinal Disease,* Sleisenger, M. H. and Fordtran, J. S., Eds., W. B. Saunders, Philadelphia, 1973, 886.
26. Rotterdam, H., Contributions of gastrointestinal biopsy to the understanding of gastrointestinal disease, *Am. J. Gastroenterol.,* 785, 140, 1983.
27. Dunne, W. T., Cook, W. T., and Allan, R. N., Enzymatic and morphometric evidence for Crohn's disease as a diffuse lesion of the gastrointestinal tract, *Gut,* 18, 290, 1977.

Chapter 11

ANIMAL MODELS OF COLITIS

Carl J. Pfeiffer

TABLE OF CONTENTS

I. INTRODUCTION

The cluster of diseases constituting inflammatory bowel disease in man has assumed great importance owing to the facts that such entities frequently are chronic, are difficult to manage clinically, may become fatal or undergo malignant transformation, often affect the young of the population at the prime of life, seem to be increasing in incidence in some countries, and in most instances have an unknown etiology. The ulcerative and inflammatory response of the intestinal wall, termed variously *ulcerative colitis, enteritis, inflammatory bowel disease* (IBD), etc. appears generally to be a nonspecific response to a large variety of initiators. Some such initiators may be identifiable, such as antibiotics, bacterial, viral, or fungal infections, dietary components, ischemic vascular changes, abdominal irradiation, etc. In many instances the pathogenetic stimuli remain unknown, as in the common syndromes of nonspecific ulcerative colitis and regional enteritis (Crohn's disease), and pseudomembranous or necrotizing colitis. Although there is a limited repertoire of pathologic changes manifested by the intestinal wall, the delineation by gross and histopathologic criteria of several of the specific IBD entities is still possible. Though considerable overlap may exist, several pathognomonic features assist in differentiating such entities as nonspecific ulcerative colitis and Crohn's disease (Table 1). Thus, presence or lack of transmural involvement, presence of granulomas, presence of crypt abscesses, fissure ulcers, spontaneous fistulae, location of onset, and distribution within the large or small intestine or rectum are but a few of the variables that aid in identification of the type of colitis at hand. From the foregoing complications, therefore, it is not surprising that animal models for inflammatory bowel disease would assume great importance in medical investigation, and that no one model could be expected to suffice for all the diverse human IBD entities. Based upon the above complex of human diseases, all of which may be made manifest by colitis, enteritis, or proctitis, and the increasing sophistication of diagnostic procedures during the past two decades, it is not surprising that any experimental animal model would be beset by problems in terminology of the experimental lesion. Is it more like human regional enteritis, more like nonspecific ulcerative colitis, or some other form of colitis?

The practicing veterinarian is also confronted by a wide variety of spontaneous inflammatory bowel disease entities, some of which may closely resemble certain human forms, and some of which may have similar known causative agents (e.g., antibiotic treatment, ischemic vascular changes, colibacillosis, etc.). Others presenting to the veterinarian may have equally obscure etiology (e.g., regional enteritis in dogs or horses, nonspecific ulcerative colitis in boxer dogs, etc.). In general the veterinarian does not encounter chronic IBD as often as the physician encounters chronic IBD in human patients. However, taking into account herd health problems, the high prevalence of calf colibacillosis, swine dysentery and other diseases that tend to occur in epidemic proportion (such as mucoid enteritis of rabbits, various forms of viral enteritis of ducks, turkeys, and chickens, etc.), and that all of these diseases are accompanied by colitis and/or enteritis, it can be acknowledged that colitis is a common veterinary occurrence. The distinction is that the majority of veterinary colitis problems are acute, frequently accompany fatal digestive tract problems, and are not treated specifically as colitis since the diarrhea, water and electrolyte losses, and survival of affected animals requires initial attention. If animals survive the initial disease onslaught, the acute colitis usually disappears with recovery. Chronic colitis in animals is less common than in humans. It was stated in 1965 that "ulcerative colitis occurs spontaneously *only* in humans",[1] but clinical veterinary case reports of chronic inflammatory bowel disease, most of which were colitis, have frequently been published. By 1976, Van Kruiningen reported[2] on the therapeutic efficacy of tylosin, a macrolide antibiotic, on 46 dogs

Table 1
DISTINCTIONS BETWEEN HUMAN NONSPECIFIC ULCERATIVE COLITIS AND REGIONAL ENTERITIS

	Ulcerative colitis	Regional enteritis
Distribution	Continuous, colon and rectum	Discontinuous, entire GI tract
Spontaneous fistulae	Not present	Common
Rectal bleeding	Common	Uncommon
Transmural inflammation	Not present	Present
Granulomas	Not present	Present
Crypts abscesses	Common	Not present
Perianal disease	Uncommon	Common
Strictures	Rare	Common
Shortening due to:	Thickened muscularis	Fibrosis

presenting in a 6-year period in Connecticut with various forms of IBD, including mucosal colitis, eosinophilic enteritis, and granulomatous colitis, entities resembling Crohn's disease, and nonspecified types of IBD. Regional enteritis has also been described in pigs, rabbits, and rats, as well as dogs.[3,4] As described in the accompanying chapter by Cimprich, a granulamatous enteritis in horses, resembling the human disease, also exists.

The usefulness of animal models representing one or more forms of human colitis would be great, and would provide for the study of etiologic mechanisms, healing, reexacerbation, possible malignant change, and therapeutic regimens. Animal models could be derived either from spontaneous varieties of colitis or from the experimental induction of lesions in suitable animals that closely resemble the human malady. As stated earlier, most animal forms of spontaneous colitis are acute and the prevalence of chronic, spontaneous cases of colitis in animals is relatively low, thus requiring the development by artificial means of inducing colitis in animals for practical exploitation of models. The present review outlines animal models of colitis of both spontaneous and experimental origin. Animal models of regional enteritis will not be emphasized, even though human regional enteritis may be manifest in the colon and/or rectum, since the accompanying chapter by Dr. Cimprich deals with granulomatous enteritis, with particular reference to the important equine model.

II. SPONTANEOUS COLITIS IN ANIMALS

In the absence of an etiologic classification for human ulcerative colitis, as well as for regional enteritis, these diseases in humans are characterized and differentiated on the basis of histopathologic processes. Therefore, spontaneous forms of colitis in animals can be compared by the same criteria. None of the spontaneous inflammatory lesions in the colon of animals has had the total characteristic histopathology of human ulcerative colitis,[5] although reports on spontaneous canine IBD have shown remarkable similarity in clinical, laboratory, radiologic, and histologic features.[6]

Many years ago, Stewart and Jones[7] reported spontaneous cecal IBD in rats, an inflammation that was mainly perivascular in location, with accompanying periarteritis and endarteritis obliterans, and marked lymphangitis and lymphostasis. The healed ulcers were scarified and strictures were observed. A large outbreak of spontaneous colitis in Fdc(sw) mice was also reported by Ediger et al.[8] This highly fatal disease featured rectal prolapse and enlarged colon. *Citrobacter freundii* was isolated from the colon of mice affected by this colitis and, in fact, colitis was later shown to be induced experimentally in mice by these bacteria.[9] The epithelial changes observed[10] in the prolapsed rectum showed proliferation and downgrowth, with or without cyst formation, extending into the submucosa or even the muscularis. The lesions closely resembled those seen in colitis cystica in man, and the experimental enteritis cystica in the rat as induced by pedicle grafting of colonic segments onto the abdominal wall.[11]

Other species presenting with spontaneous IBD include pigs, monkeys, rabbits, and horses. The entity in adult swine more closely resembled regional enteritis of humans than nonspecific ulcerative colitis, and was a terminal ileitis.[12] Colitis in young pigs has also been reported in the veterinary literature[13-15] following infection with *Escherichia coli,* and in transmissible gastroenteritis (TGE). Ulcerative colitis-like lesions also developed spontaneously in a group of stressed, captive Siamang gibbons.[16]

In rabbits kept for meat production or laboratory use, digestive tract disorders, including enteritis, have been among the most common causes of morbidity and death. In an international comparative review of rabbit diseases, Mack[17] reported enteritis was a cause of death in 15% of cases or autopsy reports, especially in young rabbits. The disease known as spontaneous rabbit *mucoid enteritis* (*mucoid enteropathy*) was frequently the cause of this subacute, fatal diathesis. Its origin remains unknown, inflammation is not a principal characteristic of the disease, and it therefore does not closely resemble human colitis. It can also be experimentally induced by ligating the large intestines of the rabbit and can be inhibited in such preparations by intracecal injections of oxytetracycline.[18,19]

As mentioned above, canine forms of spontaneous colitis represent some of the closest analogs of human colitis. The relapsing type of colitis, found most frequently but not exclusively in boxer dogs,[20] is of particular interest in regard to human IBD. The clinical symptomology, occurrence at young age, remissions followed by exacerbations, and onset triggered by environmental, dietary changes, or pregnancy, resemble features of human, nonspecific ulcerative colitis. Lawson et al.[21] studied a number of cases of this chronic histiocytic canine colitis. The earliest discernible histologic changes were focal epithelial cell degeneration and acute inflammation occurring along the luminal surface of the large intestine. In advanced stages, the colon was denuded and the submucosa was thickened. Upon autopsy, the characteristic gross lesions were confined to the colon and rectum, varying from irregular ulceration to a diffuse or patchy mucosal thickening with only minor ulceration. The unique microscopical feature of the chronic lesion was an infiltration of the lamina propria and submucosa by large, pale macrophages whose cytoplasm contained much PAS-positive material. Crypt abscesses and pseudopolyps, often noted in human ulcerative colitis, were not features of the disease stages examined.[20] This spontaneous colitis in boxer dogs shares some of the features of both ulcerative colitis and regional enteritis and is not a perfect model for either disease.[22] It more closely resembles the intestinal colitis observed in cattle with *Mycobacterium* (johnei) infection.[20] Features of the canine IBD that are also present in human colonic IBD include cryptitis, regenerative hyperplasia, loss of PAS staining, cystic downgrowth into the submucosa, cellular responses in the lamina propria, mucosal hyperemia, congestion, ulceration, and hemorrhage.[5] In any case, the canine model of spontaneous colitis, and those of other species, does not occur regularly enough to afford a good investigative tool for the study of human colitis. Therefore, at present the experimental induction of colitis in animals offers the best prospect for provision of animal models.

III. COLITIS INDUCED BY ALTERING INTESTINAL BLOOD FLOW

A vascular hypothesis has been considered in the etiology of human ulcerative colitis.[23,24] Transient bloody diarrhea and proctitis have been observed in dogs experimentally treated with cholinergic drugs[25] or after prolonged administration of histamine or the histamine releaser, Compound 48/80. This form of colitis was short-lived, and did

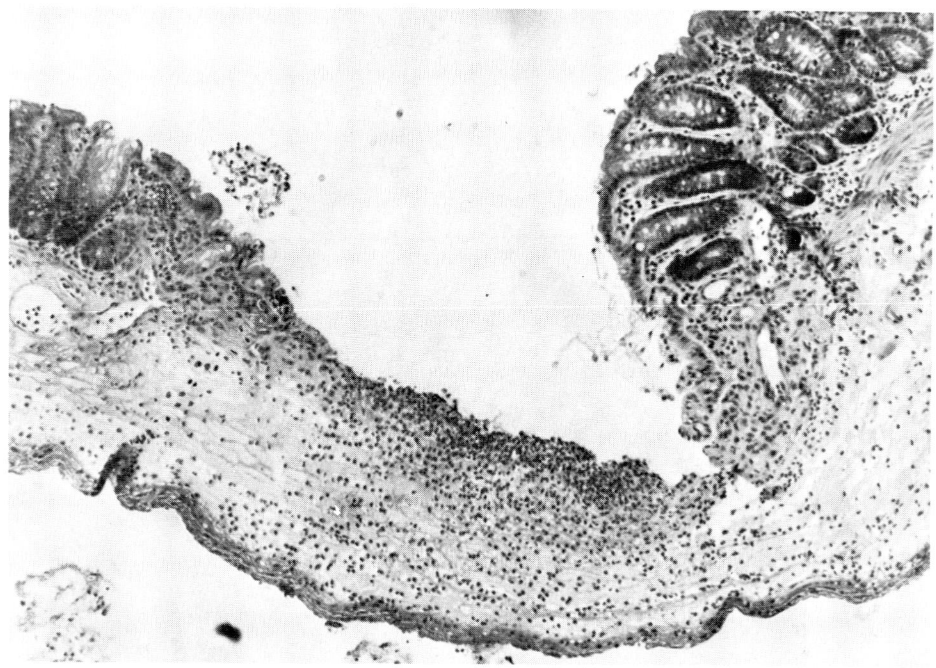

FIGURE 1.   Colonic ulceration in a rat treated with acetic acid, at 2 days after exposure, showing the acute stage of inflammation. Such lesions appear diffusely in the distal colon. Cryptitis is a common feature in this reaction.

not resemble the disease forms observed in man. In dogs, the obstruction of colonic blood flow by mechanical means induced varying degrees of mucosal ulceration, dependent upon the degree of ischemia induced.[26] These lesions resembled those observed in human ischemic colitis, and resulted in radiological "thumbprinting", occasional strictures, and full-thickness loss of mucosa, but a lesser degree of fibrosis than in human colonic lesions.

Experiments in our laboratory with cats and rats showed colonic lesions similar to the ischemic colitis of dogs, following exposure of the mucosa to the chemical irritant, acetic acid.[27,28] This organic acid was chosen because numerous previous experiments had shown that it alters colonic ionic transport and can induce semichronic gastric or intestinal ulceration.[29-32] In rats, the intrarectal instillation or serosal application of acetic acid induces within 2 to 3 days a diffuse acute colonic ulceration (Figure 1) with cryptitis, considerable submucosal edema, and full-thickness inflammation. A diagram of the early acute stages of this colonic response is shown in Figure 2. The lesions heal slowly and, probably in analogous fashion to ischemic colitis, are mediated by impaired vascularization of the mucosa. Indeed, a chronic mucosal vascular defect induced by acetic acid has been incriminated in the etiology of semichronic gastric ulceration induced by acetic acid, as well as in the clamping-cortisone ulcer.[33] This experimental method of inducing colitis has the advantages that it consistently produces a diffuse lesion in the same region where human ulcerative colitis most often occurs, it can be adapted to almost any species, and it shares some features with human IBD. On the other hand, it does not possess the tendency for chronicity and reexacerbation seen in human IBD and does not involve the complex of immunologic factors which seem to be, primarily or secondarily, of significant importance in human nonspecific ulcerative colitis. Colonic motor activity was measured in cats[28] before and after induction of colitis by the intraluminal acetic acid method. A significant reduc-

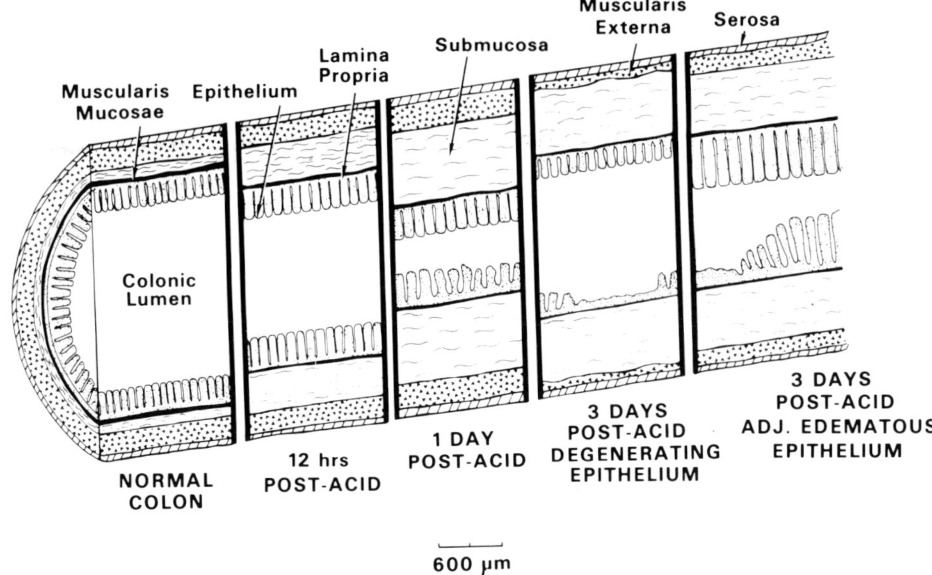

FIGURE 2.   The early sequence of events in the different layers of the rat colon in the acetic acid colitis model are shown in this diagram. Note that submucosal edema is a prominent feature.[5,27] (Prepared jointly with Dr. B. MacPherson.)

tion in both unstimulated and urecholine-stimulated activity was observed 3 days after induction of the lesion, the point at which the animals experienced the greatest ulceration and presented with diarrhea. Within 21 days postacid, the colonic motor activity of these animals in the unstimulated condition had attained a hyperactive state, while that of the stimulated condition appeared within the normal range. Salazopyrin, one of the therapeutic agents used for human ulcerative colitis,[34] was tested in a pilot trial with the rat acetic acid colitis model[35] and was found to decrease the lesion severity after a 7-day pre- and posttreatment period. Thus, this model may have some usefulness in drug testing with agents proposed for therapy in colitis.

IV. THE IMMUNOLOGY OF EXPERIMENTAL COLITIS

In humans with ulcerative colitis, histologic studies of colon tissue show changes analogous to those caused by infection due to established pathogens, similar, for example, to changes caused by bacillary dysentery.[22] Further, the autoimmunity theory (i.e., sensitivity to an endogenous colonic antigen) has aroused considerable interest in recent years since several laboratories have reported that sera from most patients with ulcerative colitis contain a γ-globulin antibody that reacts with compounds of ordinary mucosal membrane. Thus, such patients have acquired a sensitivity to their own colonic tissue. It remains unestablished whether this hypersensitivity is an etiologically primary or secondary event. The colon of the rabbit and dog has been shown to participate in Arthus, Auer, Schwartzman, and mucosal cell reactions[36,37] though such changes have not produced chronic and progressive lesions.[1,38] Delayed hypersensitivity reactions in the colon have been observed in guinea pigs[39] sensitized to 2,4-dinitrochlorobenzene (DNCB) by daily application of DNCB to the neck region. Mucosal ulceration and hemorrhage, mononuclear infiltration, crypt abscesses, depletion of mucus in crypt cells, edema, and perivascular cuffing were noted in the colon of sensitized guinea pigs. This response could be modified by altering the frequency of application of the contactant allergen and by the immunosuppressor, Immuran.[40] The guinea pig, monkey, pig, and man react identically in terms of their delayed hypersensitivity reactions.[1] In addition to guinea pigs, rabbits have been shown to present with inflammatory bowel disease, via cell-mediated immune mechanisms, with the DNCB model.[41,42] The recovery from colitis after discontinuation of DNCB treatment may indicate that the continued presence of antigen is necessary for chronic tissue damage in this T-cell-dependent model.

Nairn and co-workers[43,44] have reported an interesting animal model for human ulcerative colitis dependent exclusively on an immunologic basis. This model is based upon an immunoreactive inflammation in fetal colon implants in syngeneic adult rats. The fetal colon elicits an immunorejection reaction 7 days after its implantation under the renal capsule or in subcutaneous tissues. This is accompanied by perimural and intramural immunocytic responses, mucosal inflammation with ulceration, and immunofluorescently detectable serum antibodies in the rat. The serum autoantibodies reacted with both fetal and adult rat colon mucosa, without cross reactions with other alimentary tract tissues or adult colon mucosa of other rodents or humans. This cellular and humoral immunologic response closely mimics the reactions seen in human ulcerative colitis.

While the cause of human ulcerative colitis is not known, there is no direct evidence of its cause by microbial infection, trauma, etc., and it is potentially caused by autoimmune mechanisms. In some human alimentary tract disorders, e.g., gastric malignant states, there is a reemergence of fetal antigens,[45] so the rat fetal antigen model for colitis may be useful for further exploring the possible autoimmunologic basis for human ulcerative colitis.

Other reports of experimental colitis in animals reflecting the role of immunological processes distinct from autoimmune mechanisms have appeared over a number of years. Asherton and Holborow[46] found anti-colon autoantibodies in rabbits injected with dead bacteria in Freund's complete adjuvant. Halpern et al.[47] injected strains of live or dead *E. coli* in the footpads of rats and induced an inflammatory bowel disease with diarrhea, hemorrhage, and ulceration that was restricted to the colon. Also, Zweibaum et al.[48] immunized rats with *E. coli* and produced an experimental colitis that was similar to human ulcerative colitis in terms of symptoms, site of lesions, chronic course, and histological appearance. Repeated oral administrations of live *E. coli* was found to prevent the lesions observed by both Halpern's and Zweibaum's groups. Colonic autoantibodies were also induced in over 50% of rabbits immunized with *E. coli* derived from human patients with ulcerative colitis.[49] Although colonic mucosal ulceration was not observed in this study by Cooke and associates, histochemical enzyme analysis demonstrated an increase in glucose-6-phosphate dehydrogenase and alkaline phosphatase, which may be an early biochemical event prior to morphologic damage. *E. coli* has been associated with colitis in young pigs[13-15] and neonatal pigs monocontaminated with *E. coli* demonstrated enteritis and colitis.[50] The colitis appeared only after *E. coli* had been present in the circulatory system for a minimum of 60 hr.[51] These animal models in which *E. coli* or other bacteria, parasites, fungi, or viruses cause experimental colitis may be useful in the study of cofactors and immunology related to the etiology of human ulcerative colitis, but there is little support today to suggest that such exogenous agents are a required or independent cause of this disease in humans.

V. THE DEGRADED CARRAGEENAN MODEL FOR COLITIS

Watt and Marcus[52-58] were the initial developers of an animal model for experimental colitis by the feeding of degraded carrageenan to guinea pigs, rabbits, rats, and mice. This particular model has received widespread attention and review. Carrageenan is a sulfated polygalactoside (100,000 to 800,000 mol wt) derived from the red seaweed, *Euchema spinosum*. Its degraded form, resulting from mild acid hydrolysis, has a molecular weight of less than 30,000. This latter product was found to be more ulcerogenic to the colon of guinea pigs and rabbits than the undegraded form when given by oral administration of aqueous solutions. After 30 days of administration[59] to guinea pigs (2 to 5% solution), all animals present with intestinal lesions. A 1% solution is also effective in guinea pigs if administered for 5 months, or in rabbits if given for 3 months. The treated guinea pigs present with multiple pinpoint ulcers and hemorrhages in the cecal and colonic mucosa, enlargement of cecal and colonic lymph nodes, and increased numbers of submucosal areas of lymphoid tissue.[60] Microscopically, there are multiple crypt abscesses in the cecal and colonic mucosa, mucosal distortion, cystic dilation, lamina proprial invasion by leukocytes and lymphocytes, ulceration, and granulation tissue at mucosal and submucosal levels. The lesions are adversely affected by the gut flora, but enterobacteria-free guinea pigs are not free of carrageenan-induced colitis. Atypical epithelial hyperplasia in the vicinity of the ulceration, and pseudopolyps reminiscent of those seen in human ulcerative colitis, are evident.[61] After 5 to 6 weeks, the colonic ulcers are in various stages of healing.[58]

Detailed investigations on the assimilation of carrageenan by the alimentary tract have been undertaken by Abraham and co-workers.[62,63] It was found that this agent is either absorbed by or transported to the cecum and that the ability of the macrophage lysosomes in the lamina propria to endocytose and store carrageenan was closely related to cecal ulceration. Ulceration appeared to be initiated by the uptake of carrageenan by macrophage lysosomes, resulting in release of lysosomal enzymes with damage to surrounding tissues. When macrophage lysosomes did not endocytose the macromolecular carrageenan, ulceration did not occur in the guinea pig.[62] It is of interest that other high-molecular-weight sulfated products, such as sulfated amylopectin[57,64] and sodium lignosulfonate caused similar ulcerative lesions in the colon of guinea pigs.[58] The carrageenan-induced lesions were not prevented by dietary administration of neomycin, although the polymorphonuclear response was lessened.[65] It has recently been demonstrated that prostaglandin levels were increased in colonic tissue and the microsomal synthesis of prostaglandins from arachidonic acid was enhanced in guinea pigs treated with 3% degraded carrageenan.[66] It also has been reported[67] that the number of DNA-synthesizing cells per crypt column was increased, and the zone of proliferation was extended to the upper third of the crypt in mice with carrageenan-induced ulceration. The carrageenan model is also of interest in that carrageenan acts as a tumor promoter in the rat colorectal mucosa, since it has been established that humans with ulcerative colitis are at high risk to colon cancer.

Although the advantages vs. the limitations of the carrageenan colitis model have often been debated,[5] its reproducibility and partial similarity to human colitis make this model one of current usefulness.

VI. MISCELLANEOUS METHODS FOR EXPERIMENTAL COLITIS

Various reports have documented that colitis can be experimentally induced in animals by drug treatment, irradiation, dietary changes, or obstruction of the colon or intestinal lymphatic vessels. Colitis can be induced in hamsters by clindamycin, a process that is inhibited by the cytoprotective actions of 16,16-dimethylprostaglandin E_2.[68] The analog of clindamycin, lincomycin, also is capable of initiating colitis in both humans and hamsters.[68]

In early studies, irradiation of laboratory rats and rabbits caused an ulcerative colitis that appeared morphologically similar to human ulcerative colitis.[70,71] In 346 parabiotic rat pairs irradiated, crypt abscesses were observed in 9% of the animals. However, this model is not suitable for investigative study of human colitis (except radiation-induced colitis) because of the adverse general effects of irradiation on the animal body.

Experimental obstruction by ligation of the colon of the dog[72] or of the ileal lymphatics in various small mammals[73] produced colitis and/or ileitis. Injection of a sclerosing solution into the lymphatics of the canine mesocolon also induced an ulcerative colitis.[74] Mechanical obstruction of the rabbit colon, followed by intraarterial injection of *E. coli* endotoxin, also produced an enterocolitis.[75] None of these earlier methods have been adopted as standard models of experimental colitis.

VII. CONCLUSION

The foregoing paragraphs have been an attempt to review some of the pitfalls, problems, or advantages, of the currently known spontaneous or experimental animal models of colitis, with an emphasis toward nonspecific ulcerative colitis as observed in humans. As is clear, both the human forms of colitis and the related spontaneous diseases seen in various animal species have obscure, but apparently diverse, etiology. Because of their idiopathic origin and the relative low incidence of chronic colitis, the spontaneous animal models are intriguing but problematic for routine investigational use. Of the wide variety of experimentally induced animal models of colitis, none are ideal representatives of the human disease. However, several of the available methods have at least limited practical application because of their morphologic similarity, site of lesion, involvement of immunologic processes, responsiveness to drugs, and ready reproducibility.

REFERENCES

1. Bicks, R. O., The relationship of experimental ulcerative colitis to the human disease, *South. Med. J.*, 58, 1179, 1965.
2. Van Kruinigen, H. J., Clinical efficacy of tylosin in canine inflammatory bowel disease, *J. Am. Anim. Hosp. Assoc.*, 12, 498, 1976.
3. Rechenberg, R., Enteritis regionalis beim Hund., *Staat. Tier Gemein. Bernau.*, March 20, 1973, 352.
4. DiBartola, S. P., Rogers, W. A., Boyce, J. T., and Grimm, J. P., Regional enteritis in two dogs, *J. Am. Vet. Med. Assoc.*, 181, 904, 1981.
5. MacPherson, B. and Pfeiffer, C. J., Experimental colitis, *Digestion*, 14, 424, 1976.
6. Van Kruiningen, H. J., Canine colitis comparable to regional enteritis and mucosal colitis of man, *Gastroenterology*, 62, 1128, 1972.
7. Stewart, H. L. and Jones, B. F., Pathologic anatomy of chronic ulcerative colitis. A spontaneous disease of the rat, *Arch. Pathol.*, 31, 37, 1941.
8. Ediger, R. D., Kovatch, R. M., and Rabstein, M. M., Colitis in mice with a high incidence of rectal prolapse, *Lab. Anim. Sci.*, 24, 488, 1974.
9. Breenan, P. C., Fritz, T. E., and Flynn, R. J., *Citrobacter freundii* associated with diarrhea in laboratory mice, *Lab. Anim. Care*, 15, 266, 1965.
10. Brynjolfsson, G. and Lombard, L. S., Colitis cystica in mice, *Cancer*, 23, 225, 1969.
11. Brynjolfsson, G. and Haley, H., Experimental enteritis cystica in mice, *Am. J. Clin. Pathol.*, 47, 69, 1967.
12. Emsbo, P., Terminal or regional ileitis in swine, *Nord. Vet. Med.*, 1, 28, 1951.
13. Cross, R. F. and Kohler, E. M., Autolytic changes in the digestive system of germ-free, *Escherichia coli* monocontaminated, and conventional baby pigs, *Can. J. Comp. Med.*, 33, 108, 1969.
14. Gika, F. A., A comparative study on the pathological picture of transmissible gastroenteritis (TGE) and *E. coli* gastroenteritis in newborn piglets with special reference to the gastrointestinal tract, *Acta Vet. Hung.*, 18, 39, 1968.
15. Moon, H. W., The Association of *Escherichia coli* With Diarrheal Disease of the Newborn Pig, thesis, University of Minnesota, Minneapolis, 1965.

16. Stout, C. and Snyder, R. L., Ulcerative colitis-like lesion in Siamang gibbons, *Gastroenterology,* 57, 256, 1969.
17. Mack, R., Disorders of the digestive tract of domesticated rabbits, *Vet. Bull.,* 32, 191, 1962.
18. Greenham, L. W., Some preliminary observations on rabbit mucoid enteritis, *Vet. Rec.,* 74, 79, 1962.
19. Toofanian, F. and Targowski, S., Experimental production of rabbit mucoid enteritis, *Am. J. Vet. Res.,* 44, 705, 1983.
20. Kennedy, P. C. and Cello, R. M., Colitis of boxer dogs, *Gastroenterology,* 51, 926, 1966.
21. Lawson, T. L., Gomez, J. A., and Margulis, A. R., Vascular alterations in canine histocytic ulcerative colitis, *Invest. Radiol.,* 10, 212, 1975.
22. Mottet, N. K., *Histologic Spectrum of Regional Enteritis and Ulcerative Colitis,* Vol. 2, W. B. Saunders, Philadelphia, 1971, 1.
23. Fairburn, R. A., On the etiology of ulcerative colitis. A vascular hypothesis, *Lancet,* 1, 697, 1973.
24. Shorter, R. G. and Shephard, D. A. E., Frontiers in inflammatory bowel disease. I. The proceedings of a conference sponsored by the McReynolds Foundation, *Dig. Dis.,* 20, 540, 1975.
25. Kirsner, J. B., Experimental "colitis" with particular reference to hypersensitivity reactions in the colon, *Gastroenterology,* 40, 307, 1961.
26. Marston, A., Marcuson, R. W., Chapman, M., and Arthur, J. F., Experimental study of devascularization of the colon, *Gut,* 10, 121, 1969.
27. MacPherson, B. R. and Pfeiffer, C. J., Experimental production of diffuse colitis in rats, *Digestion,* 17, 135, 1978.
28. MacPherson, B. R., Shearin, N. L., and Pfeiffer, C. J., Experimental diffuse colitis in cats: observations on motor changes, *J. Surg. Res.,* 25, 42, 1978.
29. Okabe, S. and Pfeiffer, C. J., The acetic acid ulcer model — a procedure for chronic duodenal or gastric ulcer, in *Peptic Ulcer,* Pfeiffer, C. J., Ed., Lippincott, Philadelphia, 1971, 13.
30. Okabe, S. and Pfeiffer, C. J., Chronicity of the acetic acid ulcer in the stomach of the rat, *Am. J. Dig. Dis.,* 17, 619, 1972.
31. Okabe, S., Pfeiffer, C. J., and Roth, J. L. A., Comparison of the acetic acid ulcer model in cats and rats, *Experientia,* 27, 146, 1971.
32. Okabe, S., Pfeiffer, C. J., and Roth, J. L. A., A method of producing penetrating gastric ulcers in rats, *Am. J. Dig. Dis.,* 61, 277, 1971.
33. Pfeiffer, C. J., Ed., *Peptic Ulcer,* Lippincott, Philadelphia, 1971, 118.
34. Hazenberg, M. P., Bakker, M., Both-Patoir, H. C., Ruseler-van Embden, J. G. H., and Schröder, A. M., Effect of sulphasalazine on the human intestinal flora, *J. Appl. Bacteriol.,* 52, 103, 1982.
35. MacPherson, B. R., Development of a Model for Experimental Colitis in the Rat and Cat Using Acetic Acid, Ph.D. thesis, Memorial University of Newfoundland, St. John's, 1977.
36. Kirsner, J. B. and Goldgraber, M. B., Hypersensitivity, autoimmunity and the digestive tract, *Gastroenterology,* 38, 536, 1960.
37. Bicks, R. O. and Walker, R. H., Immunologic "colitis" in dogs, *Am. J. Dig. Dis.,* 7, 574, 1962.
38. Kirsner, J. B., Elchlepp, J. G., Goldgraber, M. B., Ablaza, J., and Ford, H., Production of an experimental ulcerative "colitis" in rabbits, *Arch. Pathol.,* 68, 392, 1959.
39. Bicks, R. O. and Rosenberg, E. W., A chronic hypersensitivity reaction in the guinea pig colon, *Gastroenterology,* 46, 543, 1964.
40. Bicks, R. O., Brown, G., Hickey, H. D., and Rosenberg, E. W., Further observations on a delayed hypersensitivity reaction in the guinea pig colon, *Gastroenterology,* 48, 425, 1965.
41. Rabin, B. S. and Rogers, S. J., A cell-mediated immune model of inflammatory bowel disease in the rabbit, *Gastroenterology,* 75, 29, 1978.
42. Rabin, B. S., Immunologic model of inflammatory bowel disease, *Am. J. Pathol.,* 99, 253, 1980.
43. Ceredig, R., Henderson, D. C., and Nairn, R. D., Experimental model of ulcerative colitis, *Nature (London),* 266, 74, 1977.
44. Nairn, R. C., Sarvas, R., Hocking,G., Kovala, M., and Rolland, J. M., Immunoreactive inflammation in fetal colon implants in syngeneic adult rats, *Am. J. Pathol.,* 96, 647, 1979.
45. deBoer, W. G. R. M., Forsyth, A., and Nairn, R. C., Gastric antigens in health and disease. Behavior in early development, senescence, metaplasia and cancer, *Br. Med. J.,* 3, 93, 1969.
46. Asherton, G. L. and Holborow, E. J., Auto-antibody production in rabbits. VII. Auto-antibodies to gut produced by the injection of bacteria, *Immunology,* 10, 161, 1966.
47. Halpern, B., Zweibaum, A., Oriol Palou, R., and Morard, J. C., Experimental immune ulcerative colitis, in *Immunology,* Grune & Stratton, New York, 1967, 161.
48. Zweibaum, A., Morard, J.-Cl., and Halpern, B., Réalisation d'une colite ulcéro-hémorrhagique expérimentale par immunisation bactérienne, *Pathol. Biol. (Paris),* 16, 813, 1968.
49. Cooke, E. M., Filipe, M. T., and Dawson, I. M. P., The production of colonic auto-antibodies in rabbits by immunization with *Escherichia coli, J. Pathol. Bacteriol.,* 96, 125, 1968.

50. Staley, T. E., Corley, L. D., and Jones, E. W., Early pathogenesis of colitis in neonatal pigs monocontaminated with *Escherichia coli*. Fine structural changes in the circulatory compartments of the lamina propria and submucosa, *Am. J. Dig. Dis.*, 15, 937, 1970.

51. Staley, T. E., Corley, L. D., and Jones, E. W., Early pathogenesis of colitis in neonatal pigs monocontaminated with *Escherichia coli*. Fine structural changes in the colonic epithelium, *Am. J. Dig. Dis.*, 15, 923, 1970.

52. Watt, J. and Marcus, R., Ulcerative colitis in the guinea-pig caused by seaweed extract, *J. Pharm. Pharmacol.*, Suppl. 21, 187, 1969.

53. Watt, J. and Marcus, R., Ulceration of the colon in guinea-pigs fed carrageenan, *Proc. Nutr. Soc.*, 29, 4, 1970.

54. Watt, J. and Marcus, R., Ulcerative colitis in rabbits fed degraded carrageenan, *J. Pharm. Pharmacol.*, 22, 130, 1970.

55. Watt, J. and Marcus, R., Hyperplastic mucosal changes in the rabbit colon produced by degraded carrageenan, *Gastroenterology*, 59, 760, 1970.

56. Watt, J. and Marcus, R., Carrageenan-induced ulceration of the large intestine in the guinea pig, *Gut*, 12, 164, 1971.

57. Watt, J. and Marcus, R., Ulceration of the colon in rabbits fed sulphated amylopectin, *J. Pharm. Pharmacol.*, 24, 68, 1972.

58. Watt, J. and Marcus, R., Progress report. Experimental ulcerative disease of the colon in animals, *Gut*, 14, 506, 1973.

59. Anver, M. R. and Cohen, B. J., Ulcerative colitis induced in guinea pigs with degraded carrageenan, *Am. J. Pathol.*, 84, 431, 1976.

60. van der Waaij, D., Cohen, B. J., and Anver, M. R., Mitigation of experimental inflammatory bowel disease in guinea pigs by selective elimination of the aerobic gram-negative intestinal microflora, *Gastroenterology*, 67, 460, 1974.

61. Mottet, N. K., On animal models for inflammatory bowel disease, *Gastroenterology*, 62, 1269, 1972.

62. Abraham, F., Fabian, R. J., Goldberg, L., and Coulston, F., Role of lysosomes in carrageenan-induced cecal ulceration, *Gastroenterology*, 67, 1169, 1974.

63. Abraham, R., Goldberg, L., and Coulson, F., Uptake and storage of degraded carrageenan in lysosomes of reticuloendothelial cells of the rhesus monkey, *Macaca mulatta*, *Exp. Mol. Pathol.*, 17, 77, 1972.

64. Marcus, R. and Watt, J., Experimental ulceration of the colon induced by non-algal sulphated products, *Gut*, 12, 868, 1971.

65. Sharrat, B. C., Grasso, P., Carpanini, F., and Gangolli, S. D., Carrageenan ulceration as a model for human ulcerative colitis, *Lancet*, 1, 192, 1971.

66. Hoult, J. R. S., Moore, P. K., Marcus, A. J., and Watt, J., On the effect of sulphasalazine on the prostaglandin system and the defective prostaglandin inactivation observed in experimental ulcerative colitis, *Agents Actions*, 4(Suppl.), 232, 1979.

67. Fath, R. B., Deschner, E. E., and Winawer, S. J., Proliferative alterations in the epithelial cells of the distal colon of mice treated with carrageenan and concurrently with levamisole or hydrocortisone, *Am. J. Gastroenterol.*, 77, 683, 1982.

68. Robert, A., Nezamis, J. E., Lancaster, C., and Hanchas, A. J., Prevention, through cytoprotection, of clindamycin-induced colitis in hamsters with 16,16-dimethyl PGE_2, *Gastroenterology*, 78, 1245, 1980.

69. Humphrey, C. D., Pittman, J. C., and Pittman, F. E., A hamster model for lincomycin colitis, *Clin. Res.*, 23, 27A, 1975.

70. Friedman, N. B. and Warren, S., Evolution of experimental radiation ulcers of the intestine, *Arch. Pathol.*, 33, 326, 1942.

71. Sommers, S. C. and Warren, S., Ulcerative colitis lesions in irradiated rats, *Am. J. Dig. Dis.*, 22, 109, 1955.

72. Glotzer, D. J. and Pihl, B. G., Experimental obstruction colitis, *Arch. Surg.*, 92, 1, 1966.

73. Kalima, T. V., Experimental lymphatic obstruction in the ileum, *Ann. Clin. Gyn. Fenn.*, 59, 187, 1970.

74. Poppe, J. K., Reproduction of ulcerative colitis in dogs, *Arch. Surg.*, 43, 551, 1941.

75. Berry, C. L. and Fraser, G. C., The experimental production of colitis in the rabbit with particular reference to Hirschsprung's disease, *J. Pediatr. Surg.*, 3, 36, 1968.

Part III
Animal Models for Congenital or Anatomic
  Maladies of the Intestinal Tract

Chapter 12

EXPERIMENTAL ISCHEMIC COLITIS IN THE DOG

J. G. W. Matthews

TABLE OF CONTENTS

I. COMPARISON OF THE EFFECTS OF ACUTE AND SUBACUTE VASCULAR OCCLUSION

For a number of years attempts have been made experimentally to render the large bowel ischemic. Boley et al.[1] carried out experiments in which they ligated the colonic arteries in dogs and also undertook other studies in which either venous or combined arterial and venous interruption was effected. They produced colonic changes, some resembling ischemic colitis in man.

Marston and co-workers[2] adopted similar techniques that involved acute ligation of the common colic, the caudal mesenteric, and the marginal arteries in the dog. The extent of devascularization ranged from acute ligation of the caudal mesenteric artery alone, to subtotal devascularization where all three arteries were ligated at once. Definite structural lesions were produced that varied in time of development and severity according to the degree of the devascularization procedure.

Boley and associates[3] investigated the effects of blockage of the vasa recta with microsphere emboli. Ceramic and glass microspheres varying in diameter from 35 to 100 μm were injected into the caudal mesenteric artery in dogs. This resulted in a spectrum of pathological change ranging from minimal mucosal edema to rapid and total intestinal necrosis, the severity of which depended on the size and quantity of the spheres injected. The larger the quantity and the smaller the spheres, the greater the damage produced.

Using the Seldinger technique, Ranniger and Scheiner[4] injected lead pellets into the cranial (superior) mesenteric artery of dogs and found that the degree of vascular embarrassment produced depended on the number of pellets introduced. If several adjacent intramural branches were occluded, the acute ischemia led to gangrene and perforation of the bowel within 15 hr in spite of collateral circulation.

De Villiers[5] perfused an isolated loop of colon in the dog with Ringer's solution, thus producing anemic anoxia. After 4 hr the normal vascular supply was restored, yet ischemic changes in the colon developed rapidly.

Marcuson et al.[6] produced ischemic change in the colon of the dog after venous obstruction. Acute ligation of the veins alone draining the colon did not lead to thrombosis, but local intravascular injection of thrombin, combined with venous ligation, readily induced venous thrombosis. Marked structural changes occurred in the colon, but there were important differences between the appearances of experimental arterial and venous lesions. In effect, this procedure led to the development of stagnant anoxia.

The present chapter describes a series of experiments we carried out to compare the effects on the colon of acute vascular interruption with the effects of a more gradual occlusion of some vessels.

A. Experimental Method

1. Group I: Acute Ligation of the Common Colic and Caudal (Inferior) Mesenteric Arteries

The common colic artery, which is the first branch of the cranial mesenteric artery in the dog, leaves the main trunk about 2.5 cm from its aortic origin. In order to expose the common colic artery, the spleen was packed into the left hypochondrium and the peritoneum over the cranial mesenteric artery was incised.

There are many lymph channels that drain into a large lymph node just to the left of the cranial mesenteric trunk. These channels had to be divided in some of the experiments so that the origin of the common colic artery could be visualized. When the trunk of the common colic artery was visualized, it was tied in two places and the artery was cut between the two ligatures.

The caudal mesenteric artery can be easily traced as it leaves the anterior wall of the

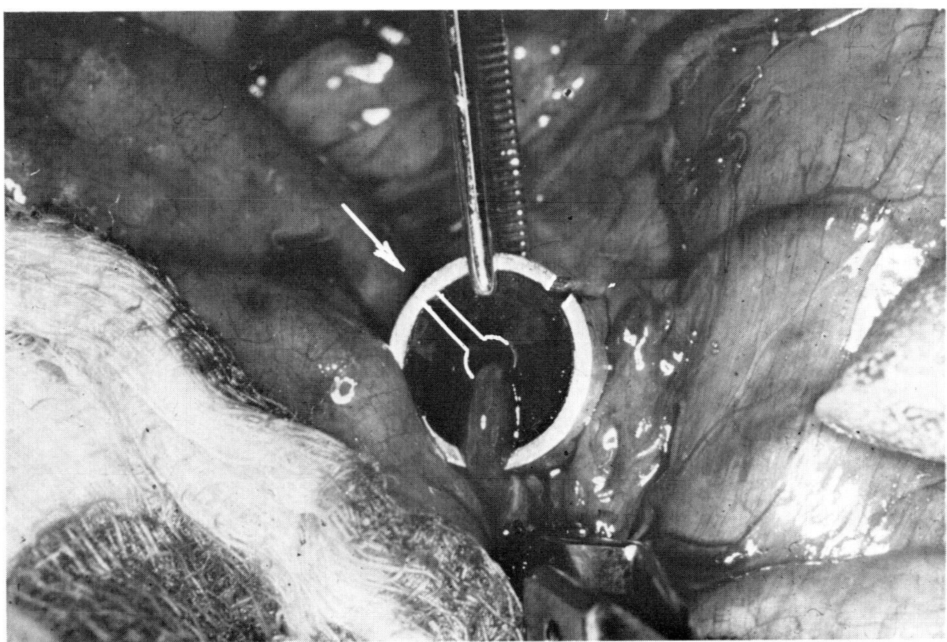

FIGURE 1.   Occlusive device, made of ameroid casein plastic, used for occlusion of caudal mesenteric artery.

distal aorta opposite the fifth or sixth lumbar vertebra. It was ligated and divided close to its origin.

2. Group II: Acute Ligation of the Common Colic and Gradual Occlusion of the Caudal Mesenteric Arteries

The common colic artery was ligated, as in Group I. An occlusive device of ameroid casein plastic was placed on the caudal mesenteric artery close to its origin from the aorta. When implanted in the body, this material absorbs fluid from the tissues, thus causing the ameroid to swell gradually. To prepare the device a 1-cm length of casein plastic was cut from a 12-mm diameter circular rod and a 2-mm diameter hole was bored through the center of the segment. A metal ring was prepared to surround the length of plastic.

After this, a narrow groove was cut in the plastic and the metal ring so that the artery of the dog could be easily placed within the device. The purpose of the metal ring was to limit swelling of the ameroid in an outward direction, thus ensuring a more definite narrowing of the central channel, resulting in compression of the artery.

When the occlusive device was placed on the artery, the metal ring was first rotated so that the artery could not slip out of the plastic, then it was squeezed with a pair of forceps to ensure that the metal ring fitted snugly around the ameroid material (Figure 1).

B. Postoperative Assessment of Dogs

In addition to assessment of the dog's general health, attention was paid to the following:

1.   Diarrhea: this was assessed on the basis of either an increase in the number of stools or an alteration in their nature to a more fluid consistency.

2.   Bleeding: this was ascertained on microscopic grounds only and the dog's feces and anus were inspected for blood.
3.   Sigmoidoscopy: sigmoidoscopy was performed using a 30-cm long instrument. This allowed inspection to almost the splenic flexure in every instance.

C. Barium Enema Examination

Before carrying out barium enema examinations, the animals were sedated with 20 to 30 mg Diazepam intramuscularly, or were lightly anesthetized using either ketamine hydrochloride with Diazepam or Immobilon. When the X-ray examination was being performed in the first few hours after a surgical procedure, the residual sedation from the anesthetic was usually adequate.

Barium was made up using Micropaque (92% w/w barium sulfate). Eight volumes of powder to seven volumes of water, yielding a "standard" mix, was used initially, but a more dilute mix proved to be more satisfactory. Barium was introduced into the large bowel through a Foley catheter.

D. Position of the Animal

The examination was started with the animal lying in the left lateral position. It was found that for complete screening of the dog's colon, it was necessary to turn the animal onto its back and occasionally to tilt its head in a downward direction. As the dog was turned from lying on its left side into the dorsal position, and then over onto its right side, the ascending colon and cecum usually filled with contrast.

E. Method of Recording

The whole procedure was monitored on an image intensifier and recorded on videotape. Standard radiographic plates were exposed to record particular features.

F. Results

1. Group I: Effects of Acute Ligation of the Common Colic and Caudal (Inferior) Mesenteric Artery

After acute ligation of both the common colic and caudal mesenteric arteries, all animals in this group developed evidence of ischemic disease. The interval between acute arterial ligation and the onset of diarrhea and/or bleeding varied considerably. Diarrhea was the first sign in three of the dogs, and a mixture of blood and diarrhea occurred in the remaining two. In the other dog that had bleeding, this was slight and was noted at sigmoidoscopy. Table 1 shows the variation in physical signs of ischemic colitis in this group. None of the dogs died from the disease; two were killed for pathological examination at 72 and 106 hr, respectively, after ligation of their mesenteric vessels.

During sigmoidoscopic examination the presence of fluid feces in the lumen was noted in every instance and frank bleeding was present in three dogs. A prominent feature soon after initiation of the ischemia was the increased irritability and spasm noted when the sigmoidoscope was being passed. Mucosal and submucosal changes were readily noted within a few hours of ligation of both main vessels. Mucosal edema was the earliest sign, but within a short time the mucosa became friable, granular, and hemorrhagic. Ecchymoses and mucosal swelling were prominent features, sometimes observable as early as 4 hr after the vascular ligation.

Regression of the endoscopic appearances was noted from day 3 onward, and within 10 to 21 days the mucosal appearance had returned to normal.

Spasm was common during radiological examination of the large bowel and on occasion this made the introduction of barium difficult. The earliest radiological signs were edema and swelling of the mucosal folds leading to the formation of narrow

Table 1
PHYSICAL SIGNS OF ISCHEMIC COLITIS
IN GROUP 1

Dog	Diarrhea	Bleeding	Sigmoidoscopy changes
1	+++	++	Yes
2	++	−	Yes
3	++	+	Yes
4	++	−	Yes
5	+++	++	Yes
p	<0.005	NS	<0.005

p = Statistical analysis derived using Fisher probability test.

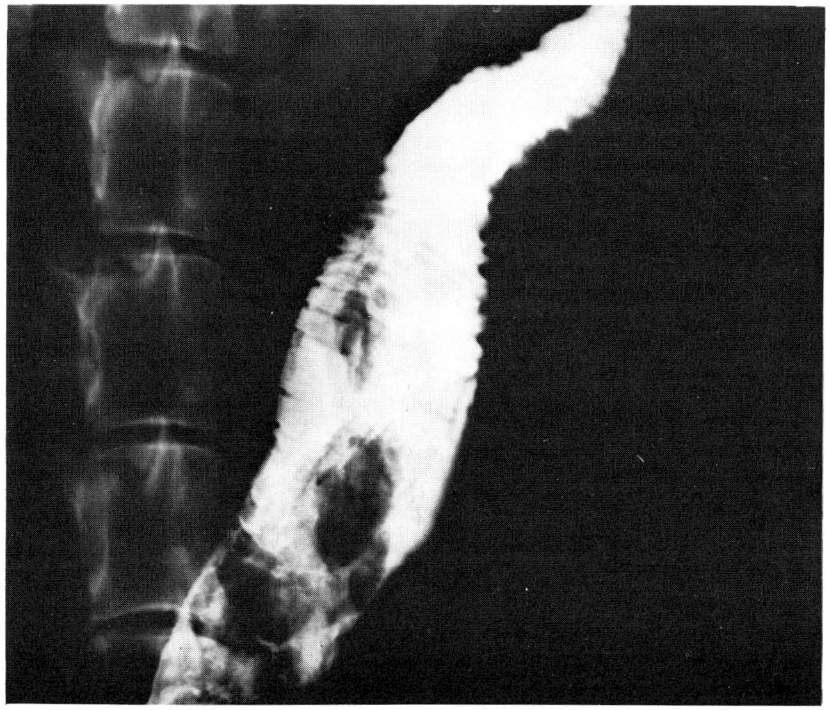

FIGURE 2.   Early radiological signs of the "spiked" or "sawtooth" margin of the bowel.

grooves between adjacent folds which, when filled with barium, gave a "spiked" or "sawtooth" margin to the bowel (Figure 2). These changes were often seen within 4 hr of vascular interruption. Subsequently, swelling of the mucosa and submucosa became more prominent and confluent. "Thumbprinting" was demonstrable as early as 12 hr after vascular occlusion, and definite "pseudotumor" formation, as shown in Figure 3, usually followed within the next 24 to 48 hr.

2. Group II: Effects of Acute Ligation of the Common Colic Artery and Gradual Occlusion of the Caudal (Inferior) Mesenteric Artery

In a series of preliminary experiments, it had been shown that the ameroid device led to complete vascular occlusion within 3 weeks of its application (Figure 4). The

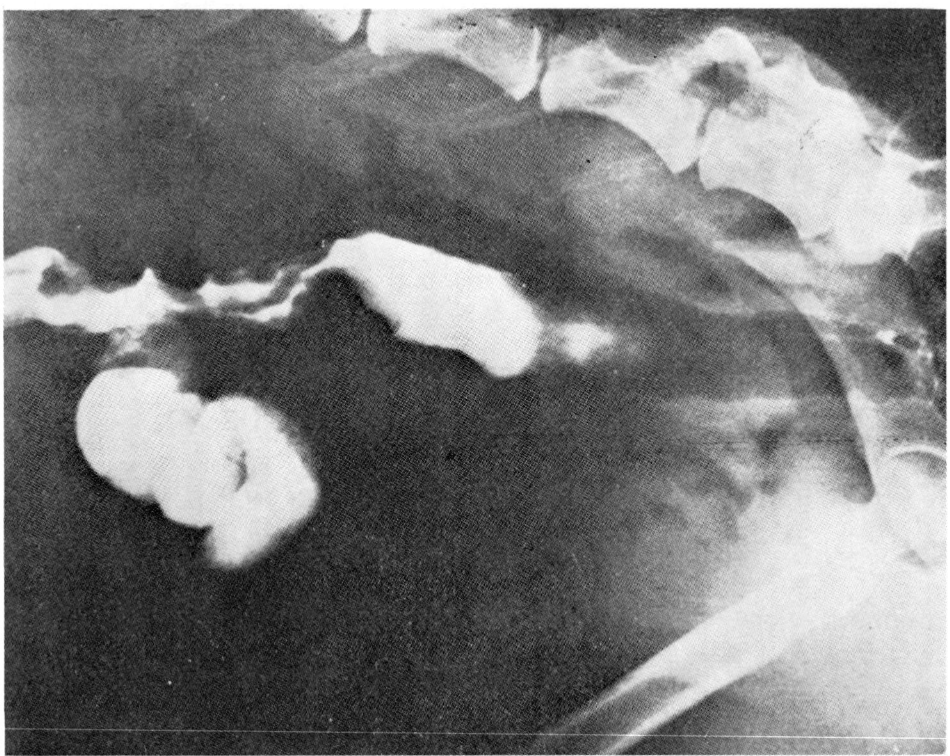

FIGURE 3.   Pseudotumor formation in the large bowel.

dogs were carefully assessed each day and there was no evidence of diarrhea or bleeding either in the kennels or on sigmoidoscopic examination.

G. Discussion

In these studies acute ligation of the two major arteries to the colon caused sufficient vascular embarrassment to lead to ischemic colitis in all five dogs. Marston et al.[2] found that not all dogs subjected to this procedure suffered from this response. In their experiments, sigmoidoscopy and barium enema examinations were performed on days 1, 14, and 42 after acute ligation. It would have been of interest to know if any pathological changes occurred in the period between day 1 and 14.

Matthews and Parks[7] reported that within the first 36 hr after acute ligation of both major arteries, bleeding was present in two dogs and diarrhea in all five. The most prominent pathological features, however, were present between days 2 and 8. After this, ulcers began to disappear and the submucosal hematomas were rapidly absorbed. Marston et al.[2] had previously shown that acute ligation of the caudal mesenteric artery alone did not usually lead to ischemic colitis, though in one case a stricture was associated with this procedure.

If two major arteries are acutely ligated, cellular anoxia occurs before the collateral blood vessels have time to open up. The acute cellular anoxia produced seems to unleash a number of mechanisms that further deplete oxygen reserves. Initially, there appears to be a breakdown of the mucosal barrier so that bacteria and other substances in the gut lumen are able to invade the bowel wall. The bacteria then evoke an inflammatory reaction in the bowel wall and this further depletes the oxygen available to the mucosal cell. Pheils[8] and Marston and associates[2] stated that the size of the occluded

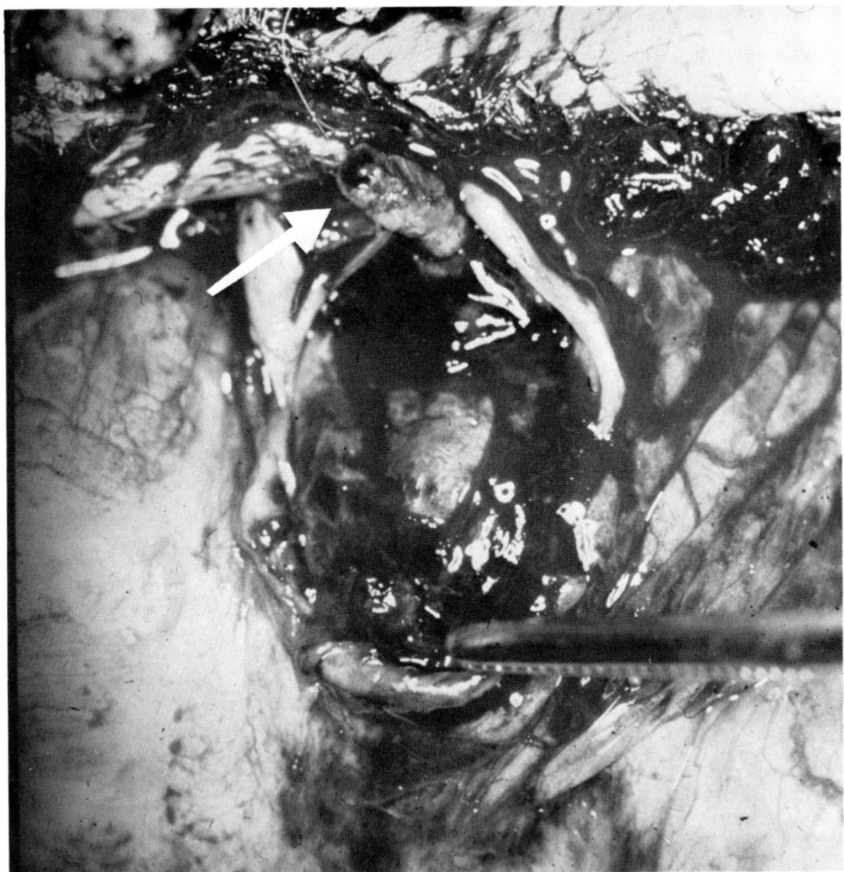

FIGURE 4.   Complete vascular occlusion induced by the ameroid device.

blood vessels, the duration of the occlusion, the efficiency of the collateral circulation, and the bacteria present in the bowel lumen were all important factors in determining the outcome of vascular occlusion.

1. Gradual Reduction in Blood Flow

In man, gradual occlusion secondary to atherosclerosis is very common in the mesenteric blood vessels[9,10] and as the arterial lumen is narrowed, according to Poiseuille's law the flow is drastically reduced. Whitaker[11] showed that with increasing age in man there was a linear decline in mean blood flow — from 120 mℓ/min in the fourth decade to a reduced level of approximately 10 to 15 mℓ/min in the eighth decade.

Matthews and Parks[7] found no evidence of ischemic colitis after acute ligation of the common colic artery or the gradual occlusion, over 2 to 3 weeks, of the caudal mesenteric artery. It appears that the dog is able to compensate for this degree of interference with the vascular supply, providing that the devascularization is gradual in onset. This suggests that the marginal artery is capable of providing adequate circulation to the dog colon even when both of its major supply arteries are occluded. These findings are to some extent comparable with those of Blalock and Levy[12] and Popovsky[13] who, by chronic techniques, occluded the mesenteric blood vessels with either Goldblatt clamps or ameroid devices without any obvious detriment. Similar work was done on the superior mesenteric artery alone by Laufman.[14] All of these workers reported the subsequent development of a profuse collateral circulation.

2. Radiological Appearances

Barium enema examination is very informative in the early stages of the disease and, indeed, mucosal edema can be detected as early as 4 hr after the production of ischemia. This usually takes the form of a fine sawtooth irregularity which over the next 24 hr changes into conventional thumbprints.

There are few reports in the literature of the time taken for experimentally induced colonic ischemia to be demonstrable by barium enema. In clinical practice most radiological investigations of this disease usually take place some days after the onset of spontaneous ischemia, due primarily to delay in considering the possibility of ischemic colitis and, secondly, because of reluctance by some workers to perform barium enema examinations in acute diseases of the colon. Thus, it is possible to miss the radiological evidence for the disease completely. In these reported experiments, all dogs with evidence of ischemic disease in barium enema examination had returned to normal within 10 to 14 days. Spasm of the colon disappeared first and thumbprinting gradually disappeared some days later. Dense thumbprints or pseudotumors were seen and these corresponded to submucosal edema, hemorrhage, and hematomas. No ulceration was seen on barium enema examination.

No strictures were noted in these studies and this was probably because the degree of devascularization on an acute basis was insufficient to lead to permanent damage of the colonic muscle with replacement fibrosis. In experiments by Marston et al.,[2] strictures were found in three animals after acute ligation of the common colic, the caudal mesenteric, and the marginal arteries.

II. ROLE OF HYPOVOLEMIA IN THE PRODUCTION OF COLITIS

From an etiological point of view, the classification of mesenteric ischemia into occlusive and nonocclusive types seems justifiable. Human patients with demonstrable vascular blockage are referred to as suffering from occlusive disease while others without blockage are classified as having nonocclusive vascular disease.

If the bowel is dependent on a diseased vascular tree, mucosal damage may develop because splanchnic vasoconstriction occurs in an effort to meet the demands from the rest of the body.[15] Among 45 patients with acute mesenteric vascular insufficiency, Britt and Cheek[16] showed that 36% were due to nonocclusive disease.

Montessori and Liepa[17] described two groups of patients who occasionally developed the signs and symptoms of ischemic colitis of a nonocclusive variety; namely (1) patients who had major surgery or trauma, and (2) patients with severe cardiovascular disease where the intestinal episode was precipitated by an acute myocardial infarction, severe congestive cardiac failure, or shock. Jensen and Smith[18] mentioned that recent abdominal surgery was the second most common factor associated with mesenteric infarction. The operation being carried out was usually either a splenectomy or removal of an abdominal neoplasm.

The severity of the colonic ischemia in nonocclusive disease may be as great as that in the occlusive variety, and Herrington[19] described a group of patients with complete mural infarction at one end of the spectrum and mild mucosal abnormalities at the other, in which no occlusion was demonstrated.

It has been suggested[20] that intestinal lesions may follow an episode of hypotension that reduces the pressure at the stenosed orifice of an artery, resulting in widespread peripheral shutdown, causing patchy necrosis of the mucosa. These ideas were again stated by Hedberg and Kirsner,[21] who described associated cardiovascular decompensation with resultant low blood flow in the mesenteric vessels. Low blood flow states may be further aggravated by the presence of a large number of adrenergic constrictor receptors in the mesenteric vessels which act to restrict flow to a greater extent, after excessive sympathetic stimulation. As early as 1919 Gessell[22] postulated that compensatory vasoconstriction resulting from shock reduced blood flow to the intestinal mucosa to such an extent that mucosal necrosis could take place. However, no attempt to investigate the hypothesis has so far been reported.

The following study was undertaken to investigate the role of reduced perfusion pressure in the etiology of ischemic colitis.

A. Experimental Method

As in the experiments in Part I, the greyhound was used. There were five dogs in each group.

1. Group I: Hypovolemia Alone

Approximately 30% (about 1137 mℓ) of the dog's blood volume was withdrawn from the femoral artery over a period of 60 min, using a Medicut cannula. The arterial pressure was monitored throughout and recorded with a pen recorder. The blood was collected in polyethylene bags containing sodium citrate and, after maintaining the hypovolemic state for 3 hr, the blood was transfused into the animal again within the next 2 hr.

2. Group II: Acute Ligation of the Common Colic Artery and Gradual Occlusion of the Caudal Mesenteric Artery, Followed 4 Weeks Later by Hypovolemia

In this group of experiments, the initial procedure was similar to that described in Section I of this chapter. The common colic artery was ligated and an ameroid occlusive device was placed on the caudal mesenteric artery to cause its gradual occlusion over the next 2 to 4 weeks. Four weeks after the operation the blood volume was reduced, as described above for Group I; that is, 30% of the blood volume was removed and hypovolemia was maintained for 3 hr before retransfusion of the dog's own blood.

3. Group III: Acute Ligation of the Caudal Mesenteric Artery With Hypovolemia Induced Immediately After Ligation Procedure

Figure 5 diagrammatically illustrates the ligation of the caudal mesenteric artery. The blood flow in the cranial mesenteric artery was measured using an electromagnetic flowmeter before the ligation of the caudal mesenteric artery, throughout the period of hypovolemia, and after restoration of blood volume. The amount of blood withdrawn and the period of hypovolemia was similar to Groups I and II.

B. Results
1. Group I: Hypovolemia Alone

When hypovolemia was induced by removal of 30% of the dog's blood volume over the period of 1 hr, the systemic blood pressure and flow in the cranial (superior) mesenteric artery were continuously monitored. None of the five animals in this group developed ischemic colitis.

In some of the experiments there were considerable changes in the mesenteric blood flow after hypovolemia, but this was paralleled by only minimal changes in the systemic blood pressure. In fact, in one animal the systemic blood pressure (systolic) actually rose from 180 to 185 mmHg, while a 76% reduction in mesenteric blood flow occurred. The effects of hypovolemia on systemic blood pressure and blood flow, as measured in the cranial mesenteric artery, are demonstrated in Table 2.

2. Group II: Acute Ligation of the Common Colic Artery With Gradual Occlusion of the Caudal Mesenteric Artery Followed 4 Weeks Later By Hypovolemia

When the initial procedure of acutely ligating one major artery and gradually oc-

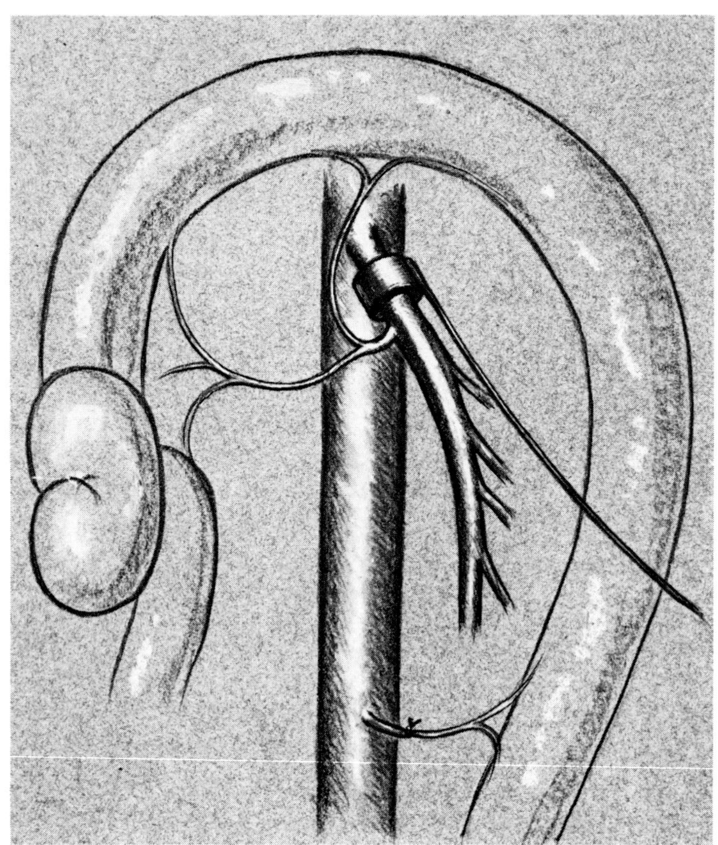

FIGURE 5.   Diagram illustrating ligation of the caudal mesenteric artery.

Table 2

PERCENTAGE REDUCTION IN SYSTEMIC BLOOD PRESSURE ASSOCIATED WITH 50 AND 75% REDUCTION IN MESENTERIC BLOOD FLOW INDUCED BY HYPOVOLEMIA

Dog	Systemic blood pressure assoc. with reduction in mesenteric flow of		% Reduction in systemic blood pressure assoc. with reduction in mesenteric flow of	
	50%	75%	50	75
1	135/100	125/80	25	30.6
2	150/105	150/110	0	0
3	180/110	185/130	0	0
4	150/105	150/110	10.9	10.9
5	130/85	110/75	13.4	26.7

cluding a second was carried out, there was no evidence of ischemic colitis, upon careful observation, during a 4-week period of recovery. At this stage, when the dogs were subjected to hypovolemia, as in Group I, signs of ischemia became detectable within a

Table 3
PHYSICAL, ENDOSCOPIC, AND RADIOLOGICAL SIGNS OF ISCHEMIC COLITIS IN GROUP II

			Typical changes on	
Dog	Diarrhea	Bleeding	Sigmoidoscopy	Barium enema
1	++	+	Yes	Yes
2	++	++	Yes	Not done
3	++	−	Yes	Yes
4	++	−	Yes	Yes
5	++	−	Yes	Yes
p	<0.005	NS	<0.005	<0.02

Table 4
PHYSICAL AND ENDOSCOPIC SIGNS OF ISCHEMIC COLITIS PRODUCED IN GROUP III

			Typical changes on
Dog	Diarrhea	Bleeding	sigmoidoscopy
1	++	−	+
2	++	+	+
3	++	+	+
4	++	+	+
5	−	+	+
p	<0.02	<0.02	<0.005

p = Statistical significance derived using Fischer probability test.

matter of a few hours. Table 3 summarizes the physical, endoscopic, and radiological changes in all five dogs at the stage at which hypovolemia was produced.

Barium enema examinations were performed on all except one animal which had already started to bleed per rectum 3 hr after hypovolemia had been induced. In the other four dogs, early mucosal edema was noted within the first 4 hr of the completion of blood withdrawal.

3. Group III: Acute Ligation of the Common Colic Artery Plus Immediate Hypovolemia

In this set of experiments, when only the major artery was ligated and immediate hypovolemia induced, all the dogs showed marked evidence of large-bowel ischemia, although one did not have diarrhea. However, sigmoidoscopy and barium enema were carried out, which confirmed the diagnosis of ischemic colitis in this dog. Table 4 summarizes the physical and endoscopic signs of ischemic colitis in this group.

The segments of colon affected by ischemia were more confined in Group III than in Group II. The localized nature of the lesion typically encountered in Group III is shown in Figure 6. Although the pathological changes were concentrated in a single area, vesicles, ulceration, hemorrhage, and submucosal hematomas were still prominent features (Figure 7).

The stages noted on sigmoidoscopy progressed from early vesicular formation first to ulceration within the vesicles, then smaller submucosal hematomas, and finally to pseudotumor formation depicted diagrammatically in Figure 8 A to D.

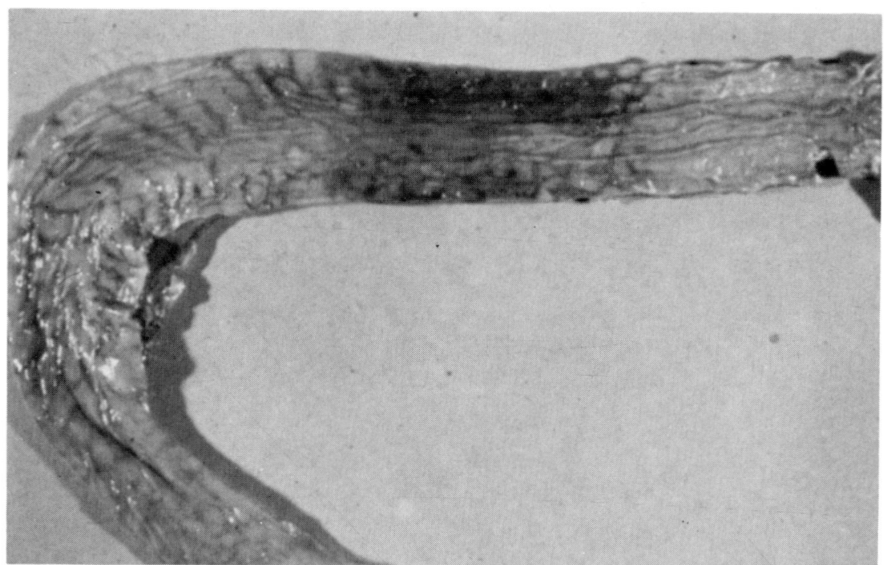

FIGURE 6.   Note localized nature of lesion, as observed in a dog of Group III.

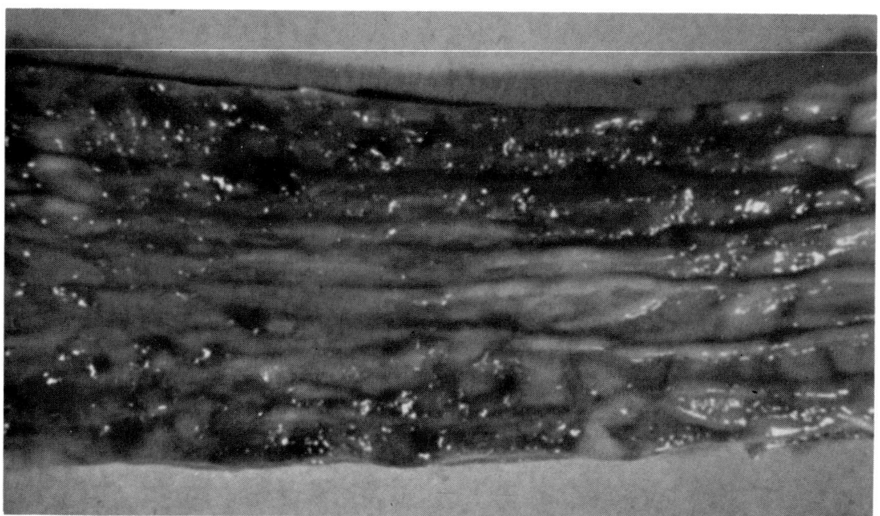

FIGURE 7.   Submucosal hematomas, ulceration, and vesicles were prominent features in areas affected by ischemia.

Within 4 hr of induced ischemia of the colon, it was possible to demonstrate changes on barium enema examination. The earliest change was increased irritability of the colon and this was often manifest by the presence of a stripping wave, as shown in Figure 9A. The spasm associated with the stripping wave was usually short-lived and when the barium distended the colon a sawtooth pattern indicative of early mucosal edema was present (Figure 9B).

During the next 48 to 72 hr the changes demonstrated by barium enema varied with the degree of ischemia. In some instances, when the physical signs and sigmoidoscopic evidence of ischemic colitis were not marked, the sawtooth appearance tended to diminish slowly. Figure 9D demonstrates changes at 3 days in the same animal as shown

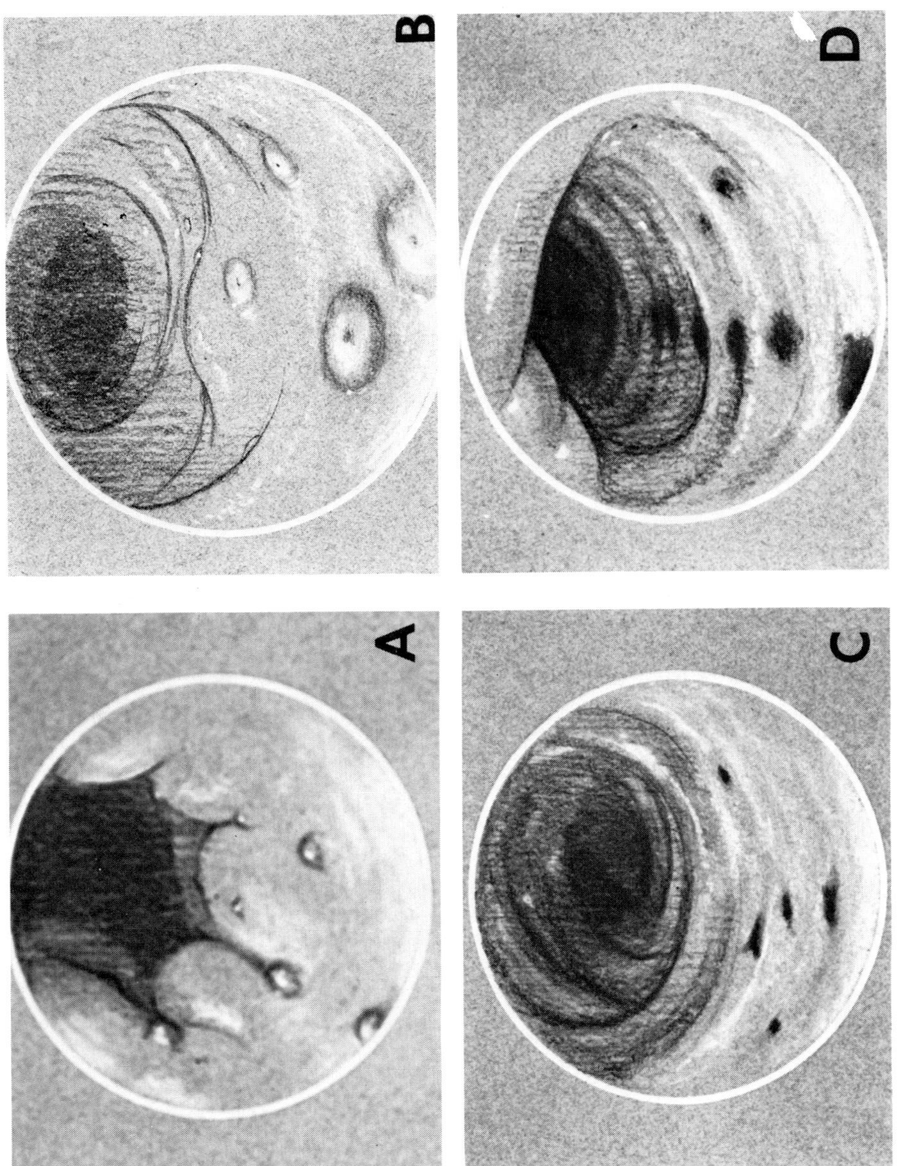

FIGURE 8.   This diagram illustrates the progressive stages (A to D) of the ischemic colon as visualized by sigmoidoscopy.

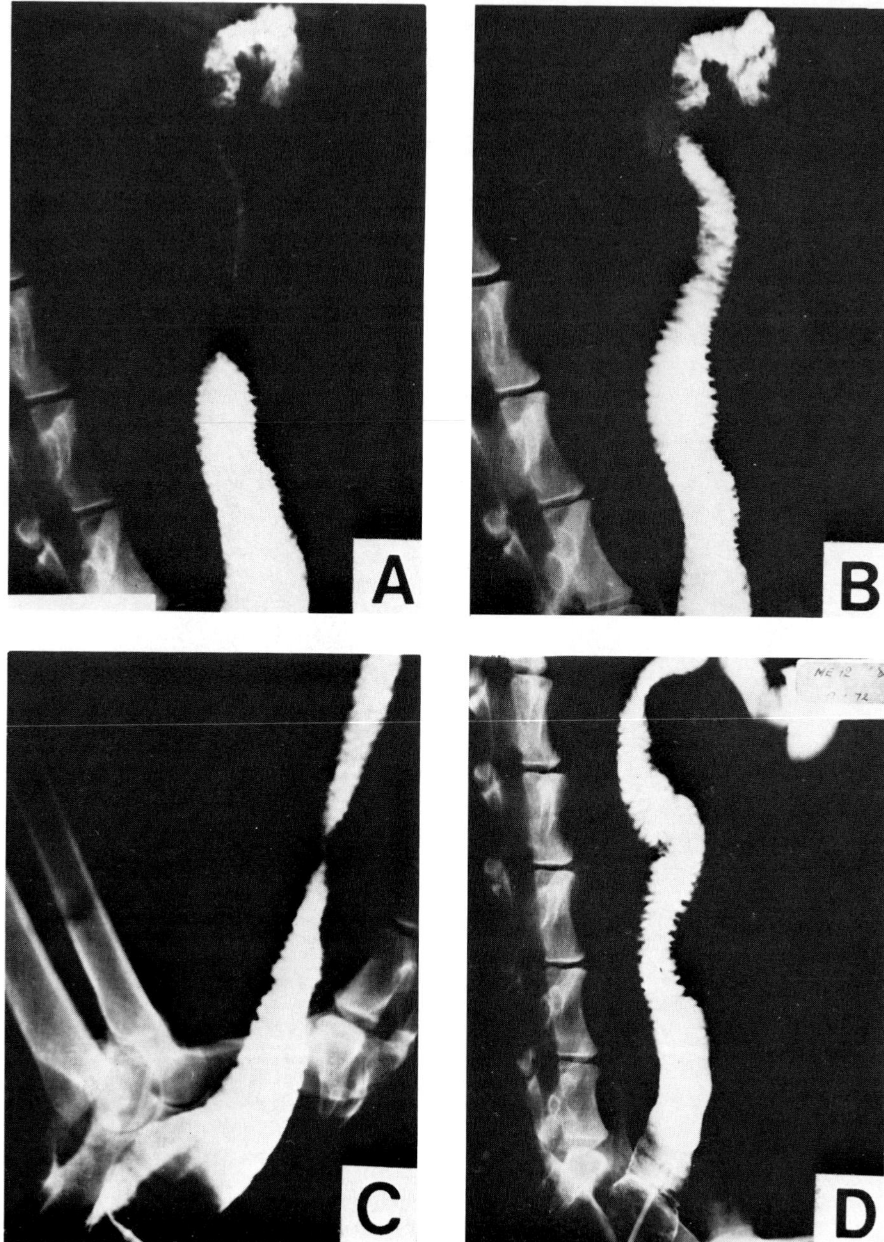

FIGURE 9.   (A)"Stripping wave"; (B) "stripping wave" filling out to "sawtooth" pattern; (C) lower portion of the colon shown in Figure 9B; and (D) shortening of the colon at 3 days, in the same animal as in A, B, and C above.

in Figures 9A to C. One of the most notable features was shortening of the colon after ischemia, and this feature is shown in Figure 9D.

In animals which had the common colic artery ligated, hypovolemia occasionally resulted in radiological changes in the terminal small bowel within the first 36 hr. Among these changes a shallow sawtooth abnormality was consistently featured, and the appearances in the small bowel and colon were not unlike those seen in malabsorptive diarrhea in man, rather than in ischemic colitis (Figure 10).

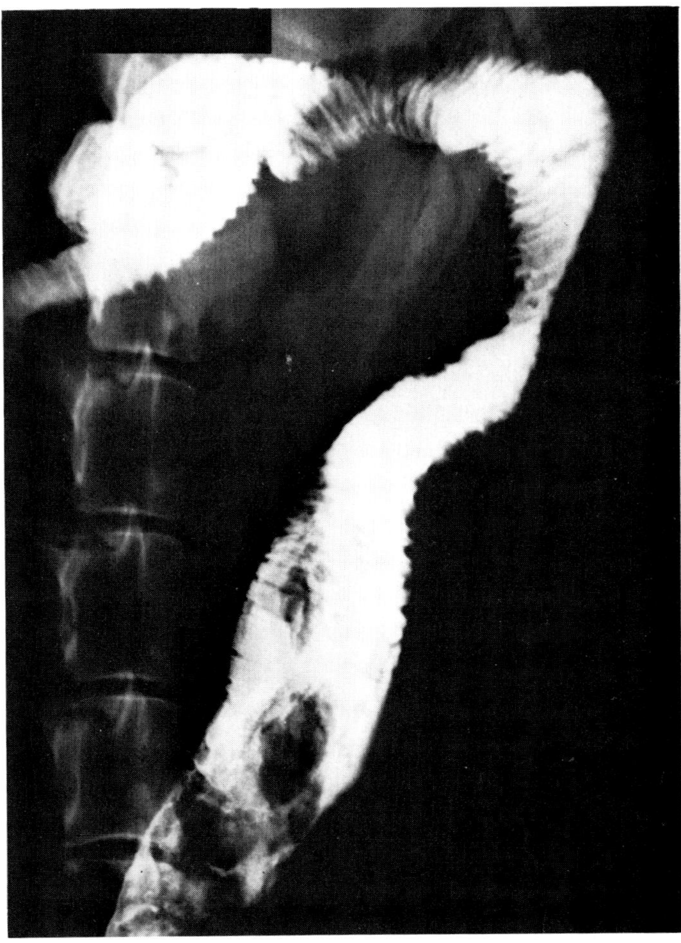

FIGURE 10. A shallow "sawtooth" abnormality was consistently found radiographically in the small bowel of dogs with common colic artery ligation and hypovolemia.

In animals with more severe ischemic involvement of the colon, other features such as the more conventional thumbprinting and pseudotumors became demonstrable. These features were shown after barium enema was carried out on day 3 after induced ischemia (Figure 11). From days 3 to 7 the most marked evidence of ischemic involvement was the development of large pseudotumors with marked edema (Figures 12 and 13). In the majority of animals that had two arteries occluded, the ischemic process induced by subsequent hypovolemia often led to involvement of the rectum. In all of the animals that had barium studies, the radiological features of ischemic colitis disappeared within 14 days.

C. Discussion
1. Blood Flow
a. General Considerations
The flow of a fluid through a tube is governed mainly by three factors: quantity, pressure, and resistance. Poiseuille resolved these factors into a formula to show that the quantity of fluid flowing through a tube depended on the pressure difference at

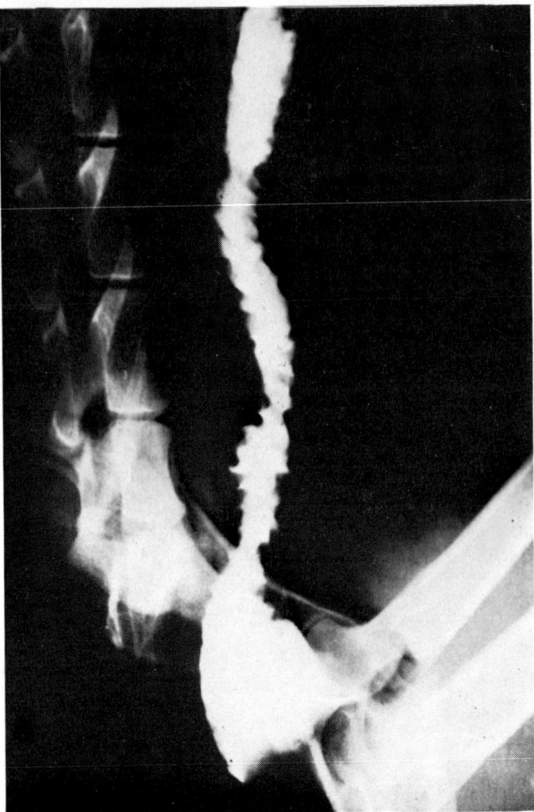

FIGURE 11.　''Thumbprinting'' and "pseudotumors" were evident in the colon of dogs with severe ischemia.

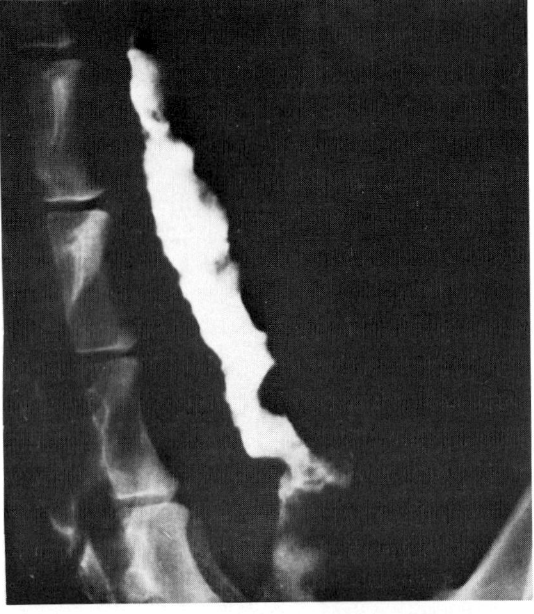

FIGURE 12.　Marked edema and large "pseudotumors" were apparent at 5 days after onset of ischemic colitis.

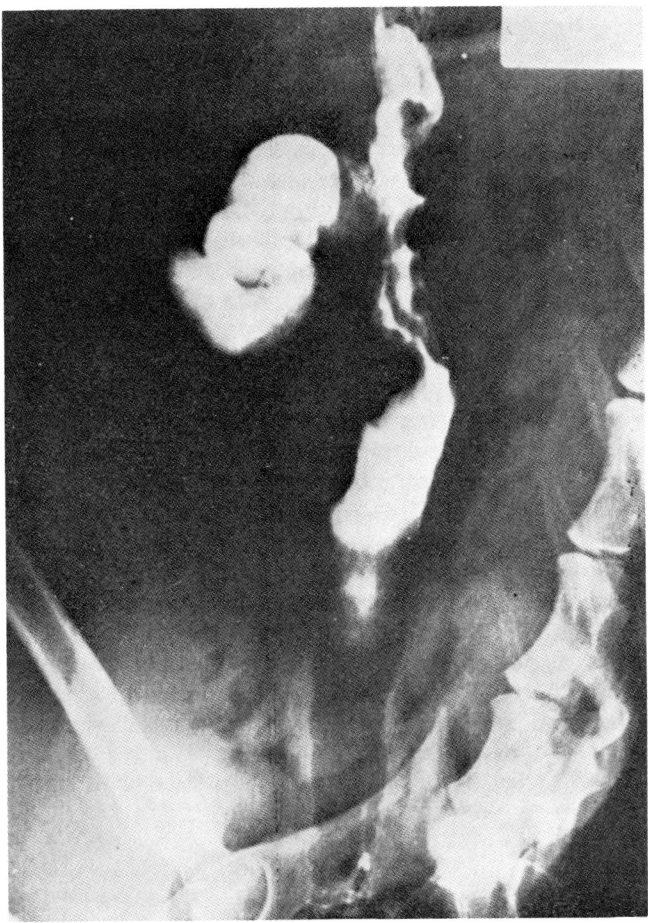

FIGURE 13.   Marked edema and large "pseudotumors" were apparent from day 3 to 7 after ischemia.

either end and the resistance factors relating to both the tube and the viscosity of the fluid. However, blood does not fall into the category of a Newtonian fluid, which is defined as a liquid that does not vary with the rate of shear and remains constant at different rates of laminar flow. Consequently, its viscosity characteristics are referred to as anomalous.

Factors affecting anomalous viscosity are hematocrit, shear rate, radius and length of tube, and temperature. Turbulence is a factor only in very large blood vessels and in the heart; otherwise, laminar flow occurs in the nondiseased peripheral vascular system.

For blood vessels of medium size, according to Poiseuille's law, blood flow varies directly with the fourth part of the radius of the lumen. Therefore, if the viscosity of the blood, loss of energy through friction, and length of the blood vessel concerned are constant and the diameter of the vessel concerned is constant, then the diameter of the vessel is the critical factor in determining the volume of blood flow.[23] Perfusion through mesenteric blood vessels is therefore influenced by two factors: (1) the diameter of the blood vessels, and (2) the activity of natural, distant regulators in the sympathetic nervous system that further alter their size.

Selkurt et al.[24] have shown that the effective radius of the vessel varies with intraluminal pressure and that the important factors influencing vascular resistance are (1) critical closure; that is, at some small arteriovenous pressure difference, the blood vessels close, (2) passive expansion of blood vessels, and (3) anomalous viscosity of the blood.

With low perfusion pressures all three factors are important, whereas, in the middle pressure range, passive expansion of blood vessels and viscosity are important. The chief factor contributing to the continued decrement of vascular resistance at high perfusion pressures is anomalous viscosity. In this case, if the factors affecting anomalous viscosity are constant, then the phenomena of critical closure and passive expansion of blood vessels are of prime importance.

The Law of Laplace states that transmural pressure

$$P_{TM} = \frac{\text{Tension in the vessel wall}}{\text{Radius}}$$

Thus, when the intravascular pressure drops below a certain point, critical closure may occur and the vessel will collapse. Marston et al.[25] have stated that the size of the occluded blood vessels, the duration of the occlusion, the efficiency of the collateral circulation, and the bacteria present in the bowel lumen are all important factors in determining the outcome of vascular occlusion.

An important additional factor that governs the outcome of vascular occlusion is the condition of the general circulation.[26] This is particularly important because, even if the collateral blood vessels do open up, blood must be supplied to them with a suitable head of pressure for adequate perfusion to occur. The cardiac output may drop considerably because of fluid loss secondary to mucosal ischemia, resulting in further strain on the general circulation.[27]

b. Microcirculation

The effects of low mesenteric blood flow in dogs have been described by Matsumoto et al.[28] Their experiments involved the continuous observation of the bowel wall and mesentery in shock. With the aid of a microscope they showed that at preshock levels there was no definite change in the microcirculation. As the blood pressure was lowered there was slowing of the blood flow in arterioles and veins and each red blood cell became visible. With reduction of 40 to 50% of blood volume, arterioles were maximally constricted and flow became very slow, the venules were full, and the cells were rolling or striking against the walls. Platelet aggregates were seen and they lodged at bifurcations of blood vessels, occluding the flow.

In earlier work, Grayson and Mendel[29] showed that in low-flow states in the mesenteric circulation there was stagnation in capillaries with distension at the venous end, in effect causing vascular obstruction and subsequent pooling of blood. In the present studies, small microthromboses occurred in the blood vessels of the lamina propria and this vascular interruption tended to initiate a process of ulceration with considerable inflammatory infiltrate. These findings are similar to those of Rosati and Augur[30] who described multiple fibrin thrombi in the capillaries and venules of the lamina propria and submucosa in a patient with ischemic enterocolitis secondary to the effects of pheochromocytoma.

In the second group of animals, in which the blood volume was reduced 4 weeks after the acute ligation of the common colic artery and the gradual occlusion of the caudal mesenteric artery, all five animals developed signs of ischemic colitis. Before blood flow was reduced by hypovolemia there was sufficient perfusion of the colon to keep it healthy and there were no signs of large-bowel ischemia. However, the further encroachment caused by hypovolemia on an already impaired circulation was sufficient to cause ischemic disease in every instance.

As described above, thrombosis occurs with low-flow states and microvascular thrombosis was a common pathological entity associated with the formation of vesicles and their subsequent ulceration and hemorrhage.[31]

In experimental work with dogs, Hardaway and McKay[32] demonstrated that a bleeding tendency always accompanied the episode of intravascular clotting, due to the appearance of a circulating anticoagulant such as heparin and a drop in circulating fibrinogen and platelets that have been already used up in the thrombotic process. Vascular blockage followed by bleeding, as occurs in the process of infarction, was clearly seen in the formation of ulcers in the present studies.

Low blood flow states may have a similar effect on the microvasculature as that produced by injecting microspheres into the caudal mesenteric artery of dogs.[3] In low blood flow states, as described above,[28] it was reported that platelet aggregates lodged at the bifurcations of blood vessels occluding the flow. If enough blood vessels are blocked then, logically, the most dependent part of the bowel wall — namely, the mucosa — will have insufficient oxygen and ischemia occurs. When microspheres were injected in experiments by Boley et al.[3] and Ranniger and Scheiner,[4] the microspheres lodged at the bifurcation of blood vessels. The latter authors showed that the important factor in producing ischemic disease is the quantity of microspheres injected. This is not surprising, as the microspheres must have effectively blocked most of the blood vessels in the bowel wall, resulting in hemorrhage, ulceration, and infarction.

The severe effects of the combined procedure of acute ligation of one major artery and immediate hypovolemia may be explained on the basis of acute limitation of blood flow resulting in severe impairment of perfusion through the marginal artery. The ligation of both major arteries, however, may lead to a more moderate impairment of cell function, since the integrity of the colon is maintained by the efficient marginal artery which still has a sufficient blood flow supplied by a healthy circulation.

REFERENCES

1. Boley, S. J., Schwartz, S., Lash, J., and Sternhill, V., Reversible vascular occlusion of the colon, *Surg. Gynecol. Obstet.*, 116, 53, 1963.
2. Marston, A., Marcuson, R. W., Chapman, M., and Arthur, J. F., Experimental study of devascularisation of the colon, *Gut*, 10, 121, 1969.
3. Boley, S. J., Krieger, H., Schultz, L., Robinson, K., Siew, F. P., Allen, A. C., and Schwartz, S., Experimental aspects of peripheral vascular occlusion of the intestine, *Surg. Gynecol. Obstet.*, 121, 789, 1965.
4. Ranniger, K. and Scheiner, D. L., Experimental bowel ischaemia, *Arch. Surg.*, 95, 768, 1967.
5. de Villiers, D. R., Ischaemia of the colon; an experimental study, *Br. J. Surg.*, 53, 497, 1966.
6. Marcuson, R. W., Stewart, J. O., and Marston, A., Experimental venous lesions of the colon, *Gut*, 13, 1, 1972.
7. Matthews, J. G. W. and Parks, T. G., Ischaemic colitis in the experimental animal. I. Comparison of the effects of acute and subacute vascular occlusion, *Gut*, 17, 671, 1976.
8. Pheils, M. T., Ischaemic colitis, *Med. J. Aust.*, 2, 715, 1969.
9. Griffiths, J. D., Surgical anatomy of the blood supply of the distal colon, *Ann. R. Coll. Surg.*, 19, 241, 1956.
10. Knoepp, L. F., Jr., Travieso, C. R., Jr., and Hanley, P. H., Spontaneous gangrene of the colon, with emphasis on the left colon, *South. Med. J.*, 63, 1072, 1970.
11. Whitaker, B. L., Observations on the blood flow in the interior mesenteric arterial system, and healing of colonic anastomoses, *Ann. R. Coll. Surg., Engl.*, 43, 89, 1968.
12. Blalock, A. and Levy, S. E., Gradual complete occlusion of the celiac axis, the superior and inferior mesenteric arteries, with survival of animals; effects of ischemia on blood pressure, *Surgery*, 5, 175, 1939.
13. Popovsky, J., Gradual occlusion of mesenteric vessels with ameroid clamp, *Arch. Surg.*, 92, 202, 1966.

14. Laufman, H., Gradual occlusion of the mesenteric vessels, *Surgery,* 13, 406, 1943.
15. Williams, L. F., Jr., Anastasia, L. F., Hasiotis, C. A., Bosniak, M. A., and Byrne, J. J., Nonocclusive mesenteric infarction, *Am. J. Surg.,* 114, 376, 1967.
16. Britt, L. G. and Cheek, R. C., Nonocclusive mesenteric vascular disease; clinical and experimental observations, *Ann. Surg.,* 169, 704, 1969.
17. Montessori, G. and Liepa, E. V., Ischemic colitis, *Can. Med. Assoc. J.,* 102, 377, 1970.
18. Jensen, C. B. and Smith, G. A., A clinical study of 51 cases of mesenteric infarction, *Surgery,* 40, 930, 1956.
19. Herrington, J. L., Jr., Multiple focal necrosis of the colon in the absence of occlusion of the mesenteric blood supply, *Am. J. Surg.,* 110, 981, 1965.
20. Anon., Patterns of intestinal ischaemia (leading article), *Lancet,* 2, 1222, 1964.
21. Hedberg, C. A. and Kirsner, J. B., Mesenteric vascular insufficiency. Editorial, *Ann. Intern. Med.,* 63, 535, 1965.
22. Gessell, R., Studies on the submaxillary gland. V. An automatically filling and recording spirometer, *Am. J. Physiol.,* 47, 507, 1919.
23. Derrick, J. R., Pollard, H. S., and Moore, R. M., The pattern of arteriosclerotic narrowing of the celiac and superior mesenteric arteries, *Ann. Surg.,* 149, 684, 1959.
24. Selkurt, E. E., Scibetta, M. P., and Cull, T. E., Hemodynamics of intestinal circulation, *Circ. Res.,* 6, 92, 1958.
25. Marston, A., Pheils, M. T., Thomas, M. L., and Morson, B. C., Ischaemic colitis, *Gut,* 7, 1, 1966.
26. Russell, J. Y. W., Inferior mesenteric vascular occlusion, *Br. J. Surg.,* 37, 321, 1950.
27. Marston, A., Vascular disorders of the colon, *Acta Chir. Belg.,* 66(Suppl. 2), 80, 1967.
28. Matsumoto, T., Hardaway, R. M., and McClain, J. E., Microcirculation in hemorrhagic shock with relationship to blood pressure, *Arch. Surg.,* 95, 911, 1967.
29. Grayson, J. and Mendel, D., The effects of haemorrhage and shock on the splanchnic circulation, in *Physiology of the Splanchnic Circulation,* Grayson, J. and Mendel, D., Eds., Edward Arnold, London, 1965, 114.
30. Rosati, L. A. and Augur, N. A., Jr., Ischemic enterocolitis in pheochromocytoma, *Gastroenterology,* 60, 581, 1971.
31. Matthews, J. G. W. and Parks, T. G., Ischaemic colitis in the experimental animal. II. Role of hypovolaemia in the production of the disease, *Gut,* 17, 677, 1976.
32. Hardaway, R. M. and McKay, D. G., Pseudomembranous enterocolitis, *Arch. Surg.,* 78, 446, 1956.

Chapter 13

MURINE MODELS FOR CONGENITAL MEGACOLON: HIRSCHSPRUNG'S DISEASE

J. D. Wood and Helen J. Cooke

TABLE OF CONTENTS

I. INTRODUCTION

Megacolon is the prominent characteristic of Hirschsprung's disease. In humans with this disease, the colon is distended proximal to a constricted rectosigmoid segment. The megacolon is attributed entirely to failure of propulsion of colonic contents through the terminal constricted segment, because all symptoms of Hirschsprung's disease disappear after colostomy or resection of the narrowed segment. Congenital absence or reduction in the number of enteric ganglion cells in the constricted segment underlies the pathophysiology of the disease. Hirschsprung's disease is usually suspected in cases of megacolon during early childhood; nevertheless, large intestinal obstruction and megacolon in which histologic appearance of the enteric nervous system is normal has been reported.[1] This neonatal form of megacolon is associated with atony of the bowel and absence of bowel sounds in contrast to increased sounds of motor activity in Hirschsprung's disease.

Acquired megacolon and enteromegaly at higher levels of the gastrointestinal tract also often are associated with ganglion cell aplasia in both children and adults. The acquired form may result from toxic damage to the enteric neurons by chemical agents;[2] it may occur secondary to immunological changes associated with small-cell carcinoma of the lung,[3] or with immunological changes associated with parasitic infection with *Trypanosoma cruzi* (Chagas' disease).[4,5] The prominent pathology in both the congenital and the acquired forms of the disease is luminal distension and muscular hypertrophy proximal to an obstructive, constricted segment that is devoid of ganglion cells.

The principal investigative work aimed at understanding the pathophysiology of Hirschsprung's disease has been done on animal models in which aganglionic megacolon was induced experimentally and on a mouse model in which the aganglionosis is congenital. Attempts have been made to produce aganglionosis in dogs by perfusion of the intestinal vasculature with hypoxic saline solution.[6] Similar attempts in rodents involved placing mercuric chloride in the intestinal lumen,[7] serosal treatment with surfactants such as benzalkonium chloride,[8] and by intraperitoneal administration of quinacrine.[9] Spontaneously occurring megacolon has been reported in swine; however, the etiology and pathophysiology of the disease is inconsistent with these animals being useful models for Hirschsprung's disease.[10-12] The best-confirmed and most thoroughly studied animal model for congenital megacolon is the piebald mouse. These mice inherit aganglionic megacolon as a recessive genetic trait and have symptoms that are similar in many respects to Hirschsprung's disease. The characteristics of the mouse model, along with the similarities and differences between the model and the human disease, will be the subject of the remainder of this chapter. This chapter is a more comprehensive and updated version of an earlier review by the principal author.[13]

II. HISTORY OF THE MURINE MODEL

Congenital megacolon in mice was reported first by two different laboratories in Australia, and later in America. Derrick and St. George-Granbauer[14] in 1957 reported megacolon in mice with characteristics of Hirschsprung's disease. Bielschowski and Schofield[15] described in 1960 a megacolon that was genetically related and associated with deficiency of fur pigmentation characteristic of the piebald (S/S) NYZ strain. Six years later, Lane[16] reported the appearance at the Jackson Laboratories in Bar Harbor, Maine of two autosomal recessive spotting genes, both of which produced phenotypes with reduced pigmentation in the fur and decreased numbers of ganglion cells in the distal large intestine. She named one of these strains "piebald-lethal" and the other "lethal-spotting".

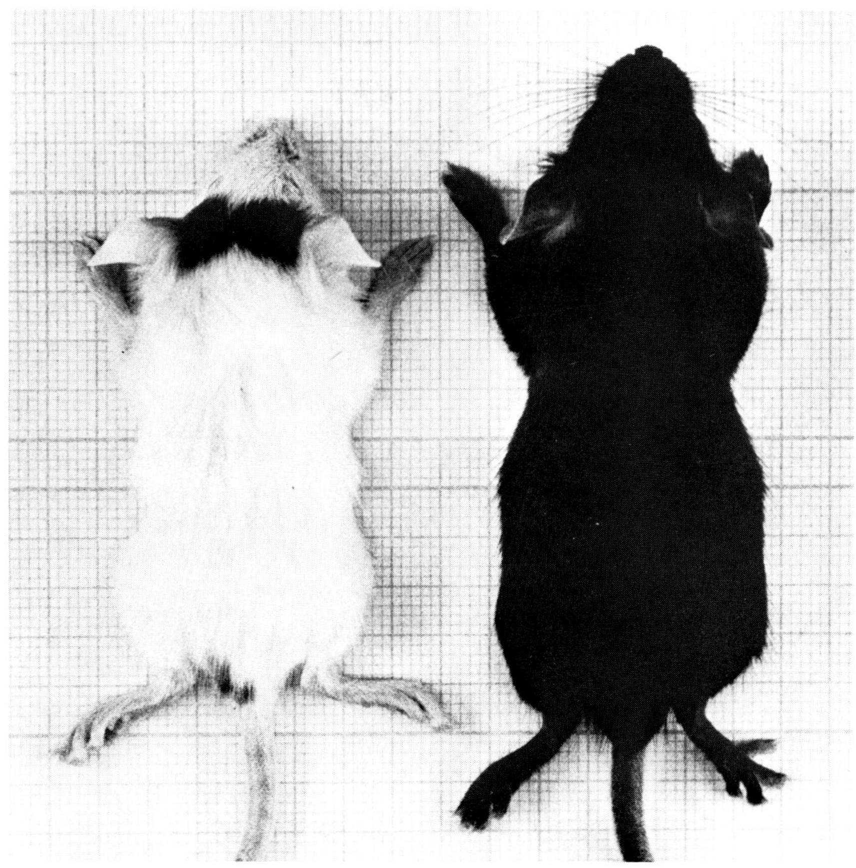

FIGURE 1.   Piebald mouse (left) and normal littermates at 24 days of age. Scale: 5 mm per large division. (From Wood, J. P., in *Spontaneous Animal Models of Human Disease,* Andrews, E. J., Ward, B. G., and Altman, N. H., Eds., Academic Press, New York, 1979, 29. With permission.)

III. GROSS CHARACTERISTICS OF THE MODEL

The homozygotes ($S^L S^L$) of the piebald lethal strain (S^L) have black eyes and white fur with an occasional patch of black pigment (Figure 1). These animals always develop megacolon (Figure 2) and die at ages ranging from a few days to several months, with median age of death at 24 days. Both the heterozygous parents and siblings have black eyes and black coat color. The lack of pigmentation permits identification at 1 or 2 days of age of the mice that will develop fecal stasis and megacolon. Piebald-lethal mice seldom survive to reproductive age, and therefore it is necessary to obtain diseased individuals by breeding heterozygous parents. The ratio of piebald to normal mice from these pairings always approximates 1:4.

The lethal spotting strain (L^s) is obtained from heterozygous parents with speckled brown coat color. The abnormal homozygous offspring ($L^s L^s$) have spotted fur with much more pigmentation than the piebald-lethal strain, and they develop megacolon. Lethal-spotted homozygotes survive longer than the piebald-lethal mice and can breed and reproduce before they die from the complications of their genetic make-up. The offspring from these homozygous crosses all develop megacolon.

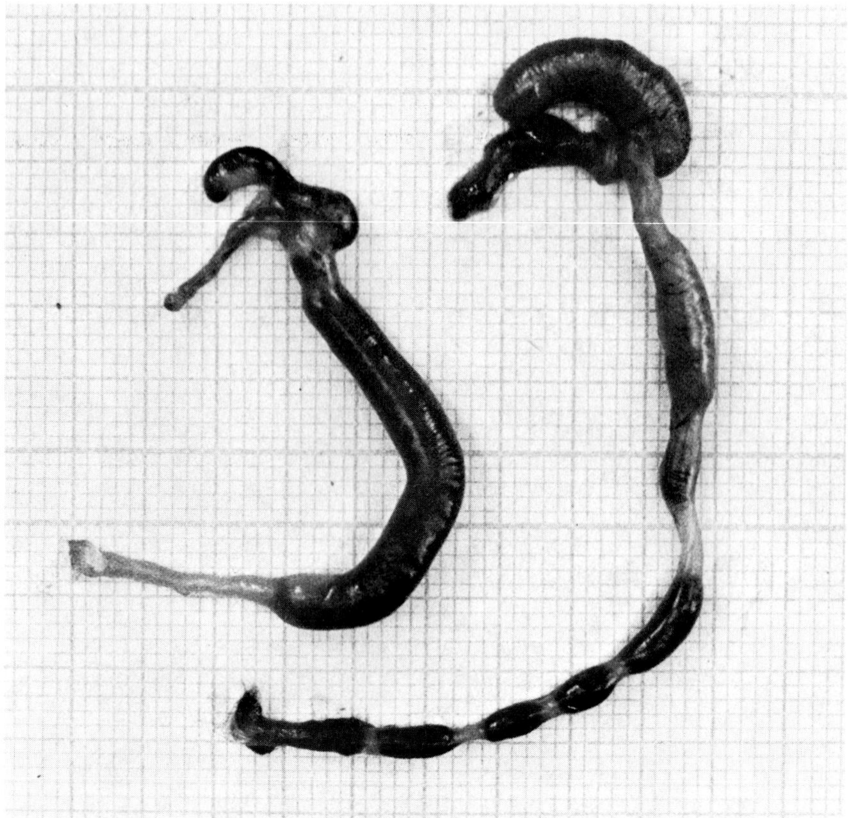

FIGURE 2.   Large intestine of piebald mouse (left) and normal littermate (right). The constricted terminal segment and impacted feces in the megacolon of the piebald mouse contrasts with formed fecal pellets in the terminal region of the large bowel of the normal mouse. Scale: 5 mm per large division. (From Wood, J. D., in *Spontaneous Animal Models of Human Disease,* Andrews, E. J., Ward, B. G., and Altman, N. H., Eds., Academic Press, New York, 1979, 29. With permission.)

IV. HEREDITARY FACTORS

Congenital megacolon in the mouse model is clearly a recessive trait that is not linked to sex chromosomes. Hereditary factors also are involved in Hirschsprung's disease. Its incidence in the general population of infants and children is 1:5000 (0.02%), whereas it occurs in siblings in 3.6% of cases.[17,18] The incidence of Hirschsprung's disease (short-segment type in which aganglionosis extends no higher than the sigmoid colon) is five to ten times higher in human males than in females. Sexual differences are not apparent for the long-segment type of the disease in which the aganglionosis extends beyond the sigmoid colon. Increased familial incidence of Hirschsprung's disease has been reported, primarily for long-segment cases.[19] Discordance and concordance for Hirschsprung's disease in monozygotic twins has been reported.[19,20] Passarge[21] suggested that Hirschsprung's disease may have a heterogeneous etiology and that it may be an example of sex-modified multifactorial inheritance in which the threshold of genes required for expression of the phenotype is lower in one sex than the other.

Hirschsprung's disease seems to be related to Down's syndrome,[18] and although it has been suggested that abnormality of chromosome 21 produces Hirschsprung's disease, no specific chromosomal studies have been reported. No gross differences are apparent between karyotypes of piebald-lethal mice and their sex-matched siblings.[75] Hirschsprung's disease occurs in conjunction with a number of other familial hereditary diseases that are believed to be related to defects in development of the embryonic neural crest.[22] Within the inbred colony maintained for production of piebald-lethal mice at the University of Nevada School of Medicine, gross abnormalities or runting, imperforate anus, and short bowel have been observed periodically over the 13-year history of the colony.

V. HISTOLOGY AND HISTOCHEMISTRY

A. Nerve and Endocrine Cells

The abnormal distribution of enteric ganglion cells in the large intestine of the mouse models is comparable with Hirschsprung's disease. In the normal mouse large intestine, ganglia are present to within about 2 mm of the anus. In the abnormal mice, ganglia are absent from both the myenteric and submucosal plexuses in the distal 1.0 to 2.5 cm of the large bowel. Occasionally, single perikarya or clusters of two or three cell somas can be observed in the aganglionic segment, and this observation has prompted some authors to suggest that "hypoganglionic" would be a more descriptive term than "aganglionic" for the abnormal terminal segment.[22,23]

The murine models and the human disease both show a cone-shaped transition zone between the constricted aganglionic segment and the proximal colon. The number of ganglion cells progressively increases in the proximal direction within the transition zone, and at the proximal margin of the zone normal-appearing ganglionic relationships between perikarya and neuropil become established. Signs of neuronal degeneration are present within the transitional zone, but there is no evidence that this transition region is a front of degeneration that is migrating in the oral direction. There are no indications of inflammatory changes in the disease.

Neurohistochemical findings for cholinergic and adrenergic nerves in the murine models do not parallel those for Hirschsprung's disease. In Hirschsprung's disease, increased numbers of nonmyelinated fibers, myelinated fibers, acetylcholinesterase-positive fibers, and adrenergic fibers occur within the external muscularis of the aganglionic segment.[24-30] The number of cholinergic fibers is reduced and no increase in sympathetic innervation can be demonstrated in the constricted segment of the lethal-spotting strain of mice.[30] In piebald-lethal mice, cholinergic fibers are reduced in the proximal aganglionic region and appear normal in the distal region of the aganglionic segment; no overgrowth of adrenergic fibers is seen in the aganglionic segment. The cholinesterase-positive fibers that are present in the aganglionic zone of both Hirschsprung's disease and murine megacolon are believed to be sacral preganglionic parasympathetic fibers rather than intramural cholinergic fibers that project downward from the ganglionic region. Cholinergic and adrenergic histochemistry within the dilated colon are not appreciably different from comparable regions of normal colon.

Histochemical findings for peptidergic neurons and endocrine cells in the piebald-lethal mouse model do parallel those for Hirschsprung's disease. Application of methods for immunocytochemical localization of bombesin, somatostatin, cholecystokinin, substance P, vasoactive intestinal peptide, and enkephalans reveal marked reduction in the numbers of peptidergic nerves in the aganglionic segment of the mouse model.[31] The number and distribution of peptidergic nerves in the megacolonic portion of the large intestine and in the small intestine of the piebald animals are not different from their normal littermates. Radioimmunoassay for total concentrations of putative peptidergic neurotransmitter substances generally confirms the immunocytochemical observations of depletion of neural peptides in the aganglionic segment. An exception to this is substance P, which is not only lower than normal in the aganglionic segment, but in the proximal colon and distal small intestine of the piebald mice as well. It is interesting that the development of substance P is generally delayed at all levels of the intestine in the piebald mice during the 15-day postnatal period.[31] This observation indicates that there are depressed concentrations of substance P in neuronal elements of the ganglionated portion of the large intestine because, in the muscularis externa, substance P is localized to nerves where it may function as a transmitter for slow synaptic modulation of neuronal excitability.[32]

Peptidergic nerves also are missing from the aganglionic segment of Hirschsprung's disease.[33] The synaptic profiles that are characteristic of peptide-containing synaptic vesicles in ultrastructural studies of normal intestine are depleted or absent from the constricted-aganglionic segment of Hirschsprung's disease.[24] This finding is related to measurements that show depletion of one particular peptide, substance P, in the constricted terminal segment in the human disease.[34]

Several lines of evidence indicate that peptidergic axons are derived mainly from intrinsic ganglion cells in the gut; consequently, the depletion of presumptive peptidergic neurotransmitters in the aganglionic segment of both the murine model and Hirschsprung's disease reflects the malformation of the intrinsic nervous system of the gut. The presence of nerve fasicles with histological and histochemical characteristics of extrinsic adrenergic and cholinergic nerves within the aganglionic segments suggests that projections of the extrinsic nerves to the gut develop normally in the disease. The overgrowth of extrinsic nerve fibers that appears to occur in the aganglionic segment in the human disease may be related to failure of the extrinsic fibers to find appropriate synaptic targets within the abnormal segment.

Biologically active peptides occur in mucosal endocrine cells of the gut as well as in the intrinsic nerves and have important significance as messenger substances in control of gastrointestinal function.[35] Examination of the mucosal endocrine cells of the piebald mouse large intestine revealed no differences between the constricted terminal segment of the diseased mice and the terminal segment of normal littermates.[31] The numbers of colonic mucosal endocrine cells that contain immunoreactive glucagon, substance P, somatostatin, or cholecystokinin are not significantly different between normal and piebald-lethal mice. This is the case also for Hirschsprung's disease in humans where normal numbers of mucosal endocrine cells are present in the aganglionic colonic segment.[36] These findings are not consistent with the earlier concept[37] that precursors of enteroendocrine cells and enteric ganglion cells have a common embryonic origin in the neural crest.

The abnormalities of gastrointestinal peptides in Hirschsprung's disease raise questions regarding the status of messenger peptides in the brain because most of the putative messenger peptides that are present in the endocrine or neuronal cells of the gut are also present in the brain. Measurements of immunoreactive substance P, bombesin, and cholecystokinin in the brains of piebald mice and their normal siblings show no significant differences in the concentrations of these peptides between the two groups of mice.[31]

B. Musculature

Hypertrophy of the muscularis externa is another prominent histological feature in both Hirschsprung's disease and the mouse model. In the piebald-lethal model, hypertrophy occurs in both longitudinal and circular muscle layers in the distended and constricted segments with no change in the normal 2:1 ratio of circular to longitudinal muscle thickness.[38]

VI. EMBRYOGENESIS OF AGANGLIONOSIS

Absence of pigmentation, abnormality of neural epithelium in the inner ear, and aganglionosis are closely linked in the murine models, and this suggests that a genetic defect in the embryonic neural crest may be the explanation for the etiology of aganglionic megacolon in the mouse.[39,40] Nevertheless, the precise nature of the defect has not been resolved. If a neural crest defect is involved, it is obvious that the defect is not incorporated into all of the crest cells because only a restricted fraction of the neural crest derivatives are abnormal. Mayer[40] suggested that abnormal sensitivity of the neural crest derivatives to environmental factors at the sites of peripheral development might account for failure of colonization by the precursor cells that migrate from the neural crest. If this were the case, then the abnormal environment would be limited to the specific areas of aganglionosis or defective pigmentation. In contrast to the view of Mayer, [40] Webster[41] and Okamoto and Ueda[42] proposed that a defect resulting in a slower migratory rate for the neural crest derivatives delayed arrival of the neuroblasts in the distal end of the developing gut and accounted for aganglionosis in the mouse model and in Hirschsprung's disease, respectively.

The hypothesis of defective migration of neural crest derivatives is based on observations of a rostral to caudal gradient in the appearance of acetylcholinesterase-positive ganglion cells during development of the gut in mice.[41] In normal mice, the embryonic gut elongates from 1 mm at 10 days to 50 mm at $15^1/_2$ days of gestation, and during this time there is a progressive appearance of acetylcholinesterase-positive cells in the caudal direction until presumptive ganglion cells are present at the distal extremity. In piebald-lethal mouse embryos, the acetylcholinesterase-positive cells appear at a slower rate and out of phase with the elongation process. One interpretation of this observation is that the precursors of ganglion cells are not present in the distal segment when the outer muscle coat is laid down and migration of the precursors stops. It is implicit in the defective migration hypothesis that all enteric ganglion cells are derived from the vagal neural crest and that none are of lumbosacral origin in both humans and in the piebald-lethal mouse strain. An attractive aspect of this hypothesis is that if these events did account for aganglionosis in Hirschsprung's disease, then it would be probable that the clinical variations of megacolon (i.e., long-segment, short-segment, ultra-short-segment and pseudo forms of Hirschsprung's disease) represent different degrees of the same migratory defect.

The defective migration hypothesis for embryogenesis of aganglionic megacolon is attractive by virtue of its simplicity; however, there are several inconsistencies that undermine its validity. First of these is that acetylcholinesterase is not a suitable marker for the appearance of primordial nerve cells in the developing gut because it is not specific for neurons and because it identifies only one of the many types of enteric neurons. More recent evidence indicates that the developing gut in mice and chicks is completely colonized by precursors from the neural crest 3 to 5 days before expression of any neurotransmitter phenotypes occurs.[43,44] A second inconsistency with the migration hypothesis is that "skip lesions", where an aganglionic segment is interposed between two ganglionated segments, can occur in Hirschsprung's disease.[45] This objection is reinforced by the absence of a rostral-caudal gradient of appearance of enteric neurons in the developing gut of rabbits, rats, and chicks.[46,47] A third difficulty with the migration hypothesis is that conclusive evidence from recent embryologic studies with chick-quail chimeras indicate that progenitors of enteric neurons in the terminal large intestine originate from both the vagal and sacral neural crest.[48,49]

The weight of evidence is shifting presently toward the defective microenvironment hypothesis as an explanation for failure of development of enteric ganglion cells in the terminal large intestine of the piebald mouse model and Hirschsprung's disease. This hypothesis supposes that the environment of the aganglionic zone is "hostile" for the development of the neuronal precursors that migrate to the area from the neural crest. There is strong evidence that the enteric microenvironment has a primary influence on development and differentiation of the enteric nervous system. The observation in chick-quail chimeras that cells taken from a region of the neural crest that would normally not give rise to enteric neuronal phenotypes will do so if transplanted to neural crest locations from which migration to the gut can occur directly indicates the importance of the microenvironment in the selection or induction of enteric neuronal phenotypes.[50] The histological appearance of the transition zone between the aganglionic and ganglionated segments of the large bowel in Hirschsprung's disease and in the murine models gives the impression that the aganglionic segment is an inhospitable environment for the intrinsic neurons of the intestine. Axons of serotonergic axons, which generally project for long distances in the aboral direction within the intestinal wall,[51] terminate sharply at the transition zone and do not project into the aganglionic region.[52] The abnormal appearance of the Schwann cells and nerve fibers within the transition zone of the colon in Hirschsprung's disease is suggestive of the occurrence of perpetual regenerative processes at the demarcation of the aganglionic segment.[24]

Results of one study suggest that progressive increase in the severity of megacolon associated with advancing age in the lethal-spotting strain of mice is paralleled by further degeneration of the already reduced number of neurons that are scattered in the aganglionic terminal segment at birth.[23] Histologic disappearance of ganglion cells between 72 and 129 days of age in a premature infant with Hirschsprung's disease has also been reported.[53] The authors of both reports suggested that the ganglion cells are congenitally abnormal in these cases and are predisposed to postnatal stress and degeneration. Nevertheless, factors related to subtle deficiencies in the microenvironment within the intestinal wall cannot be ruled out in these cases.

VII. GASTROINTESTINAL MOTOR FUNCTION

A. Motor Function In Vivo

Gastric emptying and small-intestinal transit are altered in the piebald-lethal mice relative to their siblings.[54] Gastric emptying of ^{51}Cr-labeled saline or milk test meals is significantly delayed in the conscious piebald animals relative to their normal littermates. Small-intestinal transit time for a saline meal is increased in the mice with megacolon, whereas small-intestinal transit of a labeled milk meal is not significantly changed from normal in the megacolonic mice. Similar findings have been made in mice with megacolon induced by mechanical obstruction of the terminal large intestine.[54] These findings suggest that the abnormalities in gastrointestinal propulsion in piebald-lethal mice occur secondary to fecal stasis and development of megacolon, rather than being directly related to the genetic defect that is responsible for aganglionosis in the piebald model.

B. Large Intestinal Motor Function In Vitro

Intrinsic motor function of the large intestine of piebald-lethal mice has been studied in vitro by placing artificial fecal pellets into the lumen of the bowel and photographing, on moving film, the transport of the pellet through the intestine.[55] An artificial fecal pellet placed in the oral end of the large intestine of a normal sibling is propelled to the anal end and expelled into the organ bath with a transit time of a few minutes. In the large bowel from piebald mice, after removal of the impacted feces, peristaltic propulsion transports the artificial pellets through the dilated portion of the colon; however, aboral movement always stops at the proximal margin of the aganglionic segment. After orthograde movement stops at the aganglionic transition zone, the pellets are propelled by reverse peristalsis away from the constricted segment back into the midcolon. This is followed by a recurrent pattern of forward-reverse peristalsis.

The only abnormality of motility that can be demonstrated within the megacolonic segment of the piebald mouse is an increased rate of propulsion that is probably a reflection of the hypertrophy of the muscularis externa. The neuromuscular mechanisms responsible for coordinated propulsive motility appear to be normal within the megacolon, while the distal segment is still tonically contracted and obstructive in the absence of extrinsic nervous input in vitro. Reverse peristalsis occurs in normal mouse large intestine when an obstructive ligature is placed near the terminal end, suggesting that reverse peristalsis is a general response to obstruction and is not a peculiar property of aganglionosis and megacolon. Forward-reverse cycles of peristalsis could, however, be a contributing factor to fecal impaction in the diseased mice.

Motility of the large intestine in Hirschsprung's disease has not been assessed by direct measurements of propulsive activity; however, retrograde movements of colonic contents in Hirschsprung's disease have been reported.[56] These authors reported retrograde reflux of a barium enema as far as the gastroduodenal junction.

VIII. MYOELECTRICAL ACTIVITY

Extracellular recording of electrical activity of the muscularis externa of the large bowel in vitro of both piebald-lethal and normal littermates shows typical smooth-muscle action potentials associated with electrical slow waves.[57] The only observable difference in this electrical activity between the normal and abnormal bowel is a large increase in the proportion of electrical slow waves accompanied by action potentials in the aganglionic segment.

In the normal murine large intestine in vitro, bursts of action potentials periodically originate at the oral end and propagate to the anal end of the bowel.[57] During the time intervals between the migrating spike bursts, the slow waves are not accompanied by action potentials and the circular musculature is flaccid. This periodically occurring electrical activity is reminiscent of the interdigestive migrating myoelectric complex that has been reported for several mammalian species.[58] The megacolonic region of the piebald large intestine shows the same kind of migrating electrical activity as the normal bowel, whereas, the aganglionic segment shows continuous discharge of action potentials that originate at multiple sites within the segment and propagate bidirectionally from the site of origin for only a short distance before colliding with spikes spreading from an adjacent site. The mechanical correlate of the increased discharge of action potentials is tonic contracture of the circular muscle. Superimposed on the contracture are continuous shallow waves of circular muscle contraction that originate at random sites in the segment and propagate in both oral and aboral directions from the site of origin. This electrical and mechanical activity appears to be a reflection of lack of nervous control of the autogenic musculature in the aganglionic segment. It is uncoordinated myogenic activity that is incapable of organized propulsion of the intraluminal contents.

Recordings of both electrical and mechanical activity in normal mouse large intestine shows that contraction of the longitudinal and circular muscles of the terminal 5 mm occurs in a patterned temporal sequence during a peristaltic wave. First to occur is atropine-sensitive shortening of the longitudinal muscle followed, after a latency of 8 to 12 sec, by contraction of the circular muscle. These are neurally mediated events that do not occur in the aganglionic segment of the piebald large intestine.

Electrical activity has been recorded with intraluminal electrodes from the rectosigmoid colon of children with Hirschsprung's disease.[59] These studies revealed differences between normal and diseased bowel; however, resolution with these techniques is not sufficient to permit comparison with results from the mouse model.

IX. PHARMACOLOGY

Results of organ-bath pharmacological studies on excised segments of large intestine from cases of Hirschsprung's disease and on the large intestine of the mouse models are qualitatively similar and characteristic for the intestinal musculature.[60-65] Acetylcholine is excitatory to the external muscularis and application of epinephrine evokes relaxation of the musculature of both. The response to acetylcholine is blocked by atropine, and the effects of epinephrine are prevented by β-adrenergic antagonists.

In the normal intestine of mammalian species, the sympathetic postganglionic axons synapse with ganglion cells in the myenteric plexus and only a few adrenergic axons are found within the muscle coats.[32] Both cholinergic and serotonergic nerve terminals in the myenteric plexus have α_2 adrenoceptors that function to suppress transmitter release from the terminals.[32] This connectivity, which mediates much of the influence of the sympathetic nervous system on intestinal motility, is absent in the aganglionic segment of Hirschsprung's disease and the mouse models. Noradrenergic sympathetic fibers also provide excitatory innervation to the internal anal sphincter, which appears to be functional in the aganglionic terminal segment.[24,27]

Electrical stimulation of intramural neurons of both human and mouse large intestine elicits a relaxation of the circular muscle that is followed by rebound excitation at the offset of stimulation.[66,67] This is a ubiquitous response at all levels of normal, small, and large intestine of all species tested and also within the intrinsically innervated megacolon of the mouse models.[62] This inhibitory response is mediated by intrinsic inhibitory neurons that release a transmitter substance that is neither cholinergic nor adrenergic.[68] Although this inhibitory transmitter was first postulated to be a purine nucleotide,[68] more recent evidence has implicated vasoactive intestinal peptide as the mediator;[69] however, the issue of the precise identity of the transmitter or combinations of inhibitory transmitters is unsettled. There is evidence that the intrinsic inhibitory ganglion cells have nicotinic cholinergic receptors and are activated by nicotinic agonists to release their inhibitory transmitter substance.[32,61,65]

The intrinsic inhibitory neurons are present at all levels of the gastrointestinal tract and are continuously active in nonsphincteric regions of the intestine.[70] In the internal anal sphincter, the inhibitory neurons are not continuously active, but are activated to relax the sphincter by descending neural pathways in an appropriate temporal sequence during the act of defecation. It is highly significant that these ganglion cells are reduced in number or absent in the spastic terminal segment in both the murine models and in Hirschsprung's disease.

Absence of the intrinsic inhibitory neurons explains why inhibitory responses to transmural electrical stimulation and application of nicotinic agonists do not occur or are reduced in the constricted segment in human and mouse large intestine.[60-65] Depletion of these cells and the circuitry that controls them likewise accounts for failure of sphincteric relaxation in response to distension of the rectosigmoid colon in Hirschsprung's disease.[71] In a large proportion of such children, a year or more after surgical resection of the aganglionic terminal segment, an internal anal reflexive relaxation to rectosigmoid distension appears.[71]

When the intrinsic neurons of the normal intestine are blocked by tetrodotoxin in the mouse and other species, the circular muscle layer becomes hypermotile.[57,70] After blockade of nervous function with tetrodotoxin, a greater proportion of electrical slow waves trigger action potentials, the amplitudes of the contractions associated with each slow wave are increased, and resting tone in the denervated segment increases. The contractile behavior after treatment with tetrodotoxin closely resembles that of the aganglionic segment in the murine model and in Hirschsprung's disease. This is one line of evidence which suggests that the spasticity of the aganglionic terminal segment represents myogenic contractile activity that is uncontrolled by continuous activity of intrinsic inhibitory neurons, and that absence of this inhibitory action on the autogenic musculature is the factor that underlies the achalasia and obstruction to passage of feces.

An early and often-cited hypothesis attributes achalasia of the aganglionic segment in Hirschsprung's disease to Cannon's law of denervation supersensitivity. Current findings refute this hypothesis. No increased sensitivity of the musculature of the constricted segment to acetylcholine or norepinephrine can be demonstrated in either the mouse models or in resected segments from children with Hirschsprung's disease.[27,60-62,64] There are no differences in the numbers or affinity of muscarinic cholinergic receptors between the aganglionic terminal segment and normal terminal segment of the piebald mouse model as determined by binding studies with the tritium-labeled muscarinic ligand, quinyclidinyl benzilate.[72] Some authors[73] have proposed that abnormalities of activity in the extrinsic nervous pathways to the large intestine might be a factor responsible for the contracture of the aganglionic segment. This is unlikely for the mouse because sympathetic and parasympathetic pathways are not spontaneously active after their connections with the central nervous system are cut; yet, when the abnormal intestine is isolated in an organ bath, the pathologic terminal segment is still hyperactive, constricted, and obstructive.

X. SECONDARY EFFECTS OF FECAL STASIS

Surgical treatment for Hirschsprung's disease is sometimes delayed and the disease is permitted to persist into teenage years and adulthood. In these older individuals, the characteristic symptoms are emaciation, susceptibility to infection, inhibition of growth in height, retarded intellectual development, and delayed puberty. Cases of dwarfism and sexual infantilism in adult patients have been reported.[18] Similar disturbances of growth and development are also apparent in the mouse models of megacolon. Systematic study of weight change during growth in the piebald-lethal strain shows that piebald mice weigh 6% less than normal siblings on days 1 to 4 of birth and continue to weigh less throughout their life span. Growth of piebald mice reaches a plateau at 18 to 20 days of age and the mice lose weight 1 to 2 days prior to death.[38]

The ratios of weights of various organ systems to total body weights are not significantly different between piebald mice and normal siblings, with the exception of the large bowel which shows an increase in organ weight to body weight ratio that reflects muscular hypertrophy in the diseased bowel.

The water content of the feces per gram wet weight is the same for piebald mice and their normal siblings. Sodium and potassium content of the feces is higher in piebald mice than in normal siblings. Standard clinical laboratory analysis of the blood of piebald and normal mice shows no significant difference in sodium, potassium, hemoglobin, glucose, urea, nitrogen, creatinine, total protein, albumin, bilirubin, alkaline phosphatase, cholesterol, uric acid, phosphate, and calcium.[38]

Bacteriological studies reveal no differences between piebald mice and normal siblings in kind and numbers of the aerobic and anaerobic microflora of the feces. Microorganisms cannot be cultured from the small intestine of piebald mice, and no bacterial overgrowth in the small bowel associated with fecal stasis and gross megacolon can be detected in the diseased mice.[38]

When death occurs in piebald mice that survive for 3 or more weeks, post-mortem examination always reveals a large intestine grossly distended with fecal material. Prior to death, these animals weigh 10 to 30% less than their littermates, have "scruffy" hair, and are lethargic. Diarrhea characteristic of enterocolitis is occasionally seen in younger piebald mice, but is rare in the animals that live 3 or more weeks.

The debilitation, "scruffy" fur, and lethargy that occurs prior to death can be attributed to systemic bacteremia that results when lesions in the megacolonic mucosa permit entry of bacteria from the intestinal lumen.[38] Leukocyte counts made periodically during the lives of the piebald mice show periods of abrupt increases in the numbers of white cells. During leukocytosis, blood cultures are positive for enterococci. In some mice, the white cell count returns to normal and the animal survives; in others, white count peaks, then falls below normal and the animal dies. For bacteremia to occur, the organisms must have gained access to the systemic circulation through either the lymphatic or portal system. No studies have been reported on the competence of the immune system in the murine models. Impaired immune function in children with Hirschsprung's disease has been suggested.[18]

XI. INTESTINAL ABSORPTION

Emaciation in the mice with fecal stasis and in cases of Hirschsprung's disease could be attributable to low food intake or malabsorption of nutrients from the small intestine. The latter possibility has been examined in the piebald mouse model and appears not to be the case.[74] Net fluxes of alanine, methionine, and sodium ions are two to three times greater across the small-intestinal mucosa of piebald mice in vitro than across the mucosa of normal littermates. Total electrical conductance of the tissue and transmucosal electrical potential differences are also higher than normal in the small-intestinal mucosa of piebald mice. Intestinal absorption occurring by both active and passive mechanisms, therefore, is enhanced in the megacolonic mice and is not consistent with malabsorption of these nutrients as an explanation for retarded growth in the mice.

Enhanced small-intestinal absorption in the megacolonic mice appears to be a compensatory response to fecal stasis and distal obstruction rather than being related to the genetic defect because changes in mucosal transport function in normal mice with megacolon induced by experimental anal closure at birth parallel those in the piebald mice.[74] The physiological signals that lead to altered mucosal transport in the mice with distal intestinal obstruction are unknown, although this could be related to the above-mentioned delay in gastric emptying that occurs in the mice with intestinal obstruction.

XII. CONCLUSIONS

Aganglionic megacolon occurs with high predictability in the piebald-lethal and lethal-spotting strains of mice. The recessive genetics of the disease make it possible to control the phenotype of experimental animals by selective breeding. These characteristics make the mice valuable models for basic research on both neural crest defects responsible for aganglionosis and on the effects that are secondary to malformation and malfunction of the enteric nervous system.

Although the general characteristics of the disease in the murine models resemble to a significant degree those of Hirschsprung's disease, it is not possible to state the extent to which data from the models can be applied to human disease. The histological-histochemical appearance of adrenergic and cholinergic nerve fibers in the aganglionic segment of the models is different from Hirschsprung's disease and the significance of this is uncertain. It is unlikely that the overgrowth of cholinergic and adrenergic nerve fibers is the primary factor responsible for achalasia in the terminal segment in the human disease. Uncertainty in comparing the mouse models with the human disease stems also from the inherently difficult nature of experimentation on humans, which has not produced physiological investigations with the same rigor that has been possible in controlled experiments with the mice.

Current evidence suggests that the functional obstruction in both Hirschsprung's disease and the murine models is produced by autogenic contracture of the circular muscle of the aganglionic rectosigmoid segment. The hyperactivity of the muscle reflects the absence or abnormal function of intrinsic inhibitory neurons.

Nervous coordination of gastrointestinal motor function is derived from integrative circuitry within the synaptic neuropil of the enteric ganglia that functions like an independent integrative nervous system analogous to the central nervous system. These neuronal formations process sensory information and generate output appropriate for moment-to-moment control of the musculature.[70] The intrinsic inhibitory neurons and some of the cholinergic ganglion cells are constituents of the integrated system and represent the final common motor pathways to the musculature. The function of these ganglion cells is analogous to that of efferent neurons in the central nervous system and their physiology involves more than the simple relay-distribution function that is associated with ganglion cells in other autonomic ganglia. The best interpretation of the pathophysiology of the mouse model and Hirschsprung's disease is in terms of malformation and malfunction of these neurons and their neural connectivity within the enteric nervous system.

REFERENCES

1. Kapila, L. S., Chronic adynamic bowel simulating Hirschsprung's disease, *J. Pediatr. Surg.*, 10, 885, 1975.
2. Smith, B., *The Neuropathology of the Alimentary Tract,* Williams & Wilkins, Baltimore, 1972, chap. 15.
3. Schuffler, M. D., Baird, H. W., Fleming, C. R., Bell, C. E., Malagelada, J. R., McGil, D. B., Bouldin, T., Abrams, M., and LeBauer, S., Intestinal pseudo-obstruction as the presenting manifestation of small-cell carcinoma of the lung — a paraneoplastic syndrome by a neuropathy of the gastrointestinal tract, *Gastroenterology,* 82, 1173, 1982.
4. Earlam, R. J., Gastrointestinal aspects of Chagas' disease, *Am. J. Dig. Dis.,* 17, 559, 1972.
5. Wood, J. N., Hudson, L., Jessell, T. M., and Yamamoto, M., A monoclonal antibody defining antigenic determinants on subpopulations of mammalian neurones and *Trypanosoma cruzi* parasites, *Nature (London),* 296, 34, 1982.
6. Hukuhara, T., Kotania, S., and Sato, G., Effects of destruction of intramural ganglion cells on colon motility: possible genesis of congenital megacolon, *Jpn. J. Physiol.,* 11, 125, 1965.
7. Imamura, K., Yamamoto, M., Sato, A., Kashiki, Y., and Kunieda, T., Pathophysiology of aganglionic colon segment: an experimental study on aganglionosis produced by a new method in the rat, *J. Pediatr. Surg.,* 10, 865, 1975.
8. Sato, A., Yamamoto, M., Imamura, K., Kashiki, Y., and Kunieda, T., Pathophysiology of aganglionic colon and anorectum: an experimental study on aganglionosis produced by a new method in the rat, *J. Pediatr. Surg.,* 13, 399, 1978.
9. Keeler, B., Richardson, H., and Watson, A. J., Enteromegaly and steatorrhea in the rat following intraperitoneal quinacrine (atabrine), *Lab. Invest.,* 15, 1253, 1966.
10. Osborne, J. C., Davis, J. W., and Farley, H., Hirschsprung's disease: a review and report on the entity in a Virginia swine herd, *Vet. Med. Small Anim. Clin.,* 63, 451, 1968.
11. Senk, L., Rectal stricture in the swine in intensive management, *Vet. Glas.,* 28, 829, 1975.
12. Fioramonti, J. and Bueno, L., Electrical activity of the large intestine in normal and megacolon pigs, *Ann. Rech. Vet.,* 8, 275, 1977.
13. Wood, J. D., Congenital megacolon (Hirschsprung's disease), in *Spontaneous Animal Models of Human Disease,* Andrews, E. J., Ward, B. G., and Altman, N. H., Eds., Academic Press, New York, 1979, 29.
14. Derrick, E. H. and St. George-Grambauer, B. M., Megacolon in mice, *J. Pathol. Bacteriol.,* 73, 569, 1957.
15. Bielschowski, M. and Schofield, G. C., Studies on megacolon in mice, *Aust. J. Exp. Biol. Med. Sci.,* 40, 395, 1962.

16. Lane, P. W., Association of megacolon with two recessive spotting genes in the mouse, *J. Hered.*, 57, 29, 1966.
17. Bodian, M. and Carter, C. O., A family study of Hirschsprung's disease, *Ann. Human Genet.*, 26, 261, 1963.
18. Madsen, G. M., *Hirschsprung's Disease*, Charles C Thomas, Springfield, Ill., 1964.
19. Bodian, M., Carter, C. O., and Ward, C. H., Hirschsprung's disease, *Lancet*, 1, 302, 1951.
20. Moore, T. C., Landers, D. B., Lachman, R. S., and Ament, M. E., Hirschsprung's disease discordant in monozygotic twins: a study of possible environmental factors in the production of colonic aganglionosis, *J. Pediatr. Surg.*, 14, 158, 1979.
21. Passarge, E., The genetics of Hirschsprung's disease: evidence for heterogeneous etiology and a study of sixty three families, *N. Engl. J. Med.*, 276, 138, 1967.
22. Bolande, R. P., Animal model of human disease. Hirschsprung's disease, aganglionic or hypoganglionic megacolon; animal model: aganglionic megacolon in piebald and spotted mutant mouse strains, *Am. J. Pathol.*, 79, 189, 1975.
23. Bolande, R. P. and Towler, W. F., Ultrastructural and histochemical studies of murine megacolon, *Am. J. Pathol.*, 69, 139, 1972.
24. Baumgarten, H. G., Holstein, A. F., and Stelzner, F., Nervous elements in human colon of Hirschsprung's disease, *Virchows Arch. A:*, 358, 113, 1973.
25. Gannon, B. J., Noblett, H. R., and Burnstock, G., Adrenergic innervation of bowel in Hirschsprung's disease, *Br. Med. J.*, 3, 338, 1969.
26. Garret, J. R., Howard, E. R., and Nixon, H. H., Autonomic nerves in rectum and colon in Hirschsprung's disease, *Arch. Dis. Child.*, 44, 406, 1969.
27. Kamijo, K., Hiatt, R. B., and Koelle, G. B., Congenital megacolon. A comparison of the spastic and hypertrophied segments with respect to cholinesterase activities and sensitivities to acetylcholine, DFP and barium ion, *Gastroenterology*, 24, 173, 1953.
28. Meier-Ruge, W., Lutterbach, P. M., Herzog, B., Morgen, R., Maser, R., and Scharli, A., Acetylcholinesterase activity in suction biopsies of the rectum in the diagnosis of Hirschsprung's disease, *J. Pediatr. Surg.*, 7, 11, 1972.
29. Niemi, M., Kouvalainen, K., and Hjelt, L., Cholinesterase and monoamine oxidase in congenital megacolon, *J. Pathol.*, 82, 363, 1961.
30. Webster, W., Aganglionic megacolon in piebald-lethal mice, *Arch. Pathol.*, 97, 111, 1974.
31. Vaillant, C., BûLock, A., Dimaline, R., and Dockray, G., Distribution and development of peptidergic nerves and gut endocrine cells in mice with congenital aganglionic colon, and their normal littermates, *Gastroenterology*, 82, 291, 1982.
32. Wood, J. D., Synaptic interactions in the enteric plexuses, *J. Autonomic Nerv. Sys.*, 4, 121, 1981.
33. Bishop, A. E., Polak, J. M., Lake, B., Bryant, M. G., and Bloom, S. R., Abnormalities of neural and hormonal peptides in Hirschsprung's disease, *Gut*, 21, 460, 1981.
34. Tafuri, W. L., Maria, T. A., Pitella, J. E. H., Bogdiolo, L., Hial, W., and Diniz, C. R., An electron microscopic study of the Auerbach's plexus and determination of substance P of the colon in Hirschsprung's disease, *Virchows Arch. A:*, 362, 41, 1974.
35. Dockray, G. J. and Gregory, R. A., Relations between neuropeptides and gut hormones, *Proc. R. Soc. London*, B210, 151, 1980.
36. Cristina, M. L., Lehy, T., Voillemot, N., Arhan, P. D., and Bonfils, S., Endocrine cells of the colon in Hirschsprung's and control children, *Virchows Arch. A:*, 377, 387, 1978.
37. Pearse, A. G. E., Peptides in brain and intestine, *Nature (London)*, 262, 92, 1976.
38. Brann, L., Furtado, D., Migliazzo, C. V., Baxendale, J., and Wood, J. D., Secondary effects of aganglionosis in the piebald-lethal mouse model of Hirschsprung's disease, *Lab. Anim. Sci.*, 27, 946, 1977.
39. Mayer, T. C. and Matby, E. L., An experimental investigation of pattern development in lethal-spotting and belted mouse embryos, *Develop. Biol.*, 9, 269, 1964.
40. Mayer, T. C., The development of piebald spotting in mice, *Develop. Biol.*, 11, 319, 1965.
41. Webster, W., Embryogenesis of the enteric ganglia in normal mice and in mice that develop congenital aganglionic megacolon, *J. Embryol. Exp. Morphol.*, 30, 573, 1973.
42. Okamoto, E. and Ueda, T., Embryogenesis of the intramural ganglia of the gut and its relation to Hirschsprung's disease, *J. Pediatr. Surg.*, 2, 437, 1967.
43. Rothman, T. P. and Gershon, M. D., Phenotypic expression in the developing murine enteric nervous system, *J. Neurosci.*, 2, 381, 1982.
44. Payette, R., Bennett, G. S., and Gershon, M. D., Neurofilament immunoreactivity in precursors of avian enteric neuroblasts: early commitment to a neuronal lineage, *J. Cell. Biol.*, 95, 63, 1982.
45. Kadair, B. G., Sims, J. E., and Critchfield, C. F., Zonal colonic hypoganglionosis, *JAMA*, 238, 1838, 1977.
46. Cantino, D., An histochemical study of the nerve supply to the developing alimentary tract, *Experientia*, 26, 766, 1970.

47. Keller, H., The development of the intramural nerve plexus of the gastrointestinal tract, *Anat. Embryol.*, 150, 1, 1976.
48. LeDouarin, N. M. and Teillet, M. A., The migration of neural crest cells to the wall of the digestive tract in avian embryo, *J. Embryol. Exp. Morphol.*, 30, 31, 1973.
49. LeDouarin, N. M. and Teillet, M. A., Experimental analysis of the migration and differentiation of neuroblasts of the autonomic nervous system and of neuroectodermal mesenchymal derivatives, using a biological cell marking technique, *Develop. Biol.*, 41, 162, 1974.
50. Smith, J., Cochard, P., and LeDouarin, N. M., Development of choline acetyltransferase and cholinesterase activities in enteric ganglia derived from presumptive adrenergic and cholinergic levels of neural crest, *Cell. Diff.*, 6, 199, 1977.
51. Furness, J. B. and Costa, M., Neurons with 5-hydroxytryptamine-like immunoreactivity in the enteric nervous system: their projections in the guinea-pig small intestine, *Neuroscience*, 7, 341, 1982.
52. Rogawski, M. A., Goodrich, J. T., Gershon, M. D., and Touloukian, R. V., Hirschsprung's disease: absence of serotonergic neurons in the aganglionic colon, *J. Pediatr. Surg.*, 13, 608, 1978.
53. Touloukian, B. J. and Dunean, R., Acquired aganglionic megacolon in a premature infant: report of a case, *Pediatrics*, 56, 559, 1975.
54. Pitman, K., Starr, G., Cooke, H. J., and Wood, J. D., Gastric emptying and intestinal transit in the piebald mouse model for Hirschsprung's disease, *Gastroenterology*, 82, 1258, 1982.
55. Brann, L. and Wood, J. D., Motility of the large intestine of piebald-lethal mice, *Am. J. Dig. Dis.*, 21, 633, 1976.
56. Chandler, N. W. and Zwiren, G. T., Complete reflux of the small bowel in total colon Hirschsprung's disease, *Radiology*, 94, 333, 1970.
57. Wood, J. D., Electrical activity of the intestine of mice with hereditary megacolon and absence of enteric ganglion cells, *Am. J. Dig. Dis.*, 13, 477, 1973.
58. Code, G. F., The interdigestive housekeeper of the gastrointestinal tract, *Perspect. Biol. Med.*, 22, 549, 1979.
59. Provenzale, L. and Pisano, M., Methods for recording electrical activity of the human colon *in vivo*, *Am. J. Dig. Dis.*, 16, 712, 1971.
60. Penninckx, F. and Kerremans, R., Pharmacological characteristics of the ganglionic and aganglionic colon in Hirschsprung's disease, *Life Sci.*, 17, 1387, 1975.
61. Shepherd, J. J. and Wright, P. G., The application of studies *in vitro* to the management of Hirschsprung's disease and of megacolon in adults, *Am. J. Dig. Dis.*, 13, 434, 1968.
62. Richardson, J., Pharmacological studies of Hirschsprung's disease on a murine model, *J. Pediatr. Surg.*, 10, 875, 1975.
63. Hiramoto, Y. and Kiesewetter, W. B., The response of colonic muscle to drugs: an *in vitro* study of Hirschsprung's disease, *J. Pediatr. Surg.*, 9, 13, 1974.
64. Frigo, G. M., Del Tacca, M., Lecchini, S., and Crema, A., Some observations on the intrinsic nervous mechanism in Hirschsprung's disease, *Gut*, 14, 35, 1973.
65. Beleslin, D. B., Bumbić, S., Dožić, S., and Terzić, B., Action of drugs on the human colonic preparations of Hirschsprung's disease, *Neuropharmacology*, 19, 1125, 1980.
66. Furness, J. B., An examination of nerve mediated, hyoscine resistant excitation of the guinea-pig colon, *J. Physiol. (London)*, 207, 803, 1970.
67. Wood, J. D. and Marsh, D. R., Effects of atropine, tetrodotoxin and xylocaine on rebound excitation of guinea-pig small intestine, *J. Pharm. Exp. Ther.*, 184, 590, 1973.
68. Burnstock, G., Purinergic nerves, *Pharmacol. Rev.*, 24, 509, 1972.
69. Gillespie, J. S., Non-adrenergic non-cholinergic inhibitory control of gastrointestinal motility, in *Motility of the Digestive Tract*, Wienbeck, M., Ed., Raven Press, New York, 1982, 51.
70. Wood, J. D., Intrinsic neural control of intestinal motility, *Ann. Rev. Physiol.*, 43, 33, 1981.
71. Holschneider, A. M., Börner, W., Buurman, O., Caffarena, P. F., Issendorf, H. V., Kaiser, G., Khan, O., Koepke, W., Kolb, F., Palua, M., Pickard, L., Pötzsek, R., Raffensperger, G., Scharli, A., Schnaufer, L., Waag, L., Poschl, U., and Markwalder, F., Clinical and electromanometrical investigations of postoperative continence in Hirschsprung's disease, *Z. Kinderchir.*, 29, 39, 1980.
72. Seidel, E. R., Wood, J. D., Eikenburg, B. E., and Johnson, L. R., Muscarinic cholinergic receptors in the piebald mouse model for Hirschsprung's disease, *Gastroenterology*, 85, 335, 1983.
73. Gillespie, J. S. and McKenna, B. R., The inhibitory action of nicotine on the rabbit colon, *J. Physiol. (London)*, 152, 191, 1960.
74. Cooke, H. J., Henning, H. J., Wood, J. D., and Cooke, A. R., Jejunal transport properties of piebald mouse model for Hirschsprung's disease, *Am. J. Physiol.*, 239, G123, 1980.
75. Vig, B. K., Personal communication.

Chapter 14

TORSION OF THE LARGE COLON IN THE HORSE (*TORSIO COLI ASCENDENTIS*)

B. Huskamp

TABLE OF CONTENTS

I. INTRODUCTION

The horse develops intestinal obstruction more frequently than any other domesticated species. Larger breeds of horses are more commonly involved, so that the likelihood of intestinal obstruction increases with size. This relationship has an anatomical basis. The small intestine (up to 30-m long) has a very long mesentery that allows movement of its loops into various parts of the abdominal cavity and permits intestinal entrapment in natural internal abdominal orifices (foramen epiploicum, annulus vaginalis).

Displacement and torsion are often encountered in the double horseshoe-shaped large colon (3 to 5-m long) which, apart from an attachment near the dorsal root of the mesentery, is quite freely movable. The large colon has a capacity of 60 to 130 ℓ and can rotate and turn in all directions. For this reason it is often the cause of intestinal obstruction. Even in the normal physiological state it can change its position and size depending on the degree of filling, but the pelvic flexure normally remains situated in the left abdominal region ventromedial to the spleen.

Pathological conditions of the large colon include right colonic displacement, in which the colon moves between the right abdominal wall and cecum, and left colonic displacement into the nephrosplenic space where it becomes strangulated over the nephrosplenic ligament. In both displacements, the colon can rotate 180° or more around a longitudinal axis and, as a result of turning over or of strangulation, can become partly or completely occluded.

II. TORSION OF THE LARGE COLON

Another disease of the large colon associated with mechanical ileus (intestinal obstruction) is colonic torsion along its longitudinal axis. It is by far the most dramatic equine colonic disease and due to its rapid course and fatal outcome it is an important topic of interest for the pathophysiologically oriented veterinary clinician. It is also the most common cause of ileus in the horse, comprising 19.5% in a series of 785 ileus patients (Table 1). In colonic torsion, the dorsal and ventral parts of the large intestine rotate on their longitudinal axis which is formed by the mesocolon. The direction of torsion may be lateral (80% of our cases) or medial (20%). Classification of the torsion as clockwise or counterclockwise is not precise, since the terminology depends on the position of the observer.

The degree of rotation differs from case to case. Rotation up to 90° may be regarded as within the physiological limits, that of 90 to 180° may correct itself spontaneously, while torsion in excess of 180° will never correct itself spontaneously. In exceptional cases, torsions of up to 540° have been encountered. The most frequent finding is a 360° torsion, the usual site being the region of the stomach-like dilatation, i.e., a handsbreadth in front of the cranial mesenteric root. Thus, this form involves almost the entire large colon.

The loops of colon are spirally wrapped around each other at the point of torsion (Figure 1). In rotation of up to 180° the lumen is narrowed and in cases over 240° it is totally occluded (Figure 1). In a series of 153 cases, the torsion site was near the cranial mesenteric root in 135 (88%), and in the remaining 18 it occurred at other sites, e.g., involving left longitudinal loops, diaphragmatic flexure, or at the junction of the last-named and the stomach-like dilatation.

III. CLINICAL SIGNS

Sometimes the disease starts gradually, progressing from a 180° rotation. Usually, however, it has a sudden onset, with no previous manifestations of colic.

Table 1

FREQUENCY AND OCCURRENCE OF EQUINE SMALL AND LARGE INTESTINAL OBSTRUCTION (ILEUS) IN THE TIERKLINIK HOCHMOOR, WEST GERMANY, 1979 TO 1981

Site	785 Cases	%
Duodenum and small intestine		
Gastro-duodeno-jejunitis	12	1.5
Impaction of ileum	68	8.7
Herniation through epiploic foramen	66	8.4
Mixed ileus	43	5.5
Twisting of mesentery	38	4.8
Volvulus mesenterialis	38	4.8
Volvulus nodosus	19	2.4
Pseudoligamentous hernia	18	2.3
Inguinal hernia	18	2.3
Ischemic necrosis	14	1.8
Umbilical hernia	11	1.4
Stenosis of jejunum	10	1.3
Herniation through gastrosplenic ligament	9	1.2
Omental hernia	8	1.0
Intussusception	6	0.8
Diaphragmatic hernia	5	0.6
Impaction of jejunum	4	0.5
Scrotal hernia	3	0.4
Herniation through hepatogastric ligament	3	0.4
Lipoma pendulans	2	0.3
Intramural hematoma	2	0.3
Descending mesocolic hernia	1	0.1
Total	398	50.7
Large, small colon, & cecum		
Complete torsion of large colon	135	17.2
Herniation into gastrosplenic space	78	9.9
Right dorsal displacement	44	5.6
Kinking (flexion/retroflexion) of large colon	19	2.4
Partial torsion of large colon	18	2.3
Chronic impaction of large colon incl. sand impaction	16	2.0
Enteroliths	3	0.4
Stenosis/adhesions (large colon)	3	0.4
Submucous edema (small colon)	6	0.8
Impaction of small colon	4	0.5
Intramural hematoma	3	0.4
Mesocolic rupture	3	0.4
Phytoconglobates	2	0.3
Volvulus	2	0.3
Necrosis	2	0.3
Incarceration	1	0.1
Necrosis of cecum	9	1.1
Rupture of cecum	5	0.6
Chronic impaction of cecum	3	0.4
Hypertrophy of cecum	3	0.4
Chronic tympany	2	0.3
Cecocolic intussusception	1	0.1
Internal neoplasms	14	1.8
Other cases	11	1.4
Total	387	49.3

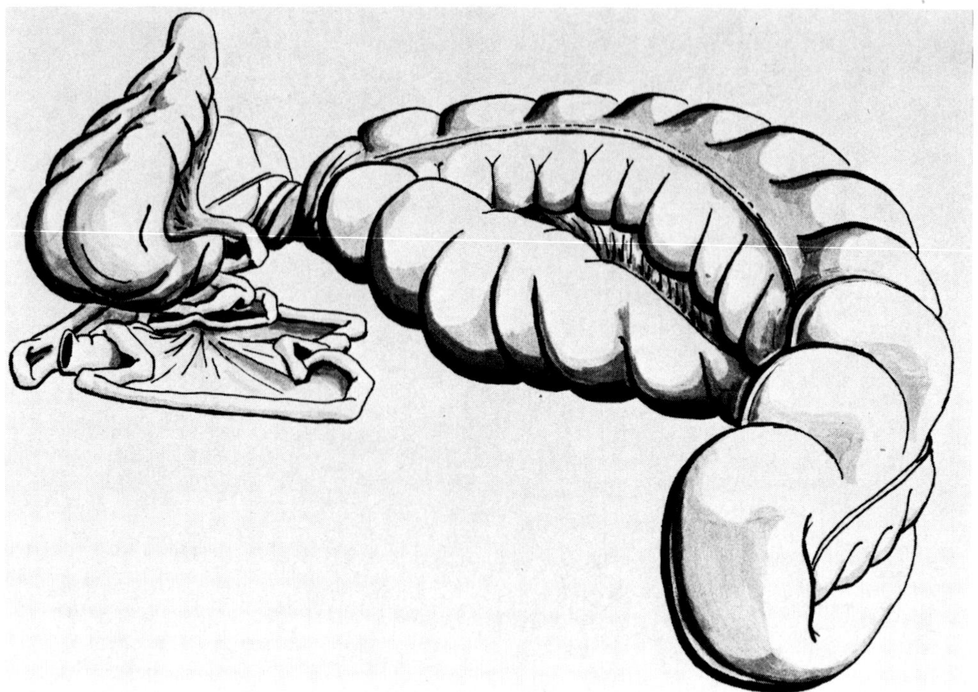

FIGURE 1.   View of the large colon to the operator standing at the left side of a horse at a midline laparotomy site with horse in dorsal recumbency (i.e., head of horse to right). Medial torsion of the entire large colon.

Colic, in this context, is a form of behavior in which the horse demonstrates evidence of pain by pawing the ground with the hooves, lying down and then standing up again, and by rolling. The colic observed in torsion of the large colon is the most spectacular of all. Affected animals crash to the ground, roll around uncontrollably, then jump up suddenly only to crash down again. Such horses are quite unpredictable in this state and endanger both grooms and veterinarians involved with the patient. A thorough clinical examination is scarcely possible. It seems that such an animal can best reduce the degree of pain during a short period by lying on its back. Even potent analgesics fail to help. Within a short period of time the horse is dripping with sweat, has very elevated pulse and respiratory rates as a result of dehydration, and has the flanks distended from gas formation in the large colon. Later the pain appears to lessen and in advanced cases may even appear to be absent. The horse then is apathetic, lies quietly on its back, and refrains from any form of movement.

IV. ETIOLOGY AND PATHOGENESIS OF TORSION OF THE LARGE COLON

Taking the example of the broodmare, which is overrepresented (52% of all cases of this condition) in our clinical material seen in the Tierklinik Hochmoor, West Germany, the course of development of the condition may be explained as follows. At the change from indoor to outdoor feeding (pasture), a period during which mares eat comparatively little hay and straw (high crude fiber feeds) but much grass (low crude fiber and high carbohydrate content), hyperactive fermentative processes occur. There is an associated excessive *Escherichia coli* and *Lactobacillus* spp. activity, with considerable gas production in the colonic lumen. The intestinal contents of the large colon are then fluid and foamy. As the intestine initially develops a degree of hyperperistalsis to propel this material forward, this atypical distension later leads to a degree of dysperistalsis that permits the intraluminal gas to induce the physiological rotation into a pathological condition in which the site of torsion is advanced to and over the stomach-like dilatation.

Factors favorable for this adverse development include the tendency to feed broodmares large volumes of foodstuffs, resulting in a very capacious colon and the potential "space" left during the post-partum months that often coincides with the period during which the mare was turned out to pasture. It is probable that initially the ventral loops of colon, which are first filled with gas, rise upward in the abdominal cavity, followed by the dorsal loops after a further increase in gas production.

V. PATHOPHYSIOLOGY

If the intestinal lumen is completely occluded, the condition is potentially rapidly fatal. Obstruction of the venous return at the site of torsion and continued arterial perfusion lead to severe hyperemic congestion and extravasation of blood, with very severe submucosal and mesocolonic edema. In addition, since the large colon is the main site of water absorption, this transport can no longer take place and dehydration quickly develops. A hemorrhagic transudate passes into the lumen as well as into the peritoneal cavity. After only a few hours the mucosa becomes necrotic, initially on the antemesenteric side. Records show that as much as 40 to 50 ℓ of transudate may be present in the colonic wall alone. If the volume of transudate in the peritoneal cavity and bowel lumen is added, the total fluid sequestration into the extracellular space will be at least 60 ℓ — an incredible amount to be withdrawn from the circulation over a brief period of 4 to 6 hr.

A very severe form of dehydration and hemorrhagic shock develops, complicated by the production of toxins which pass out from the intestinal lumen through the damaged mucosa into the general circulation. This process is accompanied by autointoxication resulting from degradation products of the bowel contents and dead tissue.

Considerable gas formation in the stenostenotic colon and the prestenotic cecum increases the intraabdominal pressure, with the consequence that the diaphragmatic pressure is increased, leading to dyspnea that may be sufficiently severe as to cause suffocation. This, in addition to the pressure on the major abdominal blood vessels, impairs cardiac function and circulation. In rare cases, bowel rupture may take place leading to a rapidly fatal peritonitis.

VI. DIAGNOSIS

The veterinary diagnosis of torsion of the large colon depends highly on the clinical picture of a dramatic and rapidly progressive colic that leads to a state of apathy and the early development of shock which soon becomes severe. In addition, a rectal examination is required which, in the horse, replaces the radiographic barium contrast studies commonly employed in man.

Rectal examination reveals tympanitic loops of large colon immediately cranial to the pelvic inlet. Their fleshy consistency is characteristic of an intramural edema, which confirms the presence of a strangulated large colon. The site of torsion cannot be determined by rectal examination.

In contrast to the frequent and acute form of torsion, a few cases have a more insidious course over a few days, and rectal examination then shows a relatively empty colon in which the small amount of ingesta does not tend to produce gas. The intraluminal pressure is therefore only slightly increased, and there is no hemorrhagic infarction

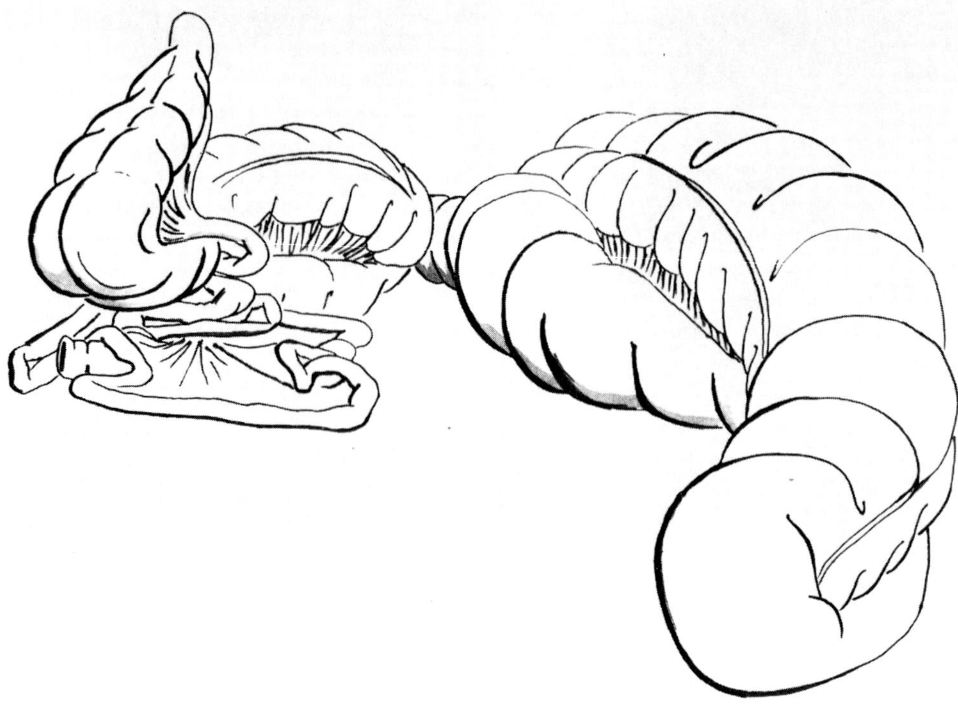

FIGURE 2.   Torsion of two thirds of the large colon. Resection is possible.

within the bowel wall. Despite marked intramural edema, this rather chronic form of torsion leads to spasmodic mild attacks of colic, but few systemic effects. This form can also be diagnosed by rectal examination, in which case edema of the bowel wall and mesocolon is ascertained by the fleshy rigid feel of the gut loops.

VII. TREATMENT

Treatment of torsion of the equine large colon is possible only by means of surgery. With the horse in dorsal recumbency, a midline laparotomy is undertaken, with the incision starting just cranial to the umbilicus and extending 30 cm or more cranially. A long incision often is needed to exteriorize the large colon. The colon is incised at the pelvic flexure and evacuated with the aid of two lengths of plastic tubing for irrigation purposes. Reposition is only possible after the colon has been emptied, due to the risk of iatrogenic rupture and the impossibility of adequate manipulation of the heavy mass of intestine. After closing the colonic incision, the colon is then replaced in the abdominal cavity. The next step depends on the direction of torsion. If it is lateral, the prestenotic colon is grasped ventrolaterally in the region of the stenosis and pulled in a lateral direction to a dorsal position. Cases of medial torsion are correspondingly manipulated medially and then dorsally. Intraabdominal handling is greatly eased by the introduction of about 10 l of sterile saline solution at body temperature. The solution reduces friction effects and enables the surgeon to manipulate the "swimming" bowel loops with ease.

In those few cases where only part of the large colon is involved in the torsion and where necrosis has developed (Figures 2 and 3) resection with anastomosis can be performed. Horses tolerate resection of up to two thirds of the large colon without difficulty and show no long-term signs of intestinal malabsorption.

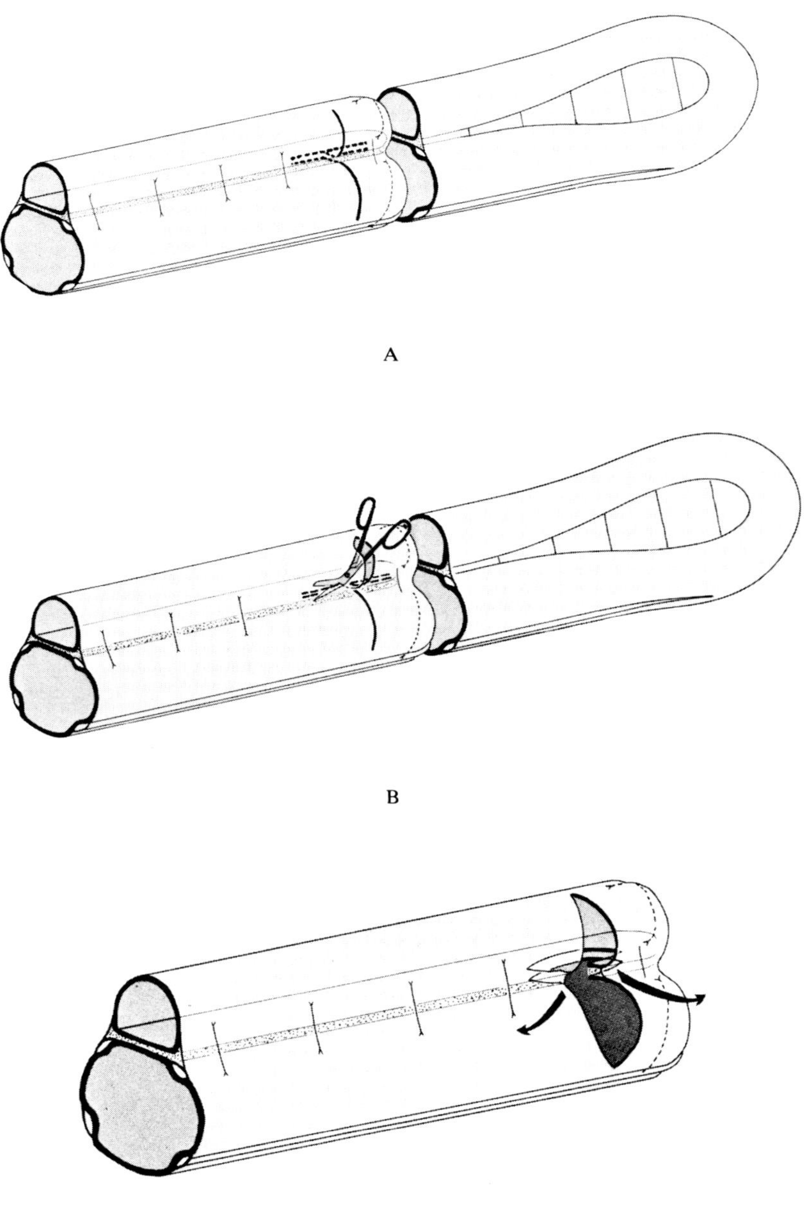

A

B

C

FIGURE 3 A to E.   Diagrams of the resection and anastomosis of the equine large colon, permitting reconstruction of a pelvic flexure.

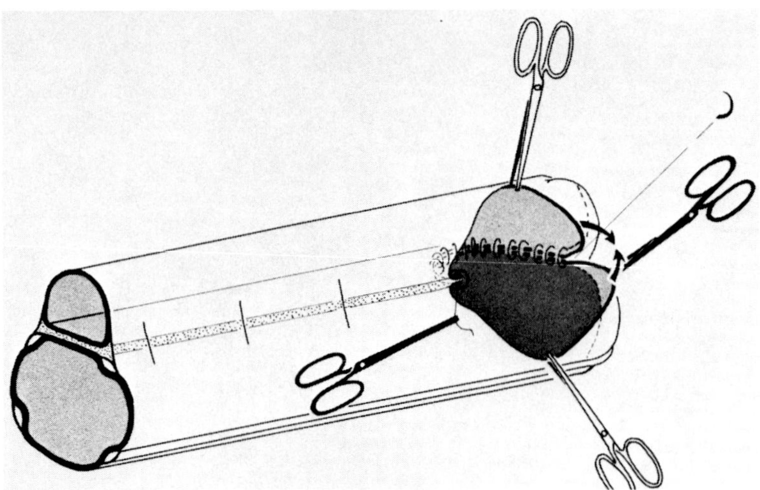

FIGURE 3D.

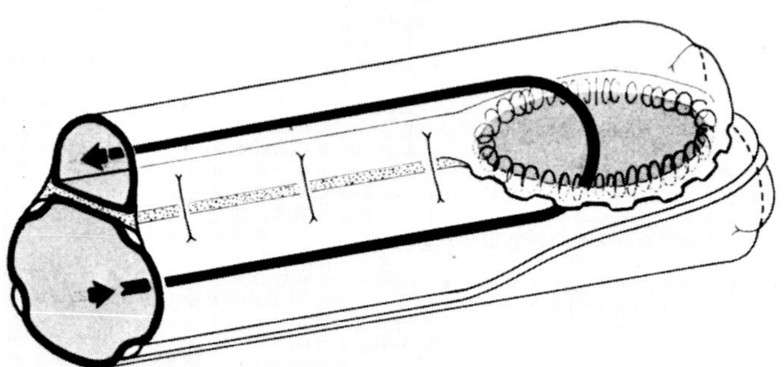

FIGURE 3E.

Chapter 15

CANINE INTESTINAL INTUSSUSCEPTION

A. David Weaver

TABLE OF CONTENTS

I. INTRODUCTION

Intussusception is an invagination or telescoping of the bowel into the adjacent portion.[1] The inner component, more proximal in prograde intussusception, is the intussusceptum, the outer distal portion, the intussuscipiens. A cross section through an intussusception shows that it comprises six layers of bowel wall. Local effects result from interference with the venous drainage from the intussusceptum leading to the development of edema, with possible eventual compromise of the arterial supply, necrosis, and gangrene with subsequent sloughing. Further significant local effects are the partial or complete occlusion of the bowel lumen and development of ileus with distension of the more proximal bowel with fluid and gas, and the development of systemic toxic signs as a result of metabolic disturbance.

Intestinal intussusception has been recorded in a variety of domestic species including the canine, feline, bovine, equine, and porcine, and in various sites including the small intestine, cecum, and colon. The veterinary literature suggests that the incidence is low in all species, but the canine appears to be most susceptible. The small intestine is the most common site. Retrograde intussusception is very rare. This chapter concerns itself only with prograde intussusception of the canine small intestine[2] and describes the clinical features of the natural disease in 32 confirmed cases examined in Glasgow University Veterinary Hospital, Scotland, over a 6-year period. These data are briefly compared with the experimental production of canine intestinal intussusception, its occurrence as a complication of canine experimental abdominal surgery, and with the natural disease in the human.

II. NATURAL DISEASE IN THE CANINE

A. Introduction: Material and History

There was no breed predilection in the 32 canines, which comprised (numbers in parentheses) German shepherds (6), Labrador retrievers (5), other purebreeds, (4), German shepherd crossbreeds (2), and other crossbreeds (15). Crossbreeds were over-represented in this study since they comprised 53%, but formed only 30% of the hospital population in the relevant period.

There were 14 males and 18 females, reflecting the hospital population. The ages ranged from 2 months to 9 years. If the 9-year-old is excluded, the mean age was 5.5 months, with 23 canines less than 6 months old.

Body weight at admission ranged from 1.5 to 34 kg, with a mean of 10.5 kg. Cases tended to become more numerous in the autumn and early winter months, as shown below:

January (1)	April (3)	July (2)	October (6)
February (1)	May (1)	August (2)	November (5)
March (0)	June (1)	September (4)	December (7)

The duration of illness at admission was 1 to 49 days, with a mean of 12 days. Twelve pups had been bought within the previous 2 weeks from a local dog home and refuge where unwanted animals were available to potential owners.

B. Clinical Features

Clinical features on presentation, together with observations of the owners, were put onto code cards (termatrex) for subsequent analysis. The signs are listed in Table 1 for the 32 canines. The most common signs were vomiting (29), diarrhea (28), and palpable mass (25). This triad was present in 19 cases (Figure B of Table 2). The triad of vom-

Table 1

SIGNS REPORTED BY OWNER (O) AND OBSERVED BY VETERINARIAN (V) IN 32 CASES OF CANINE INTUSSUSCEPTION

Case no.	Vomiting		Pain		Mucus/blood per rectum		Diarrhea		Palpable mass		Anorexia		Thirst increase		Straining	
	O	V	O	V	O	V	O	V	O	V	O	V	O	V	O	V
1	+	+	−	−	−	−	+	+	+	+	−	−	−	−	−	−
2	+	+	−	−	−	−	+	−	+	+	+	+	−	−	−	−
3	+	+	−	+	−	−	+	−	+	+	+	+	−	−	−	−
4	−	−	+	+	+	+	+	+	−	−	+	+	−	−	−	−
5	+	+	−	+	−	−	+	−	+	+	−	−	−	−	−	−
6	+	+	−	+	−	−	+	+	+	+	+	+	−	−	−	−
7	+	+	+	+	+	+	+	+	+	+	−	−	−	−	+	+
8	+	+	−	−	−	−	+	+	−	−	+	+	−	−	−	−
9	+	−	−	−	+	+	+	−	+	+	+	+	+	−	−	−
10	+	+	−	−	+	+	+	+	−	−	+	+	−	−	−	−
11	+	+	+	+	+	+	+	+	−	−	−	−	−	−	+	+
12	+	+	−	+	−	+	+	+	−	−	−	−	−	−	−	−
13	+	+	−	+	−	−	+	+	−	−	−	−	−	+	−	−
14	+	+	+	+	−	−	+	+	+	+	+	+	−	−	−	−
15	+	+	−	−	−	−	−	−	+	+	−	−	+	+	−	−
16	+	+	−	−	+	+	+	−	+	+	−	−	−	−	+	+
17	+	+	−	+	+	+	+	+	+	+	+	+	−	−	+	+
18	+	+	−	+	−	−	+	+	+	+	−	−	−	−	−	−
19	+	+	−	+	+	+	+	+	+	+	−	−	−	−	+	+
20	+	−	−	−	−	−	+	+	+	+	+	+	−	−	−	−
21	+	+	−	−	−	−	−	−	+	+	−	−	+	−	−	−
22	+	−	−	−	+	+	+	+	+	+	+	+	−	−	+	+
23	+	+	−	+	−	−	+	−	+	+	−	−	−	−	−	−
24	+	+	−	−	+	+	+	+	+	+	+	+	−	−	+	+
25	+	+	+	+	+	+	+	+	+	+	−	−	−	−	−	−
26	+	−	+	−	−	−	+	−	+	+	−	−	+	−	+	−
27	+	+	−	−	+	+	+	+	−	+	−	−	−	−	−	−
28	+	+	−	−	+	−	+	+	−	+	+	+	−	−	−	−

Table 1 (continued)

SIGNS REPORTED BY OWNER (O) AND OBSERVED BY VETERINARIAN (V) IN 32 CASES OF CANINE INTUSSUSCEPTION

Case no.	Vomiting		Pain		Mucus/blood per rectum		Diarrhea		Palpable mass		Anorexia		Thirst increase		Straining	
	O	V	O	V	O	V	O	V	O	V	O	V	O	V	O	V
29	+	−	−	−	+	+	−	−	−	−	+	+	−	−	−	−
30	−	−	−	−	−	−	+	+	+	+	−	+	−	−	−	−
31	−	−	−	−	−	−	+	+	−	+	+	+	−	−	−	−
32	+	+	−	−	+	+	−	−	+	+	−	−	−	−	+	+
Total	29		15		16		28		25		15		5		9	

Table 2

TRIAD OF DIFFERENT SIGNS IN 32 CASES OF CANINE INTUSSUSCEPTION

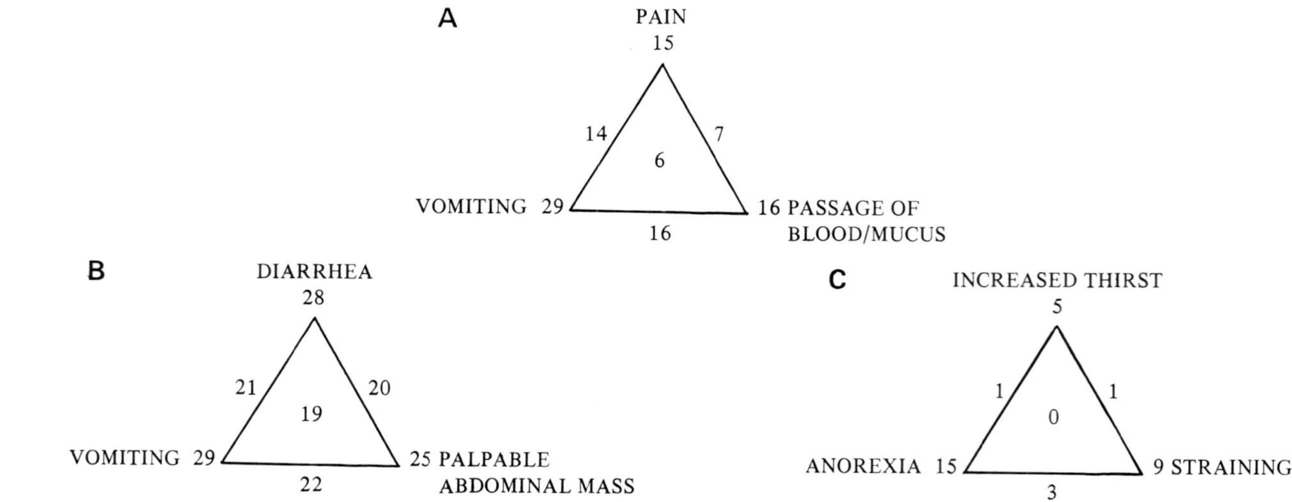

iting, pain, and the passage of blood or mucus per rectum was noted in six animals (Figure A of Table 2). Anorexia was a feature of 15 cases, with tenesmus (9) and polydipsia (5) experienced by a small minority (Figure C of Table 2).

The frequency of vomiting was highly variable and was unrelated to ingestion of fluids or solids. Hematemesis was not recorded. Diarrhea was usually characterized by the frequent passage of relatively small amounts of very watery feces. The cases that exhibited mucus and blood in the feces were not necessarily those animals that had tenesmus (Table 1).

The palpable mass was usually firm, smooth, ovoid or sausage-shaped, with a curvature of 20 to 70°. It was not very painful on pressure, but traction ventrally on the mass and associated mesentery provoked a pain response in half the cases. The position of the mass was highly variable, as was its mobility. The commonest site was the cranial dorsal quadrant, ventral and caudal to the right kidney and aorta. In such cases only minimal movement of the mass was possible. In half the cases the intussusception was freely movable in the midabdomen, occasionally being capable of being pulled to the ventral abdominal wall. In three canines the mass occupied much of the dorsal caudal portion of the abdomen and was prolapsed through the anal orifice.

Differential diagnosis was primarily from a smooth small intestinal foreign body, secondly, from gross lymphadenopathy of the mesenteric nodes associated with intestinal neoplasia (e.g., lymphosarcoma), and thirdly, from a linear foreign body that led to the development of a secondary intussusception. Cases with the intestine prolapsing through the anal orifice required differentiation from rectal prolapse.

Radiography was routinely performed. Plain lateral films (to exclude a radiopaque foreign body) were followed by a retrograde positive contrast study, using a suspension of barium sulfate injected via a Foley catheter into the distal colon. The volume of contrast medium used ranged from 20 to 100 mℓ, depending on patient size. In a few selected cases where diagnosis was still uncertain, liquid barium sulfate was given per os and films were taken at hourly intervals.

Unless the film quality was exceptionally good, it was rarely possible to confirm the presence of a small intestinal intussusception on a plain film. The radiographic features primarily tended to confirm the suggestion of a partial intestinal obstruction, with loops of gas- and fluid-filled bowel. Retrograde positive contrast study was more useful in demonstrating bowel obstruction in the ileocolic area, with little or no contrast passing proximally through the narrowed bowel lumen of the intussusceptum. In cases of mid- and lower jejunal obstruction, contrast material was able to pass retrograde through the ileocolic junction and then tended to stagnate distal to the obstruction. Hydrostatic pressure reduction was never attempted or accidentally achieved in any canine of this series.

C. Laboratory Investigation

Laboratory investigations (blood biochemistry, urine analysis, and hematology) were done in 20 cases before treatment started. The results (Table 2) showed that abnormalities were only detected in a minority of cases, namely, a raised blood urea (4/18), lowered plasma Na and Cl (1/17), raised plasma inorganic phosphate (3/18), raised alkaline phosphatase (1/16), raised SGOT (3/15), low plasma albumin and globulin (7/19), lowered packed cell volume (4/16), and a leukocytosis (9/18).

D. Site of Intussusception

The sites were as follows:

Jejunal	12	Ileocolic-rectal	3
Mid or distal ileal	4	Total cases	32
Ileocolic or ileocecocolic	13		

Table 3

SITE AND EXTENT OF INTUSSUSCEPTION IN 32 CANINES

Case no.   Jejunum   Ileum   Colon   Rectum

1
2 ●
3 ●
4 ●
5
6 ●
7
8
9/1
9/2
9/3
9/4 ●
10
11
12 ●
13
14/1
14/2
15
16/1
16/2
17 ●
18/1
18/2
18/3
19
20
21
22
23
24 ●
25/1
25/2
25/3
26
27
28/1
28/2
29 ●
30
31
32

● = Fatality
▲ = Splitting of bowel wall
n = Severe necrosis
━ = Reducible bowel
■ = Irreducible bowel

The site, the reducibility of the intussusception, the number of operations, and the outcome are shown in Table 3. The features of splitting of the bowel wall (serosa or muscularis) and of severe necrosis of the intussusceptum or intussuscipiens are also given in Table 3.

E. Surgery

Surgery was undertaken in all cases (32 canines), usually after the administration of intravenous fluids, and was invariably done under general anesthesia. Midline laparotomy was carried out through an appropriate incision extending cranially from the umbilicus. At the initial laparotomy easy manual reduction of the intussusception was possible in six instances. The affected bowel did not require further attention.

Manual reduction was carried out with difficulty in a further nine initial cases, where there was splitting of the serosa and musculature in six cases and with evidence of bowel necrosis in the other three canines. Bowel resection was carried out in this subgroup of nine animals. The remaining 17 cases were irreducible and these also underwent resection and anastomosis, usually with the end-to-end (12), occasionally end-to-side (3), or side-to-side (2) pattern.[3] Anastomotic suture material was 2/0 or 3/0 chromic catgut. The total length of resected bowel varied from 10 to 105 cm. The maximum length was in a 3-month-old Labrador retriever (case 25) in which three operations were needed as a result of recurrence of the intussusception. Six dogs had multiple operations that involved further resection at intervals up to 20 days after the initial surgery. Thus, a total of 42 operations was performed on 32 canines (Table 3).

F. Mortality and Survival

Six animals died 2 to 24 hr after the initial surgery, one from an unrelated but intercurrent disease (*Leptospira icterohemorrhagiae* infection, confirmed by pathology and bacteriology). An additional 5 died from 4 to 15 days postoperatively. Three of the latter group involved wound breakdown and severe peritonitis. Two others died from intercurrent disease (confirmed distemper). All three cases of intercurrent disease came from a local dog home where there is known exposure to distemper virus.

There were no recurrences of intussusception more than 20 days after the previous episode and 21 (65.5%) survived surgery, were discharged, and at follow-up 8 months to 4 years later were reported to be alive and well. None had a problem with diarrhea (short bowel syndrome).

III. EXPERIMENTAL DISEASE IN THE CANINE

A survey[4] of the literature of canine intussusception revealed that the condition can take a chronic course. One third of cases in which intussusception was experimentally produced by suture of an invaginated length of jejunum died within 6 days, having failed to defecate after the operation. However, the remaining two thirds of the experimental group developed a chronic form of the disease with intermittent vomiting and diarrhea, and slow weight loss. One dog survived 77 days. The authors emphasized the difference in signs seen in the first few days, characterized by complete ileus, and then later by chronic gastroenteritis. These observations contradict the opinion of Larsen,[5] who claimed that cases of nonoperated intussusception were invariably fatal within a few days.

Various abdominal experimental surgical procedures, such as canine renal transplantation, have been associated with the subsequent development of intestinal intussusception in a number of animals.[6] These experimental procedures were often prolonged and involved considerable displacement and manipulation of the bowel. Most cases developed within 1 week (and invariably within 3 weeks) of surgery — the cardinal signs being anorexia, vomiting, and passage of bloody feces. Plication of the distal ileum to the ascending colon at the initial surgical intervention failed to prevent small-bowel intussusception.[6]

IV. NATURAL DISEASE IN HUMANS

The condition is almost invariably acute in young children or infants, often 3 to 12 months old.[7] There is usually no history of related illness. The site is usually ileoileal or ileocolic. The mesenteric lymph nodes are invariably enlarged, and it has been postulated that lymphoid hyperplasia of the bowel wall is due to an adenovirus infection and that the lymphoid tissue, by protruding into the bowel wall, acts as a form of "foreign body".[8,9] In adults and some children, various forms of polyps (adenomata and lipomata), carcinomata, or an inverted Meckel's diverticulum may form the apex of the intussusception.[9] Chronic intussusception in children is uncommon.[14]

Clinical signs in infants include paroxysms of abdominal colic and severe shock with vomiting and the passage of blood and mucus ("red currant jelly"). After 24 hr, neglected cases show abdominal distension, feculent vomiting, and severe signs of toxicity due to gangrene of the intussusception and a related peritonitis.

The majority of cases in North America are treated by hydrostatic reduction using liquid positive contrast run into the rectum and colon under fluoroscopic control.[10,11] Successful reduction has been claimed in over 80% of cases so treated.[10] Operative treatment is generally practiced outside North America, and in those cases in America where hydrostatic pressure fails. Usually a simple manipulative reduction without resection is sufficient.[12] Mortality is low in the majority of cases which are treated within 24 hr of the onset of clinical signs. Recurrence is uncommon.

Chronic intussusception in children may be difficult to diagnose.[1] Postoperative intussusception is an infrequent but important complication of surgical procedures performed on infants and children and classical signs are not seen.[14] Pain is not of the periodic character, a bloody stool is rare, and an abdominal mass not palpable. The etiology of most cases is unknown, but a disturbance of peristalsis following mild operative trauma is thought to be the probable cause.[14] Older children and adults with postoperative intussusception often have associated local pathology such as Meckel's diverticula, inverted appendiceal stumps, or intestinal submucosal hematomas.[24]

V. DISCUSSION

In both the canine and human subject the etiology of most cases of intestinal intussusception remains obscure. A change of environment or feeding pattern in both species at the age of 2 to 9 months probably plays a contributary role. In the canine it has been thought that severe intestinal infection with parasites such as roundworms (e.g., *Toxocara canis*) may be significant, but in this series severe roundworm infestation was rarely encountered.

Common factors contributing to intussusception following experimental surgery were a recent dietary change following weaning, malabsorption with diarrhea following total pancreatectomy, and an upper respiratory tract infection.[6] Associated hypermotility of gut and mesenteric adenitis with enlargement of Peyers patches have been hypothetical factors contributing to the onset of intussusception.[6]

As in the human, a number of benign and malignant neoplasms in the adult dog have been found occasionally to contribute to the development of intussusception.[15,16] Small intestinal neoplasms are by no means rare in the canine and while some may be diffuse (e.g., lymphosarcoma), many are discrete, and the proportion of them associated with intussusception is extremely small, probably under 0.5%.

Similarities in the natural condition in the canine and human subject include the predominance of the young age group, as well as the site of the lesion. Differences include the more dramatic and potentially fatal course of the disease in babies and young infants, compared with the more protracted course in the canine, and the relative success of hydrostatic pressure or manual reduction in the human subject.

There has been no explanation for a statistically significant drop in the incidence of acute intussusception cases in children,[17] while figures are not available for the canine.

The long duration of signs (4, 5, and 7 weeks) in some cases of this clinical series suggests that they may have been cases of chronic intussusception. No relationship could be found between the duration of signs and the length of the intussusception or the ability to reduce it manually. Some cases had experienced a course of illness up to 16 days, yet the intussusception was reducible manually. Since others required resection as a result of adhesion formation and yet had a course of illness as short as 2 to 3 days, it seems that in some longstanding cases the intussusception had developed only a few days before presentation. In one instance (case 6) there had been intermittent prolapse of the small intestine through the anus for at least 10 days before presentation.

The intramural pressure of the intussusception is liable to play an important part, not only in the development of a severe degree of intestinal obstruction (ileus) and, therefore, on the rapidity of development of toxic signs, but it can also account for this variation in the duration and character of signs. It is hypothesized that some cases may develop a short and relatively nonobstructive form of intussusception with mild signs, which later progresses physically into a longer and more occluding lesion. No relationship was noted between the degree of intestinal obstruction per se in short (<15 cm overall length) vs. longer forms of intussusception.

The two forms of disease, acute and chronic, seen in an experimental canine series[4] may possibly be attributed to a technical inability to ensure production of a standard model, so that although a standard length of jejunum was sutured into the succeeding portion of bowel, the degree of intestinal obstruction produced was evidently variable from case to case.

The relatively minor effects of canine intestinal intussusception of the natural series, in terms of adverse changes in body fluids, are probably attributable to the fact that obstruction was only partial in most cases. Additionally, the site tended to be the distal jejunum or ileum (Table 3), so that vomiting was not so prolonged or severe as it might have been in the event of duodenal obstruction. Most dogs continued to drink water. Plasma albumin is known to decrease following major trauma or operation,[19] but the fall in globulin is difficult to explain. Most patients were young, and their values would therefore be lower than the adult figures. The effect of water conservation is reflected in the high specific gravity of urine in four of nine recorded cases.

In the canine clinical cases the greatest proportion of resected intestine was estimated to be 105 cm in a 3-month-old Labrador retriever, equivalent to a 44% reduction, and two cases of 43 cm, one in a 4-month-old crossbred, equivalent to 21%, the other in a 4-month-old cocker spaniel, equivalent to 25% loss. The calculations are based on the estimate[21] that the length of the small intestine is approximately 3.5 times the length of the dog. Although visually extensive, it must be appreciated that the major length of the small intestine was retained.

The long-term effects of resection of a considerable length of canine small intestine have been studied,[22] and relatively minor changes were seen in the follow-up period of 3 months following resection of half of the small intestine.

The recovery rate in this series was almost twice as high as the 35% recorded elsewhere.[16] The American series included many cases that died or were destroyed on humane grounds and which, therefore, did not undergo surgery. The better success rate may also be due to the intensive care taken in the Glasgow series, in which problems of poor surgical technique (leading to leakage of bowel contents and peritonitis) were a minor problem.

VI. SUMMARY

Canine intestinal intussusception is sporadically encountered, usually in young animals aged 2 months to 2 years. In puppies it is sometimes associated with dietary changes in the new owner's home. It is rare in the adult, where intestinal neoplasia or a linear foreign body (thread, string) may predispose. In 32 canines the cardinal signs were vomiting, diarrhea, and the presence of a palpable mass. Pain, an elusive sign in young animals, and the passage of bloody mucus were inconsistent signs. The sites of intussusception were jejunal (12 cases), mid or distal ileal (4), ileocecal or ileocecocolic (13), or ileocolorectal (3). At laparotomy many cases could not be manually reduced, and resection was required in 26 cases. Recurrence was seen in six canines. The recovery rate was 65.6%. No chronic problems were encountered.

The canine and human syndromes are briefly contrasted. In most cases of canine intestinal intussusception, as in human infant intussusception, the etiology appears to be obscure, with a number of contributing factors playing a part in the provocation of this intestinal physiological abnormality.

REFERENCES

1. Dorland, W. A., *Dorland's Illustrated Medical Dictionary*, 26th ed., W.B. Saunders, Philadelphia, 1981, 676.
2. Weaver, A. D., Canine intestinal intussusception, *Vet. Rec.*, 100, 524, 1977.
3. Markowitz, J., Archibald, J., and Downie, H. G., *Experimental Surgery*, Williams & Wilkens, Baltimore, 1964, 96.
4. Cermak, K., Sankovic, F., and Pajtl, M., Einige Beobachtungen bei experimenteller Dunndarminvagination beim Hund, *Arch. Exp. Vet. Med.*, 20, 553, 1966.
5. Larsen, L. H., Stomach and small intestine, in *Canine Surgery*, Archibald, J., Ed., American Veterinary Publications, Santa Barbara, Calif., 1965, 517.
6. Dutoit, D. F., Homan, W. P., Reece-Smith, H., McShane, P., French, M. E., Denton, T. G., and Morris, P. J., Canine intestinal intussusception following renal and pancreatic transplantation, *Vet. Rec.*, 108, 34, 1981.
7. Ravitch, M. M., Intussusception, in *Pediatric Surgery*, Vol. 2, Mustard, W. T., Ed., 1969, 914.
8. Ellis, H. and Calne, R. W., in *Lecture Notes on General Surgery*, 5th ed., Blackwell Scientific, Oxford, 1977, 197.
9. Walter, J. B. and Israel, M. S., in *General Pathology*, 5th ed., Churchill Livingston, Edinburgh, 1979, 283.
10. Gierup, J., Jorulf, H., and Livaditis, A., Management of intussusception in infants and children: a survey based on 288 consecutive cases, *Pediatrics*, 50, 535, 1972.
11. Wayne, E. R., Campbell, J. B., Burrington, J. D., and Davis, W. S., Management of 344 children with intussusception, *Radiology*, 107, 597, 1973.
12. Dennison, W. M. and Shakar, M., Intussusception in infancy and childhood, *Br. J. Surg.*, 57, 679, 1970.
13. Macauley, D. and Moore, T., Subacute and chronic intussusception in infants and children, *Arch. Dis. Child.*, 30, 180, 1955.
14. Rees, B. I. and Lari, J., Chronic intussusception in children, *Br. J. Surg.*, 63, 33, 1976.
15. Larsen, L. H. and Bellenger, C. R., Stomach and small intestine, in *Canine Surgery*, Archibald, J., Ed., American Veterinary Publications, Santa Barbara, Calif., 1974, 583.
16. Wilson, G. P. and Burt, J. K., Intussusception in the dog and cat: a review of 45 cases, *J. Am. Vet. Med. Assoc.*, 164, 515, 1974.
17. Pollet, J. E. and Hems, G., The decline in incidence of acute intussusception in childhood in northeast Scotland, *J. Epidemiol. Commun. Health*, 34, 42, 1980.
18. Steyn, J. and Kyle, J., Epidemiology of acute intussusception, *Br. Med. J.*, 1, 1760, 1961.
19. Frawley, J. P., Howard, J. M., Artz, C. P., and Anderson, P., Investigation of serum protein changes in combat injuries: systemic response to injury, *Arch. Surg.*, 71, 605, 1955.
20. Glenert, J., Jarnum, S., and Riemer, S., Albumen transfer from blood to gastrointestinal tract in dogs, *Acta Chir. Scand.*, 124, 63, 1962.
21. Miller, M. E., *Anatomy of the Dog*, W. B. Saunders, Philadelphia, 1964, 685.
22. Bukzek, A., Sycinski, Z., Trojniak, T., and Utzig, J., Wplyw rozleglych resekcji jelita cienkiego na ksztaltowanie sie poziomubialka, hemoglobiny, czerwonych i bialych krwinek oral ciezaru ciala psow (Effect of extensive resection of the small intestine on serum protein, hemoglobin, red and white cell counts, and weight in dogs), *Weterynaria (Wroclaw)*, 30, 203, 1973.
23. Tank, E. S., Postoperative intussusception, *J. Urol.*, 123, 603, 1980.
24. Burke, M., Intussusception in adults, *Ann. R. Coll. Surg. Engl.*, 59, 150, 1977.

Part IV
*Experimental Animal Preparations to Assess
Function and Metabolism of the Intestines
During Pathologic States*

Chapter 16

THE EXPERIMENTAL RAT BLIND LOOP PREPARATION: A MODEL FOR SMALL-INTESTINE BACTERIAL OVERGROWTH IN MAN

Charles E. King and Phillip P. Toskes

TABLE OF CONTENTS

I. INTRODUCTION

Bacteria present in abnormal quantities in the small intestine can interfere with normal digestion and absorption of ingested nutrients. Development of this small-intestine bacterial overgrowth occurs due to failure of one or more of the mechanisms that normally maintains a proximal small-bowel flora of less than 10^5 organisms per milliliter of intestinal secretions.[1] The mechanisms include killing of ingested bacteria by acid in the stomach; propulsion of bacteria to the colon by normal small-bowel motor function; bacteriostatic effects of luminal constituents such as bile salts, mucus, immunoglobulins, and products of bacterial metabolism; and the prevention of circulation of colonic contents into the small intestine.[1-3]

Nutrient malabsorption in the setting of small-intestine bacterial overgrowth is called the blind loop, stagnant loop, or stasis syndrome.[1,2] Regardless of the etiology, bacteria in the lumen of the small bowel may have deleterious effects on the digestion and/or absorption of ingested nutrients. In addition, injury to the mucosa due to the presence of the bacterial overgrowth may lead to excessive passage of nutrients or serum constituents into the lumen of the small intestine (reverse direction of the absorptive process), magnifying deleterious effects that digestive or absorptive abnormalities have on nutrient assimilation.[1] Prior to the last 10 to 15 years, malabsorption of fat and cobalamin (vitamin B_{12}) were the primary recognized manifestations of the blind loop syndrome.[2] Since then, it has been better appreciated that malabsorption of other nutrients (carbohydrate, protein, water/electrolyte) may occur solely or in combination with the more classic manifestations.[1] The subject of this review, the experimental rat blind loop model, has aided in advancing knowledge regarding these newly recognized effects of bacterial overgrowth, including development of a much better understanding of the pathophysiologic events. This better understanding of the syndrome has raised even more questions regarding the interactions of bacteria and the gut, which will undoubtedly maintain the significance of the experimental model for years to come.

II. EXPERIMENTAL MODELS

Although alteration of small-bowel motility by treatment with ganglionic blockers has been reported as a method to induce acutely bacterial overgrowth,[4] this method has not been used frequently as an experimental model because of inconsistent results.[5] In addition, the medical therapy model has an undue risk of side effects from the therapy and requires frequent parenteral administration of the agent, which is impractical for long-term studies.[4,5]

Partial gastrectomy, especially when vagotomy and/or gastrojejunal anastomosis is part of the procedure, is a frequent cause of bacterial overgrowth in the human.[1] Although performance of various ulcer operations in dogs has been attended by a variable incidence of small-intestine bacterial overgrowth, use of dogs is expensive and impractical for study of a large number of animals.[6] Alternative use of these ulcer therapy operations in the small rodent is often impractical because of the size of the organs involved and difference in gastric secretion/anatomy of the rat, which does not contain acid-secreting mucosa in the cephalad half of the stomach (as does the human).

The model easiest to create and most widely used for the bacterial overgrowth syndromes is the jejunal self-filling blind loop model.[7] Cameron and co-workers,[7] in a classic study of the development of macrocytic anemia, developed the experimental rat self-filling blind loop model. In their experiments they demonstrated that self-filling blind loops in the mid or upper jejunum were attended by the development of macrocytic anemia.[7] These changes were not seen in rats having self-filling blinds placed in the distal small intestine nor in rats in which the blind loops were constructed in a self-

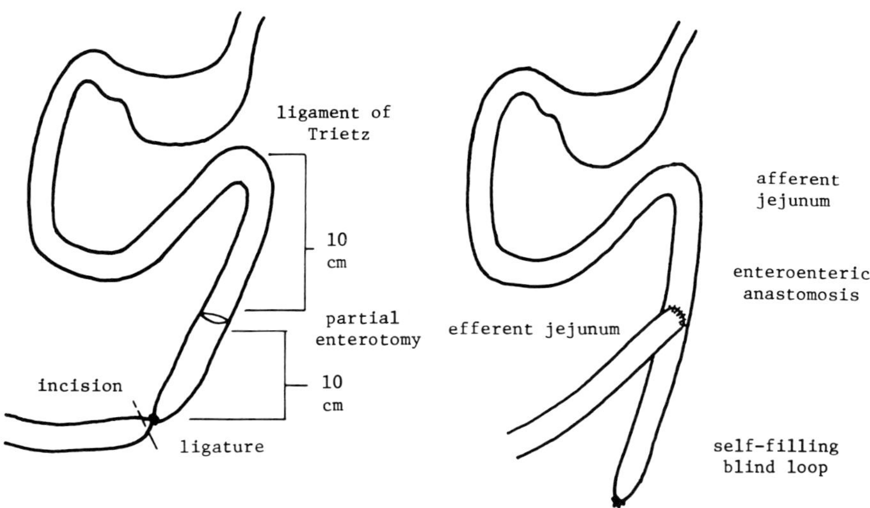

FIGURE 1. Stepwise creation of the jejunal self-filling blind loop. On the left side, a partial enter-otomy has been made 10 cm distal to the ligament of Treitz, while bowel ligation and incision was made 20 cm distal to the ligament of Treitz. On the right side, enteroenteric anastomosis was performed at the proximal aspect of the self-filling blind loop, bringing the efferent jejunum in continuity with the afferent jejunum and blind loop.

emptying fashion.[7] As depicted in Figure 1, the currently used modification of this model entails creation of a blind loop beginning 10 cm distal to the ligament of Treitz. The blind loop is surgically constructed so that small-bowel motility keeps the loop preferentially filled. This self-filling jejunal blind loop, after maturation, serves as a continuous contaminating source of bacteria to the absorptive small bowel distal to the surgical blind loop. This stagnant loop thus acts similarly as the dysfunctional afferent loop of a patient with a gastrojejunal anastomosis, as the collective stagnant diverticuli of the subject with small-bowel diverticulosis, and/or as the stagnant small intestine of the subject with a motility disorder such as scleroderma or intestinal pseudo-obstruction.[1] Although this model has been used occasionally in the dog,[8] its primary use as an experimental model of bacterial overgrowth has been in the laboratory rat.

III. SURGICAL CONSTRUCTION

Rats are prevented from eating food 8 hours prior to the surgery to assure a food-free small intestine in the operating field (minimizing peritoneal soiling by luminal contents). Because of the nocturnal eating habits of the rat, this requires overnight abstinence from food, even if the surgery is to be performed the next afternoon. Because of the sensitivity of the rat to water deprivation, water *ad libitum* is allowed up to the time of surgery and not withheld once recovery from the anesthesia is apparent postoperatively.

The abdominal hair is shaved and a left paramedian incision made from below the ribcage to approximately two thirds the distance to the pubic area. After covering the skin with a slit 4 × 4 gauze pad wetted with irrigating saline, the small bowel is gently lifted out of the peritoneal cavity until either the ileocecal junction or the ligament of Treitz is located. The small bowel is then moistened with saline and replaced in the peritoneal cavity except for approximately 30 cm beginning at the ligament of Treitz, which is laid in a semicircular fashion on the wetted gauze. At a point 10 cm distal to the ligament of Treitz, a horizontal incision approximately one third the circumference of the bowel is made on the antimesenteric side of the jejunum (Figure 1). At a point 20 cm down from the ligament of Treitz, a ligature of 3-0 or 4-0 suture is tied around the bowel and the bowel severed distal to the ligature. The free (distal) end is then anastomosed to the enterotomy 10 cm distal to the ligament of Treitz.

Approximation of small-bowel segments and placement of well-spaced sutures are aided by placement of a 2- to 3-cm-long roll of dry absorbable Gelfoam® into the lumen of one of the bowel segments to be anastomosed; the roll is then partially "milked" into the other bowel segment to bridge the area to be anatomosed. Suturing of the enteroenterotomy is accomplished by placement of interrupted sutures at the three nonmesenteric quadrants, plus placement of a continuous running suture beginning and ending at the mesenteric border of the distal segment of the enteroenterotomy. The ligated end of the bowel loop has thus become the blind end of a 10-cm jejunal loop that preferentially fills in a peristaltic fashion.

Although one could prophylactically place antibacterial solution in the peritoneum following surgery, we have not done so and have had no trouble with peritonitis/undue peritoneal adhesions despite use of clean but not necessarily sterile technique during the procedure. Following closure of the peritoneum/muscle and skin with interrupted sutures/clips, the animal is returned to regular caging and allowed water upon awakening; solid food is allowed the next day.

Because removal of the 10-cm segment of bowel for creation of the jejunal blind loop could lead to compensatory changes of the digestive/absorptive function of the small intestine distal to the blind loop,[9] a surgical control group is required for experimental blind loop studies. The usual control is that in which the 10-cm jejunal blind loop is constructed so that aboral motility moves toward, rather than away from the ostium of the jejunal blind loop. This self-emptying (as contrasted to self-filling) jejunal blind loop is constructed in a similar fashion as the self-filling blind loop, except that for the procedure the ligature tying off the jejunum is placed 10 cm distal to the ligament of Treitz, the jejunum is circumferentially incised proximal to this ligature, and the partial enterotomy/enteroenteric anastomosis made 20 cm distal to the ligament of Treitz. Studies in our laboratory have demonstrated that absorption of various nutrients (cobalamin, xylose, fat) in the self-emptying blind loop model remains normal.[10-13] In addition, bacterial cultures and histology of the small intestine is similar to unoperated control animals.[10-14]

IV. MANIFESTATIONS OF THE EXPERIMENTAL BLIND LOOP SYNDROME

A. Gross Anatomy

Upon initiation of feeding, passage of luminal contents into the self-filling blind loop leads to stagnation and growth of the loop to 1.5 to 2.5 times in length and 3 to 4 times in diameter the size of the adjacent afferent and efferent jejunum.[13] Contents of the blind loop take on the appearance and odor of liquid feces and account for the ability of the loop to continuously contaminate the adjacent small bowel with an overgrowth of bacteria.

On occasion, experimental animals will have a poorly developed self-filling blind loop, especially early in the experience of the investigator performing the surgery. In these rare failures, stenosis at the ostium of the blind loop has led to diminished flow of luminal contents (which acts as a culture medium for bacteria in the loop) into the blind loop. Development of this stenosis at the blind loop ostium usually is due to either improper size of the enterotomy (receiving site of the proximal end of the blind loop), use of too much suture material at the enteroenteric anastomosis (with secondary foreign body stenosis), or inadequate sealing at the anastomosis due to improper suturing which is followed by leakage of luminal contents and secondary excessive peritoneal reaction.

In a similar fashion, improper suturing at the enteroenteric anastomosis of the self-emptying blind loop can lead to partial obstruction to the normal jejunal flow of luminal contents and stagnation/bacterial overgrowth occurring in the duodenum and proximal jejunum.

Because of these rare "opposite-response" findings in the failed self-filling loop (less overgrowth than usual) or the failed control self-emptying loop animals (more bacterial overgrowth than usual), assessment of the anatomic status of the surgical blind loop is necessary at the time of experimental study or post-mortem, especially early in the experience of the investigator.

B. Bacteriology

Content of bacteria in the proximal jejunum of the unoperated experimental rat contains 10^6 to 10^7 aerobes and anaerobes per milliliter of intestinal fluid, with anaerobes usually slightly predominant.[10-14] Coprophagy by the rat leads to somewhat higher counts than in the normal human jejunum, which usually contains $<10^5$ organisms per milliliter and very limited numbers of coliforms and anaerobes. Creation of a self-filling blind loop in the jejunum leads to a 1- to 2-log increase in aerobes in both the blind loop and efferent jejunum and a 2- to 3-log increase in the blind loop and 1- to 2-log increase in the efferent jejunum of anaerobic organisms.[10-14] The usually higher degree of bacterial growth in the blind loop than the efferent jejunum reflects the fact that although continuously seeded by blind loop contents/bacteria, the efferent small bowel more easily than the stagnant loop propels bacteria to the colon. We have noted that this quantitative change in the flora occurs as early as 3 days postoperatively,[12] although most studies with the rats are done no earlier than 2 weeks after construction of the blind loop.[11,13]

C. Histology

Light microscopy of the mucosa of rats with jejunal self-filling blind loops demonstrates villous deformity (shortening, broadening, fusion of villi) with associated hyperplasia of glandular cysts.[14] These changes are most prominent in the self-filling blind loop, but are also seen to a lesser degree in the jejunum distal to the blind loop. Electron microscopy reveals a variable degree of cytoplasmic degeneration and alteration (shortening, swelling, blistering) of the microvilli.[14,15] These changes are seen in many cells of the efferent jejunum, including ones that appear normal by light microscopy.

D. Brush Border Enzymes

Analysis of lactase, sucrase, and maltase levels in mucosal homogenates has demonstrated a moderate to marked decrease in both the blind loop and the efferent jejunum.[10,16-18] Histochemical staining for brush border alkaline phosphatase and leucine aminopeptidase has also revealed depressed levels of these enzymes in the self-filling blind loops.[14,18] Forstner's laboratory has demonstrated that these changes are related to enhanced turnover of mucosal surface glycoproteins,[17] with the turnover being most rapid at the most exposed surface of the brush border.

E. Absorption

A major impact of the experimental rat blind loop model has been in the study of absorption of various nutrients. With this model, the degree of malabsorption that can occur with various nutrients (e.g., fat, cobalamin, monosaccharides) has been delineated.[10-12,18,19] Even more importantly, ability to manipulate the animal with various therapeutic regimens has demonstrated the importance of different parts of the overgrowth flora on the malassimilation of various nutrients.[11,12,20] Use of the experimental model has allowed experimental manipulation that has distinguished the coexisting pathophysiologic events of intraluminal bacterial catabolism of substrate and altered mucosal absorption.[11,20] The mucosal injury component has been shown to have a delayed and/or incompletely reversible nature.[13] In addition, an additive burden to protein and iron assimilation has been seen with excessive passage of labeled serum protein and hemoglobin iron to the gut lumen.[13,21]

V. POSTTHERAPY STUDIES

In studies of small-intestine bacterial overgrowth, correction of the malabsorption following antimicrobial therapy is evidence that bacterial overgrowth is the cause of the malabsorption.[1,2] Use of selective antimicrobial therapy (e.g., selectively affecting aerobic or anaerobic overgrowth) has been used to demonstrate the predominant importance of parts of the flora for various types of nutrient malabsorption.[11,12,20] The selective therapy can either be initiated at the time of performance of the blind loop surgery,[12] or it may be initiated following development of bacterial overgrowth.[11,20] In the latter case, therapy is begun following demonstration of a functional abnormality, in which case the experimental animal serves as its own pretherapy control. Use of selective antimicrobial therapy beginning at the time of blind loop surgery serves as an effective (and much simpler) alternative to monocontamination experiments of germ-free animals with selective organisms.

In studies requiring complete reversal of bacterial overgrowth (e.g., investigations evaluating a slowly reversible manifestation of mucosal injury), long-term antimicrobial therapy is not always adequate for completely correcting the bacterial overgrowth and/or functional abnormalities.[13] An alternative therapy entails surgical extirpation of the jejunal blind loop.[13,22] This surgical therapy not only removes the blind loop as a site for contamination of the remaining small intestine, but also removes the blind loop as a participating site in a functional abnormality (e.g., as a site for serum protein loss or as one initiating abnormal motor responses).[13,22]

The experimental blind loop syndrome can also be combined with other manipulations of the gastrointestinal tract, such as performance of an ileal conduit for biliary diversion, in the evaluation of pathogenetic mechanisms in the syndrome.[18,23] Ability of the investigator to perform successfully a second operation (e.g., performing blind loop surgery in biliary-diverted animals or extirpation of the blind loop) depends on the skill and expertise in performing the first operation, which minimizes surgical deformity and adhesions.

VI. SUMMARY

The self-filling blind loop rat model for small-intestine bacterial overgrowth offers an inexpensive, reproducible, and relevant model of a relatively frequent, clinically important human problem. The technique for creation of the jejunal blind loop is easily learned and the procedure is well tolerated by the experimental animal. Although the self-filling blind loops grow to considerable size, their presence and the healed surgical areas still allow easy follow-up abdominal manipulation, such as performance of a second surgical procedure or placement of perfusion catheters for in vivo studies of small-bowel absorption. As interest in the interaction of the gut with the intestinal microflora expands, this model takes on increased importance as an experimental model for human disease.

REFERENCES

1. King, C. E. and Toskes, P. P., Small intestine bacterial overgrowth, *Gastroenterology*, 76, 1035, 1979.
2. Donaldson, R. M., Jr., Small bowel bacterial overgrowth, *Adv. Intern. Med.*, 16, 191, 1970.
3. Gorbach, S. L., Intestinal microflora, *Gastroenterology*, 60, 1110, 1971.
4. Dixon, J. M. S. and Paulley, J. W., Bacteriological and histological studies of the small intestine of rats treated with mecamylamine, *Gut*, 4, 169, 1963.
5. Summers, R. W. and Kent, T. H., Effects of altered propulsion on rat small intestinal flora, *Gastroenterology*, 59, 740, 1970.
6. Greenlee, H. B., Gelbart, S. M., DeOrio, A. J., Francescatti, D. S., Paez, J., and Reinhardt, G. F., The influence of gastric surgery on the intestinal flora, *Am. J. Clin. Nutr.*, 30, 1826, 1977.
7. Cameron, D. G., Watson, G. M., and Witts, L. J., The experimental production of macrocytic anemia by operations on the intestinal tract, *Blood*, 4, 803, 1949.
8. Kim, Y. S., Spritz, N., Blum, M., Terz, J., and Sherlock, P., The role of altered bile acid metabolism in the steatorrhea of experimental blind loop, *J. Clin. Invest.*, 45, 956, 1966.
9. Gleeson, M. H., Dowling, R. H., and Peters, T. J., Biochemical changes in intestinal mucosa after experimental small bowel by-pass in the rat, *Clin. Sci.*, 43, 743, 1972.
10. Giannella, R. A., Rout, W. R., and Toskes, P. P., Jejunal brush border injury and impaired sugar and amino acid uptake in the blind loop syndrome, *Gastroenterology*, 67, 965, 1974.
11. Toskes, P. P., King, C. E., Spivey, J. C., and Lorenz, E., Xylose catabolism in the experimental rat blind loop syndrome: studies including use of a newly developed d-[^{14}C]-xylose breath test, *Gastroenterology*, 74, 691, 1978.
12. Welkos, S. L., Toskes, P. P., Baer, H., and Smith, G. W., Importance of anaerobic bacteria in the cobalamin malabsorption of the experimental rat blind loop syndrome, *Gastroenterology*, 80, 313, 1981.
13. King, C. E. and Toskes, P. P., Protein-losing enteropathy in the human and experimental rat blind-loop syndrome, *Gastroenterology*, 80, 504, 1981.
14. Toskes, P. P., Giannella, R. A., Jervis, H. R., Rout, W. R., and Takeuchi, A., Small intestinal mucosal injury in the experimental blind loop syndrome: light- and electron-microscopic and histochemical studies, *Gastroenterology*, 68, 1193, 1975.
15. Gracey, M. J., Papadimitrious, J., and Bower, G., Ultrastructural changes in the small intestines of rats with self-filling blind loops, *Gastroenterology*, 67, 646, 1974.
16. Gracey, M., Thomas, J., and Houghton, M., Effect of stasis on intestinal enzyme activities, *Aust. N.Z. J. Med.*, 5, 141, 1975.
17. Jonas, A., Flanagan, P. R., and Forstner, G. G., Pathogenesis of mucosal injury in the blind loop syndrome: brush border enzyme activity and glycoprotein degradation, *J. Clin. Invest.*, 60, 1321, 1977.
18. Menge, H., Kohn, R., Dietermann, K. H., Lorenz-Meyer, H., Riecken, E. O., and Robinson, J. W. L., Structural and functional alterations in the mucosa of self-filling intestinal blind loops in rats, *Clin. Sci.*, 56, 121, 1979.
19. Donaldson, R. M., Jr., Studies on the pathogenesis of steatorrhea in the blind loop syndrome, *J. Clin. Invest.*, 44, 1815, 1965.
20. King, C. E., Lorenz, E., and Toskes, P. P., The pathogenesis of decreased serum protein protein levels in the blind loop syndrome: evaluation including a newly developed ^{14}C amino acid breath test, *Gastroenterology*, 70, 901, 1976.
21. Giannella, R. A. and Toskes, P. P., Gastrointestinal bleeding and iron absorption in the experimental blind loop syndrome, *Am. J. Clin. Nutr.*, 29, 754, 1976.
22. Justus, P. G., Fernandez, A., Martin, J. L., King, C. E., Toskes, P. P., and Mathias, J. R., Altered myoelectric activity in the experimental blind loop syndrome, *J. Clin. Invest.*, 72, 1064, 1983.
23. King, C. E., Snook, L. B., and Toskes, P. P., Development of mucosal injury in the blind loop syndrome: effect of deconjugated bile salts on the genesis of protein-losing enteropathy, *Gastroenterology*, 80, 1192, 1981.

Chapter 17

USE OF HYDROGEN GAS (H_2) ANALYSIS TO ASSESS INTESTINAL ABSORPTION: STUDIES IN NORMAL RATS AND IN RATS INFECTED WITH THE NEMATODE, *NIPPOSTRONGYLUS BRASILIENSIS*

Edward A. Carter

TABLE OF CONTENTS

I. INTRODUCTION

In recent years, analysis of H_2 production has been used successfully to demonstrate the presence and the extent of carbohydrate malabsorption.[1-4] Under normal conditions, orally administered carbohydrates such as lactose or sucrose are hydrolyzed and absorbed in the small intestine. If hydrolysis and absorption do not occur, unabsorbed carbohydrate reaches the colon where bacteria are able to utilize and oxidize the unabsorbed sugar. One of the products of colonic bacterial metabolism is H_2, part of which escapes in the flatus, while part equilibrates with the blood and escapes from the lungs. The released H_2 may be detected in the flatus or breath by gas chromatographic techniques. The present report provides data on the use of H_2 analysis to monitor both protein as well as carbohydrate absorption in normal rats and in rats with nematode-induced malabsorption.

II. METHODS

A. Animals

Male Sprague-Dawley rats (Charles River Breeding Labs, Wilmington, Mass.) weighing approximately 300 to 500 g were used throughout this study. All rats were fed Purina laboratory chow (Purina, St. Louis, Mo.) and water *ad libitum*. Approximately 5000 *N. brasiliensis* larvae were injected subcutaneously into the rats 14 to 17 days prior to absorption studies. This number of larvae has been shown previously to produce partial villus atrophy in segments of the small intestine harboring the mature worms.[5,6] The method of maintaining the life cycle of *N. brasiliensis* in the laboratory has been described previously.[6] Normal (control) or infected rats were fasted for 18 hr and were then given glucose, sucrose, xylose, lactulose, bovine serum albumin, or casein hydrolysate by gavage. Each animal was then immediately placed in a separate H_2 and $^{14}CO_2$ collecting system diagrammatically represented in Figure 1. In one set of experiments, fasted normal rats were anesthetized with ether and their cecum identified at laparotomy. While still anesthetized, one group received carbohydrate or protein by direct injection into the cecum, while the other group received the carbohydrate or protein by gavage. The incisions in both groups were closed. Each rat was then placed in a separate closed recirculating animal chamber (Figure 1). The entire procedure (from initiation of anesthesia to the closing of the incision) lasted no more than 5 min.

B. Uptake By Gut Sacs In Vitro

Fasted rats were sacrificed by cervical dislocation. Then 8-cm sections of the small intestine were removed, rinsed with 20 mℓ of ice-cold saline, everted, and the ends tied to form closed sacs.[7,8] Gut sacs were filled with 1.0 mℓ buffer that contained 125 mM NaCl, 10 mM fructose, 30 mM Tris HCl (pH 7.4), and 10 mM of either 3-O-(methyl-^{3}H)-D-glucose (60 to 90 μCi/mmol) or 1-(carboxyl-^{14}C)aminocyclopentane-1-carboxylic acid, (40 to 60 μCi/mmol), the buffer adjusted to contain sufficient radioactivity to provide 20,000 cpm/mℓ. Both isotopes were obtained from New England Nuclear Co., Boston. Subsequently in this paper, 3-O-(methyl-^{3}H)-D-glucose will be referred to as 3-O-methylglucose, while 1-(carboxyl-^{14}C)-aminocyclopentane-1-carboxylic acid will be referred to as cycloleucine. The filled gut sacs were placed in 10 mℓ of the same buffer (as that inside each sac) in 50 mℓ Erlenmeyer flasks. The flasks and their contents were incubated at 37°C for 90 min in a shaking water bath (100 strokes/min) under 100% O_2. After incubation, the sacs were removed, cut open, and drained. Aliquots of buffer (0.1 mℓ) inside and outside each sac were added to 10 mℓ of Aquasol 2, and the radioactivity measured by liquid scintillation spectrometry. Data are expressed as the ratio of the radioactivity inside the sac (serosal surface) to that outside the sac (mucosal surface).

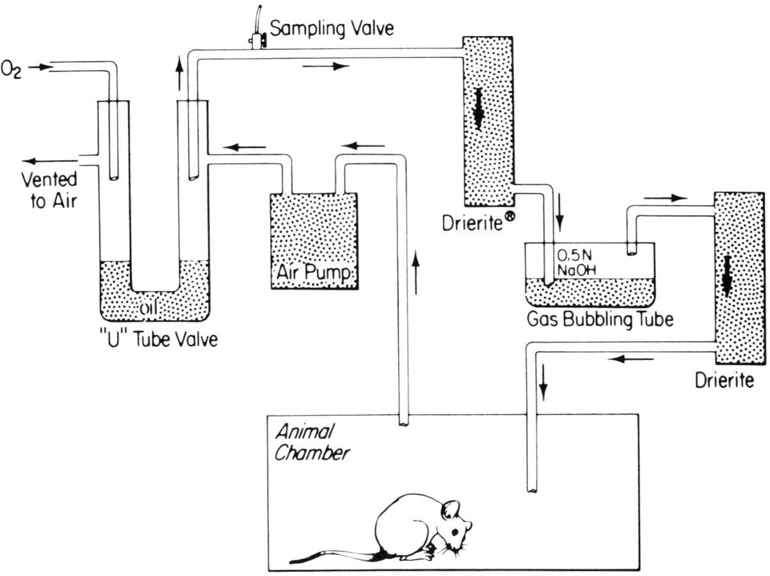

FIGURE 1. Diagrammatic representation of the system used for in vivo H_2 and $^{14}CO_2$ collection from rats.

C. H_2 Production In Vitro

H_2 production by rat fecal homogenates was assessed according to Perman et al.[9] Fasted rats were sacrificed by cervical dislocation. The cecum and colon of each rat were removed and their contents emptied. A mixture was made of the colonic and the cecal contents of several rats. This mixture was immediately weighed and homogenized in a Waring blender in a volume of phosphate buffered saline (PBS) equal to three times the weight of the fecal sample, for 1 min at a rheostat setting of 100. One milliliter of the fecal homogenate was added to 1 mℓ of PBS containing either glucose, sucrose, xylose, lactulose, bovine serum albumin, or casein hydrolysate, each at a concentration of 12.5 g/100 mℓ, in a 50-mℓ glass centrifuge tube. In preliminary experiments it was established that maximal H_2 production was achieved by the fecal homogenate from these concentrations of substrates. The control tube received 1 mℓ of fecal homogenate and 1 mℓ of PBS containing no additional substrate. The contents in each tube were gassed with N_2 for 1 min, after which each tube was capped and placed in a 37°C water bath for 1 hr. A needle attached to a 50-mℓ syringe was then inserted through the cap of each tube. Approximately 40 mℓ of water was injected into each capped tube via a second needle and syringe inserted through the cap, forcing gas from the tube into the empty syringe. The needle and syringe containing the gas sample were removed and the collected gas then analyzed for H_2 as described below.

D. H_2 Production In Vivo

H_2 production by rats was determined using a closed recirculating animal chamber system similar to the one described by Gumbmann and Williams[10] (Figure 1). The animal chamber consisted of a 30-cm Desaga vacuum desiccator (Catalog No. 2510450-k, Brinkmann Instruments, Inc., Westbury, N.Y.) connected to an air pump (Whisper 300, Willinger Bros., Inc., Ft. Lee, N.J.). At the beginning of each experiment, the cover to the animal chamber was opened and the rat placed inside (Figure 1). The cover to the animal chamber was then replaced and the air pump started. Initially, the oil levels in the two arms of the U-tube valve were equalized by adjusting the flow of O_2. Air was drawn via the pump from the animal chamber into a column of Drierite® to remove water. Thereafter, the air was drawn into a gas-bubbling tube containing 0.5 N NaOH to remove CO_2 and then into a second Drierite® column to remove water. The treated air was pumped back into the animal chamber. Consumption of O_2 by the rat plus removal of the CO_2 produced by the rat resulted in a slight negative pressure within the animal chamber. This negative pressure caused O_2 to bubble through the U-tube valve into the airflow of the otherwise closed animal chamber system. Thus, the N_2 and O_2 content of the chamber remained constant, while the H_2 produced was quantitatively collected. The rats were maintained in these jars for a total of 6 hr. At 90-min intervals, samples of air were withdrawn from the sampling valve and analyzed for H_2 as described below.

E. H_2 Analysis

H_2 content was determined with a Carle gas chromatograph (ACG-111, Anaheim, Calif.) equipped with thermistors using argon as the carrier gas. Quantitation of the H_2 content was achieved by the method we have used routinely for breath H_2 analysis of patients. A gas mixture containing a known amount of H_2 (Liquid Carbonic Crop., Tewksbury, Mass.) was used to standardize the system. The H_2 content of the test sample was determined from the ratio of the peak height of the test sample (with the same retention time as the H_2 standard) to the peak height of the H_2 standard. This ratio was multiplied by the H_2 concentration (in parts per million, ppm) of the standard provided by the manufacturer. Our system accurately measures H_2 concentrations greater than 10 ppm. The final concentrations of H_2 for either the in vitro or in vivo experiments were determined using van der Waals equation, $PV = nRT$, where P is in atmospheres, V is the volume of the air space in liters, n is in moles, R is 0.08206 $\ell/$atm$/$mol$/$degree, and T is in degrees Kelvin.

F. $^{14}CO_2$ Production In Vivo

In experiments with D-(U-^{14}C)xylose (5 mCi/mmol, Amersham, Arlington Heights, Ill.), $^{14}CO_2$ was collected in 0.5 N NaOH (Figure 1). At 90-min intervals, the gas-bubbling tube in the system was quickly removed and replaced by a fresh tube containing NaOH. Duplicate 0.5-mℓ samples of the NaOH solution were added to duplicate 15-mℓ aliquots of Aquasol 2 and the radioactivity of the samples was measured by liquid scintillation spectrometry.

G. Additional Tests

Lactase and sucrase activities in small-intestinal homogenates were determined by the method of Messer and Dahlquist,[11] except that the assays were carried out in two steps as previously described.[12] Alkaline phosphatase activity in small-intestinal homogenates was assayed according to the method of Weiser.[13] Serum xylose was determined chemically.[14] Protein content was measured by the method of Lowry et al.[15] Student's *t*-test was used to assess the significance of differences between means of the various studies.

III. RESULTS

A. In Vitro and In Vivo H_2 Production

One objective of the present study was to determine whether H_2 analysis could be utilized to monitor both carbohydrate and protein absorption in normal rats and rats infected with the nematode *Nippostrongylus brasiliensis*. Initial experiments were designed to determine whether H_2 was produced by rat fecal homogenates from carbohydrate or protein (Figure 2). Following the addition of glucose, sucrose, xylose, or lactulose to the fecal homogenates, large amounts of H_2 were produced. The amounts

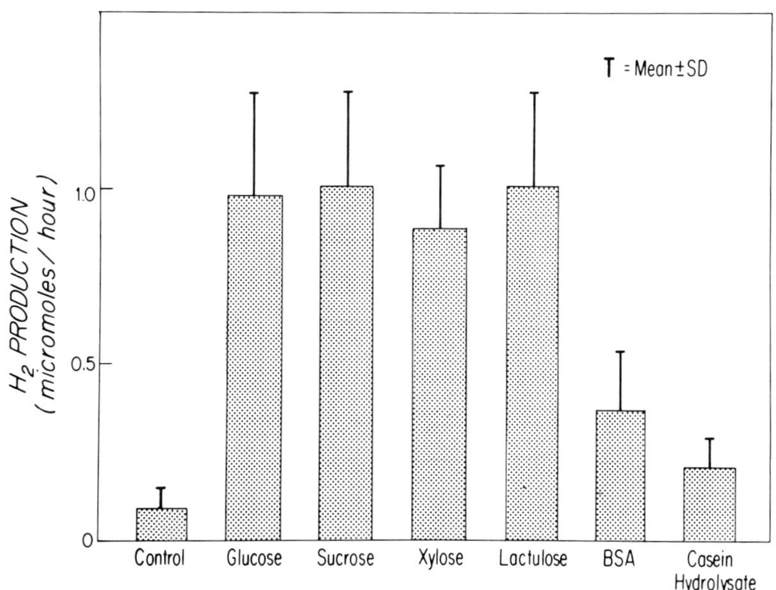

FIGURE 2. H₂ production in vitro by rat fecal homogenates after various additions. Conditions for preparing the fecal homogenates and for determining H₂ production are described in Section III. The results are the average of six experiments. BSA stands for bovine serum albumin.

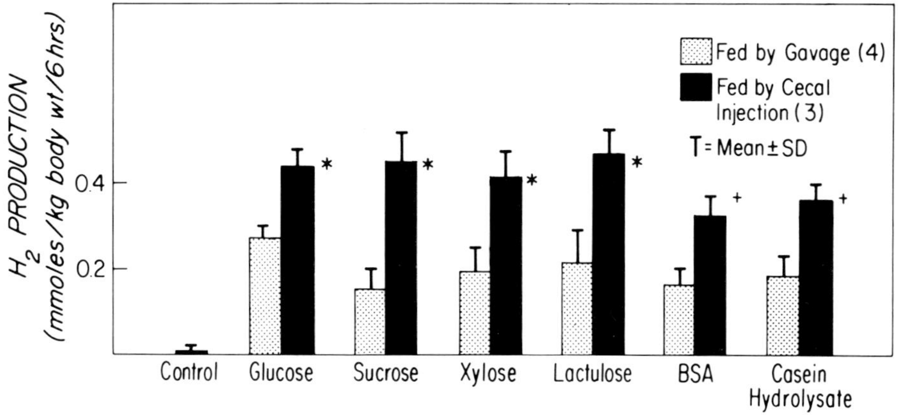

FIGURE 3. H₂ production in vivo by normal rats following administration of various substances by gavage or cecal injection. Normal rats, fasted 18 hr, were subjected to laparotomy as described in Section III and then given the indicated nutrients, either by gavage or cecal injection, at a dose of 2 g/kg, 25% w/vol. The controls were normal rats subjected to laparotomy, but not given carbohydrate or protein by gavage or cecal injection. The carbohydrates were dissolved in water; bovine serum albumin (BSA) and casein hydrolysate were dissolved in water with 1.38 g of sodium bicarbonate per 100 mℓ. H₂ was determined on samples of air withdrawn from the closed recirculating animal chamber system was described in Section III. The numbers in parentheses indicate the number of rats fed by gavage and the rats fed by cecal injection by * ($p < 0.01$) or + ($p < 0.05$).

of H₂ produced exceeded those obtained from fecal homogenates incubated without additional substrate (Figure 2, control). H₂ was also produced after the addition of protein (either bovine serum albumin or casein hydrolysate) to the fecal homogenates. The absolute amount of H₂ produced from the bovine serum albumin or casein hydrolysate was considerably less ($p < 0.01$) than the H_2 produced from the carbohydrate (Figure 2).

In vivo H_2 production was determined in normal rats after administration of carbohydrate (glucose, sucrose, xyclose, lactulose) or protein (bovine serum albumin or casein hydrolysate) by gavage or cecal injection at laparotomy (Figure 3). Essentially no H_2 was produced by the control rats (Figure 3, control). Significantly more ($p < 0.05$ or $p < 0.01$) H_2 was produced after the cecal injection of the carbohydrates or proteins than after these same substances were given by gavage (Figure 3). It should be noted that less ($p < 0.05$) H_2 was produced from bovine serum albumin or casein hydrolysate than from the carbohydrates regardless of whether the substances were administered by gavage or by cecal injection. These data suggest that H_2 can be produced by rat colonic bacteria from either the carbohydrates or the proteins used in these experiments.

B. Intestinal Absorption in Normal and Nematode-Infected Rats

Infection of rats with *N. brasiliensis* leads to the development of partial villus atrophy in segments of the small intestine harboring the worms.[5] The typical histology of the normal rat jejunum is shown in Figure 4A. This should be contrasted to the histology of the nematode-infected rat jejunum shown in Figure 4B, where there is blunting of the villi and infiltration of the lamina propria.

Intestinal brush border enzyme activity was determined with preparations from fasted normal and nematode-infected rats 14 to 17 days after a primary infection. Lactase, sucrase, and alkaline phosphatase were significantly reduced in nematode-infected rats compared with normal rats ($p < 0.05$ or $p < 0.01$) (Table 1, A).

Everted intestinal gut sacs of fasted normal and nematode-infected rats were tested for their ability to transport 3-*O*-methylglucose or cycloleucine from the mucosal to the serosal surface (Table 1, B). In both normal and nematode-infected rats, the uptake of 3-*O*-methylglucose was maximal in jejunal sacs while cycloleucine uptake was maximal in ileal sacs. There was a significant decrease in uptake of 3-*O*-methylglucose and cycloleucine by gut sacs from nematode-infected rats compared with normal rats ($p < 0.05$ or $p < 0.01$) (Table 1, B).

Following the administration of D-(U-^{14}C)-xylose by gavage, less D-xylose was detected chemically in the blood of the nematode-infected rats than in the blood of normal rats (Table 1, C) ($p < 0.05$). Consistent with this finding, suggesting impaired malabsorption, was the observation that more $^{14}CO_2$ was produced from this substrate by the nematode-infected rats compared with the normal rats (Table 1, C).

In the next series of experiments, H_2 production in vivo by fasted normal and nematode-infected rats was determined after lactulose or water were given by gavage (Figure 5). After administration of water, H_2 evolution was not detected during 7.5 hr of observation in either normal or nematode-infected rats (Figure 5). However, in both normal and nematode-infected rats, H_2 was generated following the administration of lactulose with no significant difference being observed in the amount of H_2 produced by either the normal or nematode-infected rats.

Hydrogen production was also examined in normal and nematode-infected rats following administration of various carbohydrates or proteins by gavage. Glucose, sucrose, or xylose administration to normal rats resulted in H_2 production during the 6-hr collection period; the amount produced by the nematode-infected rats under the same conditions was always greater ($p < 0.01$) (Figure 6). Compared with the carbohy-

FIGURE 4.   (A) Cross-sectional view of jejunum of normal rat ($\times$ 150). (B) Cross-section of the jejunum of a rat infected 15 days earlier with 5000 larvae of *N. brasiliensis*. Note blunting of villi and infiltration of lymphocytes and plasma cells in the lamina propria. The separation of the mucosa and muscular layer of the intestine is artifactual ($\times$ 110).

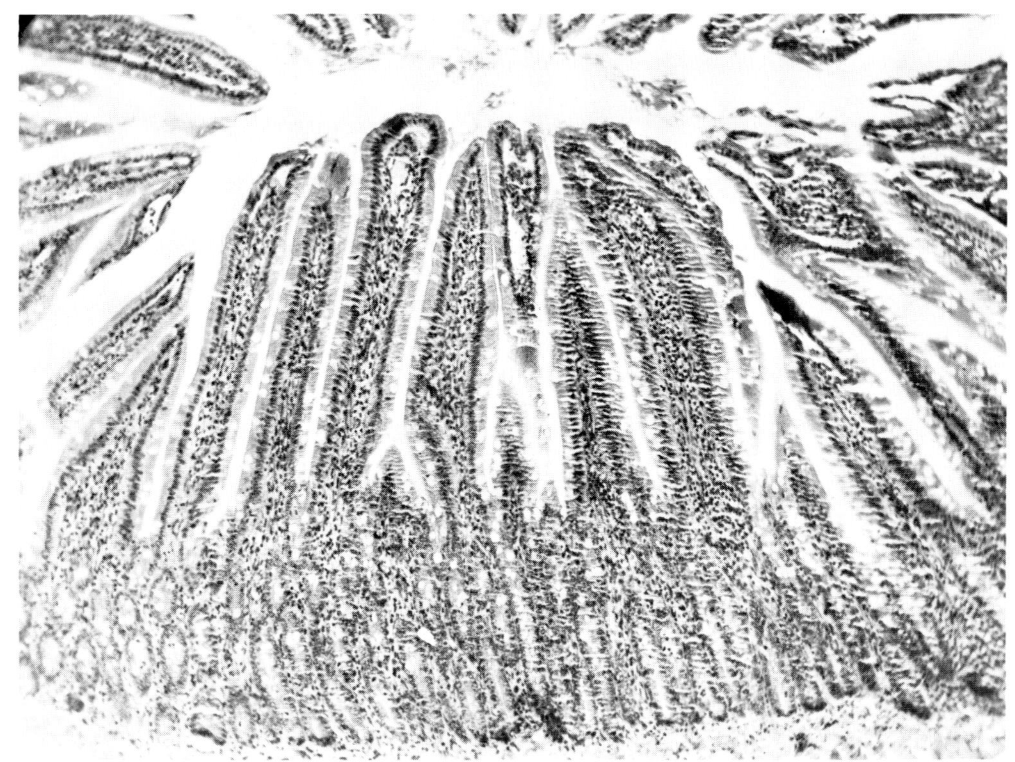

FIGURE 4A.

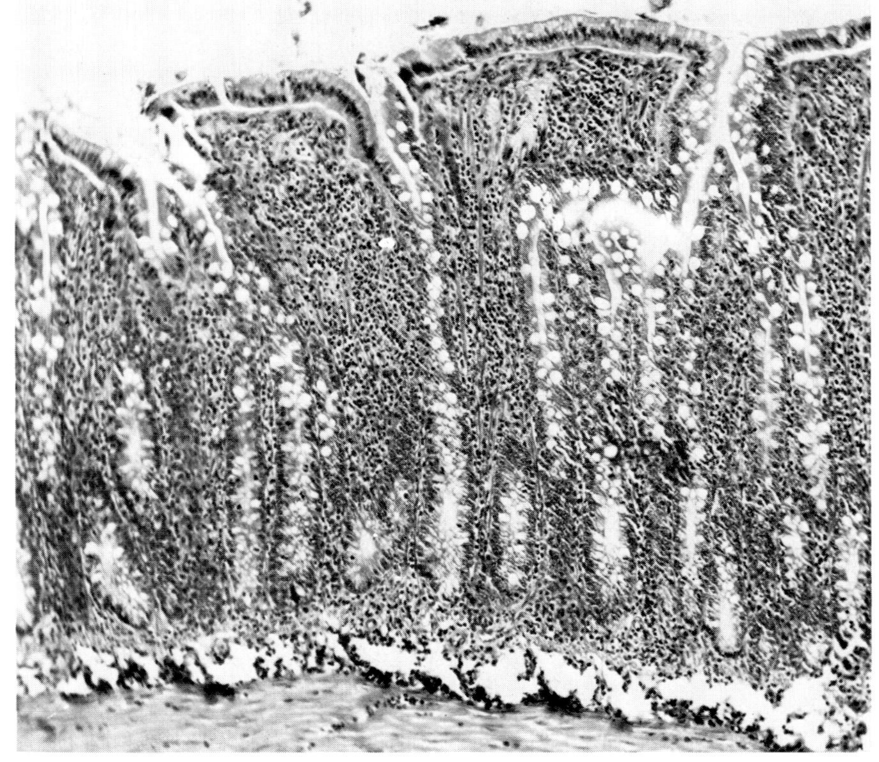

FIGURE 4B.

Table 1
EXAMINATION OF INTESTINAL FUNCTION IN NORMAL AND
N. BRASILIENSIS-INFECTED RATS

| | Results (mean ± SD) | | |
Assay	Normal rats	Nematode-infected rats[a]	p
A. Intestinal brush border enzyme activities			
[ΔOD·(mg protein)$^{-1}$ min^{-1}]			
1. Lactase	0.07 ± 0.02	0.04 ± 0.01	<0.01
2. Sucrase	0.15 ± 0.05	0.10 ± 0.04	<0.05
3. Alkaline phosphatase	0.13 ± 0.03	0.07 ± 0.01	<0.001
B. Intestinal gut sac uptake[c]			
(serosal/mucosal ratio)			
1. 3-*O*-methylglucose	4.3 ± 0.3	3.4 ± 0.2	<0.05
2. Cycloleucine	4.3 ± 0.3	3.1 ± 0.2	<0.01
C. D-xylose absorption[d]			
1. Serum levels (mg%)	35 ± 10	16 ± 5	<0.05
2. Recovery as $^{14}CO_2$ (% dose)			
a. 1.5 hr	0.03 ± 0.01	0.20 ± 0.1	<0.001
b. 3.0 hr	0.26 ± 0.03	0.75 ± 0.3	<0.01
c. 4.5 hr	1.4 ± 0.04	2.3 ± 0.3	<0.05

[a]   Rats were infected with approximately 5000 *N. brasiliensis* larvae 14 to 17 days prior to sacrifice.

[b]   The intestine of nine pairs of fasted normal or nematode-infected rats were washed and scraped. The mucosal scrapings were homogenized and the enzyme activities determined in duplicate by conventional methods.[11-13]

[c]   Small-intestinal everted sacs were prepared from five pairs of normal and nematode-infected rats and gut sac transport was determined as in Methods.

[d]   Three pairs of normal and nematode-infected rats were fasted 18 hr and given D-[U-^{14}C]xylose by gavage at a dose of 2 g/kg, 25% w/vol, in water. Serum D-xylose levels were determined chemically 6 hr after administration of the D-[U-^{14}C]xylose by gavage. The percent of radioactivity recovered as $^{14}CO_2$ was calculated by a method similar to that of Toskes et al.[16] The counts recovered in the NaOH solution at the indicated time intervals were divided by the counts originally given to the animals.

drates, less H_2 ($p < 0.05$) was produced by normal fasted rats following administration of bovine serum albumin or casein hydrolysate; however, here the amount of H_2 produced was also greater in the nematode-infected rats ($p < 0.05$).

IV. DISCUSSION

The purpose of the present study was to determine whether H_2 analysis could be utilized to monitor the absorption of either carbohydrate or protein in normal rats and in rats infected with the nematode, *Nippostrongylus brasiliensis*.

Initially, we attempted to determine whether H_2 could be produced by fecal homogenates in vitro from either carbohydrate or protein. We observed that rat fecal homogenates produced H_2 from the carbohydrates glucose, sucrose, xylose, and lactulose as well as from the proteins bovine serum albumin and casein hydrolysate. Essentially the same amount of H_2 was produced from any of the carbohydrates tested, confirming reports by Bond and Levitt[1] and Perman et al.[9] However, the amount of H_2 generated from bovine serum albumin or casein hydrolysate was always less than that produced from the carbohydrates. Calloway et al.[17] previously reported that H_2 was generated by human ileal and colonic contents in vitro from carbohydrate and amino acid; they also noted that less H_2 was produced from amino acid than from carbohydrate.[17]

The reduced ability of fecal homogenates to generate H_2 from protein substrates may

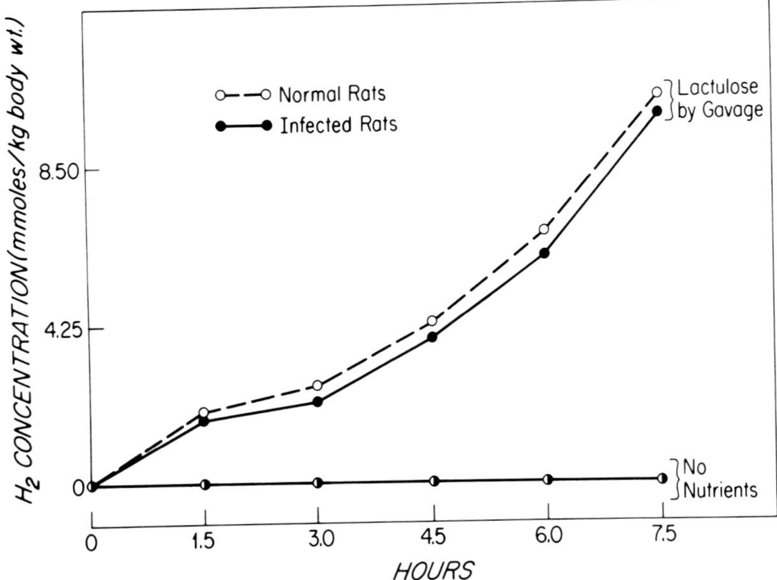

FIGURE 5. H_2 production in vivo by normal rats and nematode-infected rats following administration of lactulose or water by gavage. Normal rats or rats infected with *N. brasiliensis* 14 to 17 days earlier were fasted 18 hr and then given either lactulose (2 g/kg, 25% w/vol, water) or water by gavage. H_2 was determined on air samples removed from the closed recirculating animal chamber system described in Section II. There were four animals in each group.

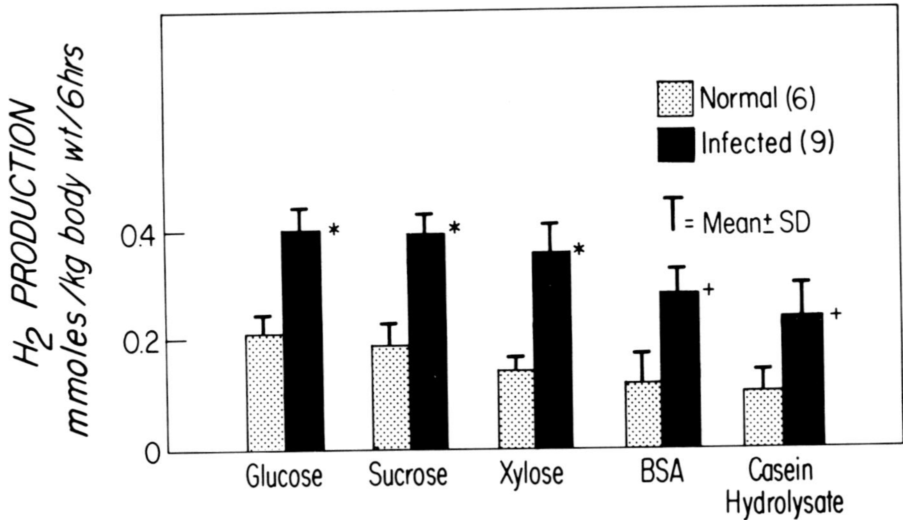

FIGURE 6. H_2 production by normal and nematode-infected rats following administration of nutrients by gavage. Normal rats or rats infected with *N. brasiliensis* 14 to 17 days earlier were fasted 18 hr and given the nutrient by gavage at a dose of 2 g/kg, 25% w/vol. The glucose, sucrose, and xylose were dissolved in water. Bovine serum albumin and casein hydrolysate were dissolved in water with 1.38 g of sodium bicarbonate per 100 mℓ H_2 was determined on samples of air withdrawn from the closed recirculating animal chamber system described in Section III. The statistical significance of difference between the normal and the nematode-infected rats is indicated by * ($p < 0.01$) or + ($p < 0.05$).

be a reflection of the type or number of bacteria in the rat feces and which may also vary from species to species. In preliminary experiments, we have found that H_2 production from glucose by adult human fecal homogenates was ten times greater than from rat fecal homogenates.

We subsequently tested the hypothesis that enhanced delivery of carbohydrate and protein substrates to the large intestine of the rat would lead to an increase in the production of H_2. There are several earlier studies showing that the enhanced delivery of carbohydrate to the large intestine does result in increased production of H_2.[1-3,18] Injection of carbohydrate or protein substrates into the cecum of normal rats led to the production of more H_2 than when these substrates were given by gavage. These findings are not surprising since one would expect carbohydrates or proteins administered by gavage to undergo partial or complete digestion, thus limiting the amount of substrate available for H_2 production by reducing colonic bacteria.

We also attempted to determine to what extent H_2 production reflected impaired absorption and mucosal cell function. For this purpose we used a closed recirculating animal chamber system similar to that described by Gumbmann and Williams.[10] These investigators used the chamber to study H_2 production by rats given oligosaccharide-free bean residue or the purified oligosaccharides raffinose or stachyose.[19] They observed that oligosaccharide feeding led to increased production of H_2 in vivo. It was suggested that the oligosaccharides could not be degraded by intestinal enzymes and were thus subject to oxidation by colonic bacteria.[19]

It has been shown that rats infected with *N. brasiliensis* exhibited diminished glucose, maltose, Na^+, Cl^-, and water transport as well as reduced intestinal cell activities of maltase and alkaline phosphatase.[20] Symons[21] also reported that in nematode-infected rats there was significantly less digestion and absorption of ^{131}I-labeled egg albumin. In the present study, impaired intestinal function in the nematode-infected rats was reflected by (1) decreased intestinal brush border enzyme activity, (2) decreased uptake of 3-*O*-methylglucose and cycloleucine by gut sacs, and (3) decreased absorption of D-xylose. Since the sucrase, lactase, and alkaline phosphatase are localized predominantly in the microvillus membrane of intestinal epithelial cells, reductions in the activities of these enzymes probably reflect the overall impairment in small-intestinal function in the nematode-infected rats. These decreased enzyme activities could reflect a reduction in the function of individual villus cells, a decrease in the number of villus cells, or both. A decrease in the number and function of villus cells may account in part for the diminished uptake of nutrients in nematode-infected rats observed in the present study and previous studies by others.[5,20,21]

In the present study, significantly more H_2 was generated after the gavage administration of carbohydrate (glucose, sucrose, and xylose) or protein (bovine serum albumin and casein hydrolysate) to rats infected with *N. brasiliensis* compared with normal rats. The increased production of H_2 in vivo by the nematode-infected rats after the separate administration of glucose, sucrose, xylose, bovine serum albumin, or casein hydrolysate was associated with intestinal dysfunction determined by small-intestinal brush border enzyme analysis, gut sac uptake, and D-xylose absorption. The most likely explanation for the increased production of H_2 in vivo by the nematode-infected rats after nutrient administration was the increased delivery of undigested and/or unabsorbed substrate to the colonic bacteria. However, in the present experiments there was no difference in H_2 production by either normal or nematode-infected rats when given lactulose — a nondigested, nonabsorbed carbohydrate. Analysis of H_2 production in humans after lactulose administration has been used as an index of intestinal transit time.[1,18] Thus, our data with lactulose suggest that there was no difference in the intestinal transit time of the normal rats as compared to the nematode-infected rats. Launiala[22] however, has suggested that unabsorbed sucrose and mannitol increase the small-intestinal flow rate and mean transit time. Hence, it is possible that the unabsorbed carbohydrate (other than lactulose) and protein used in this study led to an accelerated transit time through the small intestine of the nematode-infected rats.

The results of the present study suggest that H_2 analysis was useful in the overall assessment of the impaired intestinal absorption of carbohydrate and protein in rats. H_2 analysis may also be of value to assess whether some nutrients may be absorbed better than others in patients who present with complicated feeding problems.

V. SUMMARY

The in vitro and in vivo production of hydrogen gas (H_2) from various carbohydrate or proteins has been examined in normal rats and in rats infected with the nematode *Nippostrongylus brasiliensis*. Normal rat fecal homogenates were capable of producing H_2 in vitro from glucose, sucrose, xylose, lactulose, bovine serum albumin, or casein hydrolysate. Direct injection of glucose, sucrose, xylose, lactulose, bovine serum albumin, or casein hydrolysate into the cecum of normal rats resulted in approximately twice as much H_2 production in vivo than when these same carbohydrates or proteins were administered to the normal rats by gavage. Partial small-intestinal villous atrophy was produced by infecting rats with the nematode *N. brasiliensis*. Impaired small-intestinal cell function and evidence of malabsorption in the nematode-infected rats included: (1) decreased activity of intestinal cell lactase (-43%), sucrase (-33%), and alkaline phosphatase (-46%); (2) decreased gut sac uptake of 3-*O*-(methyl-^{3}H)-D-glucose (-21%) or 1-(carboxyl-^{14}C)-aminocyclopentane-1-carboxylic acid (-28%); and (3) increased ($+64$ to 561%) $^{14}CO_2$ production after D(U-^{14}C)xylose administration. These rats produced approximately twice as much H_2 after gavage administration of glucose, sucrose, xylose, bovine serum albumin, or casein hydrolysate compared with normal rats. The present study suggests that H_2 analysis may be useful in the evaluation of small-intestinal malabsorptive states in rats.

REFERENCES

1. Bond, J. H. and Levitt, M. D., Use of breath hydrogen (H_2) in the study of carbohydrate absorption, *Am. J. Dig. Dis.*, 22, 379, 1977.
2. Perman, J. A., Barr, R. G., and Watkins, J. B., Sucrose malabsorption in children: noninvasive diagnosis by interval breath hydrogen determination, *J. Pediatr.*, 93, 17, 1978.
3. Douwes, A. C., Fernandes, J., and Degenhart, H. J., Improved accuracy of lactose tolerance test in children, using expired H_2 measurements, *Arch. Dis. Child.*, 53, 939, 1978.
4. Cook, G. C., Breath hydrogen after oral xylose tropical malabsorption, *Am. J. Clin. Nutr.*, 33, 555, 1980.
5. Oglivie, B. M. and Jones, V. W., Parasitological review. *Nippostrongylus brasiliensis:* a review of immunology and host parasite relationship in the rat, *Exp. Parasitol.*, 29, 138, 1971.
6. Wilson, R. J. M. and Bloch, K. J., Homocytotropic antibody response in the rat infected with the nematode, *Nippostrongylus brasiliensis*. II. Characteristics of the immune response, *J. Immunol.*, 100, 622, 1968.
7. Wilson, T. H. and Wiseman, G., The use of sacs of everted small intestine for the study of the transference of substances from the mucosal to the serosal surface, *J. Physiol. (London)*, 123, 116, 1954.
8. Martin, D. L. and DeLuca, H. F., Influence of sodium on calcium transport by the rat small intestine, *Am. J. Physiol.*, 216, 1351, 1969.
9. Perman, J. A., Modler, S., and Olson, A. C., Effects of pH on carbohydrate consumption and hydrogen production by colonic bacteria, *Pediatr. Res.*, 14, 508, 1980.

10. Gumbmann, M. R. and Williams, S. N., The quantitative collection and determination of hydrogen gas from the rat and factors affecting its production, *Proc. Soc. Exp. Biol. Med.*, 135, 1171, 1971.
11. Messer, M. and Dahlquist, A., A one-step ultramicro method for the assay of intestinal disaccharides, *Anal. Biochem.*, 14, 376, 1966.
12. Garvey, T. Q., Hyman, P. E., and Isselbacher, K. J., Gamma-glutamyl transpeptidase of rat intestine: localization and possible role in amino acid transport, *Gastroenterology*, 71, 778, 1976.
13. Weiser, M. M., Intestinal epithelial cell surface membrane glycoprotein synthesis. I. An indicator of cellular differentiation, *J. Biol. Chem.*, 248, 2536, 1973.
14. Roe, J. H. and Rice, E. W., A photometric method for the determination of free pentoses in animal tissues, *J. Biol. Chem.*, 173, 507, 1948.
15. Lowry, O. H., Rosenbrough, N. J., Farr, A. L. et. al., Protein measurement with the Folin phenol reagent, *J. Biol. Chem.*, 193, 365, 1951.
16. Toskes, P. P., King, C. E., Spivey, J. C. et al., Xylose catabolism in experimental rat blind loop syndrome. Studies, including use of a newly developed D-[^{14}C]-xylose breath test, *Gastroenterology*, 74, 691, 1978.
17. Calloway, D. H., Colasito, D. J., and Mathews, R. D., Gases produced by human intestinal microflora, *Nature (London)*, 212, 1238, 1966.
18. Rhodes, J. M., Middleton, P., and Jewell, D. P., The lactulose hydrogen breath test as a diagnostic test for small-bowel bacterial overgrowth, *Scand. J. Gastroenterol.*, 14, 333, 1979.
19. Wagner, J. R., Becker, R., Gumbmann, M. R. et al., Hydrogen production in the rat following ingestion of raffinose, stachyose and oligosaccharide-free bean residue, *J. Nutr.*, 106, 466, 1976.
20. Symons, L. E. A. and Fiarbarn, D., Pathology, absorption, transport, and activity of digestive enzymes in rat jejunum parasitized by the nematode *Nippostrongylus brasiliensis*, *Fed. Proc. Fed. Am. Soc. Exp. Biol. Med.*, 21, 913, 1962.
21. Symons, L. E. A., Pathology of infestation of the rat with *Nippostrongylus muris* (Yokogawa). V. Protein digestion, *Aust. J. Biol. Sci.*, 13, 578, 1960.
22. Launiala, K., The effect of unabsorbed sucrose and mannitol on the small intestinal flow rate and mean transit time, *Scand. J. Gastroenterol.*, 39, 665, 1968.

Chapter 18

PRAOMYS (MASTOMYS) NATALENSIS AS AN ANIMAL MODEL IN HISTAMINE-INDUCED DUODENAL ULCERS

Syun Hosoda, Motokazu Suyama, Seiji Yamada, and Toshiko Saito

TABLE OF CONTENTS

I. INTRODUCTION

Praomys (Mastomys) natalensis, commonly called the multimammate mouse, is a wild rodent belonging to the family Muridae. Intermediate in size and in several other respects between a mouse and a rat, it is the most widely distributed and one of the most common rodent species in Africa, ranging from Knysna on the southern coast to Eritrea in the northeast and Morocco in the northwest.[1,2]

In 1951, *Mastomys* was first introduced to the scientific community because of its high and uniform susceptibility to plague.[3] Subsequent work pointed out its further usefulness for infection experiments of certain parasitic diseases caused by Protozoa and Schistosoma.[1,4] Meanwhile, Oettlé reported that *Mastomys* spontaneously develop a high incidence of stomach tumors, which was diagnosed as adenocarcinoma of the glandular stomach.[5] This discovery greatly stimulated the interest of scientists in the fields of cancer and aging research, and led to extensive use of *Mastomys* in a number of institutes and laboratories on a worldwide scale.[6,7] In fact, there is increasing evidence that *Mastomys* develop a wide variety of spontaneous neoplastic and non-neoplastic diseases resembling those occurring in humans.[6,7]

Among neoplastic diseases in *Mastomys,* the important entity of gastric cancer has been reconsidered by two groups of pathologists. Both groups proved that this neoplasm was an argyrophilic carcinoid, based on the histochemical finding with Sevier-Munger's silver stain.[8,9] Thus, it became clear that *Mastomys* is the only mammal other than humans to develop carcinoids at high incidence. Snell and Stewart[8,10] pointed out that the most conspicuous effect on the host of the *Mastomys* gastric carcinoid, either primary or transplantable, was the development of severe duodenal ulcer(s) due to the hypersecretion of gastric acid. A similar lesion had already been documented as an unexplained perforation of the duodenum complicated in *Mastomys* with carcinoma of stomach, in the first report by Oettlé.[5] Snell and Stewart kindly provided us with 16 *Mastomys* bearing a transplant of gastric carcinoid. Because of the similarity of this tumor to human carcinoid, we initially sought to demonstrate 5-hydroxytryptamine and its precursor 5-hydroxytryptophan in the tumor tissues, but failed to detect any of these substances. The body of the stomach, which is the site of the primary carcinoid(s) in *Mastomys,* contains a greater concentration of histamine than the antrum,[11-13] whereas the antrum is the main source for gastrin extraction.[14] This, and the finding that some gastric carcinoids of humans produce fair amounts of histamine,[15,16] prompted us to examine the possibility that histamine might be produced by the transplantable gastric carcinoid of *Mastomys.* As was expected, we could demonstrate large amounts of histamine in homogenates of all growing transplants and appreciable activity of specific histidine decarboxylase, an enzyme catalyzing the conversion of 1-histidine to histamine from the microsome-free supernatant.[17,18] These findings strongly suggest a link between the production of histamine by the carcinoid cells and the development of duodenal ulcers through the hypersecretion of gastric acid.

During our study of histamine in the urine of *Mastomys* bearing either primary or transplantable gastric carcinoid, we found that the tumor-bearing *Mastomys* excreted increased amounts of histamine in their urine and the urinary levels of histamine paralleled the intensity of the duodenal ulcers.[19,20] About the same time, we encountered by happenstance a newly devised and commercially available apparatus — the Alzet osmotic minipump — which delivers small amounts of various chemicals at a steady rate for a week. We readily recognized the similarity between the self-powered, continuous-delivery infusion of the chemical of choice from the apparatus and the autonomic liberation of histamine from carcinoid cells. Therefore, an attempt at experimental production of duodenal ulcers in *Mastomys* was made by constant infusion of exogenous histamine, using the osmotic minipumps. The results obtained indicated that

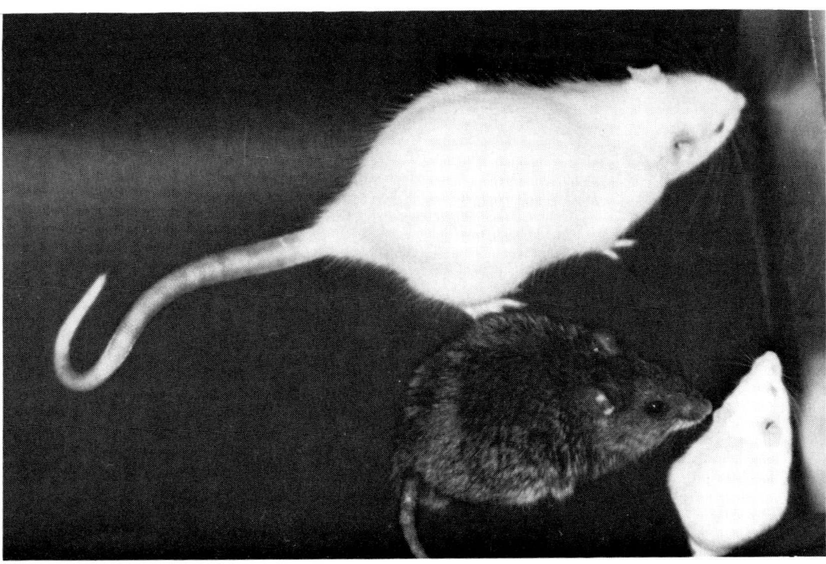

FIGURE 1. From top to bottom: Wistar-King A rat, *Praomys (Mastomys) natalensis,* and BALB/c mouse.

Mastomys is more susceptible to the induction of duodenal ulcers by histamine than other rodents such as the mouse, rat, and guinea pig.[21] Thus, *Mastomys* also proves valuable as an animal model for the study of the etiology and treatment of duodenal ulcer disease in humans.

In this study, the results presented earlier in the original paper are reported[21] and some unpublished data are added from our recent experiments, including the effects of drugs other than histamine on the formation of duodenal ulcer(s) and the inhibition of ulcer development by certain agents, including peptide hormones and vagotomy.

II. MATERIALS AND METHODS

Mastomys used in this study were descendants of three pairs of the Tokyo colony in the 16th generation by sibling mating of the Tohoku colony[6,19] that were descendants of family B from the colony at the Small Animal Section, Veterinary Resources Branch, Division of Research Services, National Institutes of Health, Bethesda, Md.[22] They have been maintained by random breeding in our laboratory since 1975 (Figure 1).

The chemicals used were purchased from the following sources: histamine dihydrochloride (Katayama Chemical Co., Osaka), tetragastrin and somatostatin (Protein Research Foundation, Osaka), pentagastrin and human synthetic gastrin I (Imperial Chemical Industries, Alderley Park, England), cysteamine monohydrochloride (Tokyo Kasei Kogyo Co., Tokyo), morphine hydrochloride (Takeda Chemical Industries, Osaka), atropine sulfate (Merck, Darmstadt, Germany), secretin (Eisai Co., Tokyo), and VIP (Peninsula Laboratories, San Carlos, Calif.). Carbachol was a generous gift from Wakamoto Pharmaceutical Co. (Tokyo), cimetidine from Smith, Kline & French Laboratories (Welwyn Garden City, England), probanthine from Dainihon Pharmaceutical Co. (Osaka), and GIP (200 μg) from the National Institute of Arthritis, Metabolism and Digestive Diseases (Bethesda, Md.).

All experiments except those with gastrin peptides were performed on 6-month-old *Mastomys* (body weight range: 78 to 80 g in males, 48 to 50 g in females), 6-month-old

DBA/2 female mice (body weight range, 23 to 26 g), 1.5-month-old Sprague-Dawley-derived Charles River CD female rats (body weight range, 140 to 150 g), 1-month-old Hartley male guinea pigs (body weight range, 250 to 270 g), and 2.5-month-old female Mongolian gerbils (body weight range, 55 to 60 g). Throughout the period of observation, the animals were given standard commercial food pellets and water *ad libitum.* The aqueous solutions of histamine dihydrochloride at the desired concentrations were infused through one or two Alzet osmotic minipumps (Alza Corp., Palo Alto, Calif.) implanted subcutaneously in the dorsal region of each animal. The minipump has a reservoir volume of 170 $\mu\ell$ (model 1701) or 200 $\mu\ell$ (model 2001), and its nominal pumping rate is 1 $\mu\ell$/hr; thus, it delivers histamine solution continuously for up to 1 week. The animals in which this minipump was implanted were killed on day 7, unless they became moribund due to the perforation of duodenal ulcer(s) into the peritoneal cavity, with resultant generalized peritonitis.

Urine was collected twice over a 24-hr period, with a special metabolic cage, 2 days before the infusion of histamine and on the day before death.[23] Only in the group of *Mastomys* to which the largest doses of histamine (15 mg/kg/24 hr) were given urine was collected twice (2 days before and 1 day after the infusion), because of their high mortality before day 7 due to the perforated duodenal ulcer(s). The amounts of histamine excreted in the urine were determined by the method of Oates et al.[24] The intensity of duodenal lesions was graded using a scale of 0 to 3 as described by Szabo,[25] where 0 = no ulcer, 1 = superficial mucosal erosion, 2 = deep ulcer or transmural necrosis, and 3 = perforated or penetrated (into the pancreas or liver) ulcer.

Mastomys used for the infusion of various gastrin peptides were 1.5-month-old males with body weights of about 30 g. Tetragastrin, 1 mg, was dissolved in 2 mℓ of 0.1% aqueous solution of sodium bicarbonate, and 1 mg of human synthetic gastrin I in 1 mℓ of the same bicarbonate solution. *Mastomys* were fasted overnight. On the following morning, the secretagogues were infused through one or two minipumps in the manner similar to the histamine infusion. Throughout the infusion, food and water were withheld. After 48 hr, the animals were killed and examined for ulceration.

The experiment for cysteamine-induced duodenal ulcer of *Mastomys* was carried out by two subcutaneous injections of cysteamine monohydrochloride in 5% aqueous solution (0.1 or 0.2 g/kg) at 9:00 a.m. and 5:00 p.m. on a single day.[25] Throughout the period of observation, the animals were given food pellets and water *ad libitum.* After 48 hr, they were killed and necropsied for ulceration.

Vagotomy was performed under anesthesia with Somnopentyl (Pitman-Moore, Inc., Washington Crossing, N.J.). Following an epigastric incision, the terminal branches of both vagi were exposed and cut just beneath the diaphragm. About 1 month after the vagotomy, they were used for the infusion experiment of histamine.

The pilot experiment for possible suppression of histamine-induced duodenal ulcers in *Mastomys* was performed by means of either free drinking of cimetidine in 0.3% aqueous solution in place of water, or two subcutaneous injections at 9:00 a.m. and 5:00 p.m. of 4% aqueous solution of cimetidine. This solution was adjusted to pH 6.5 with 1 *N* HCl (0.4 g/kg/24 hr) over 7 days for the animals implanted with an osmotic minipump, releasing 15 mg of histamine per kilogram per 24 hr (i.e., an ample amount to produce duodenal ulcers).

III. RESULTS

A. Histamine-Induced Acute and Chronic Duodenal Ulcers

In the preliminary experiment, we confirmed that *Mastomys* implanted with an osmotic minipump filled with water, 0.1% aqueous solution of sodium bicarbonate, or 0.1 *N* HCl solution for a week showed no particular pathologic lesions in their stomach

Table 1

PRODUCTION OF DUODENAL ULCERS BY CONSTANT INFUSION OF HISTAMINE IN *MASTOMYS* AND OTHER RODENTS AND THEIR URINARY HISTAMINE LEVELS

| | | | Histamine base | | | |
| | | | Amount excreted in urine (μg/24 hr) | | Duodenal ulcer | |
Species	Sex	Amount infused (mg/kg/24 hr)	Before infusion	During infusion	Incidence (positive/total)	Severity
Mastomys	M	5	0.32 ± 0.11[a]	50.1 ± 14.7[a]	6/10	1.8 ± 0.8[a]
Mastomys	M	10	0.31 ± 0.12	80.3 ± 19.0	9/10	2.3 ± 0.7
Mastomys	M	15	0.30 ± 0.10	112.7 ± 24.9	10/10	2.8 ± 0.4
Mastomys	F	15	0.25 ± 0.09	69.8 ± 18.4	10/10	2.8 ± 0.4
Mouse	F	100	55.3 ± 13.7	479.9 ± 63.5	0/10	0
Rat	F	100	47.3 ± 15.4	2796.9 ± 230.9	0/10	0
Guinea pig	M	15	6.8 ± 2.1	260.1 ± 30.9	0/10	0.4 ± 0.2

[a] All values are mean ± SD.

and duodenum; the animals could tolerate a single subcutaneous injection of 50 mg of histamine per kilogram of body weight without the formation of gastroduodenal ulcers.

Table 1 shows the amounts of histamine excreted in the urine before and during the infusion as well as the incidence and intensity of duodenal ulcers induced in *Mastomys* and other rodents. In the *Mastomys* group, the duodenal ulcers were produced in a dose-related manner. The duodena, unless perforated, were markedly distended due to the accumulation of abundant mucinous milky juice which gave a low pH (2.0 to 3.0) as indicated by the pH test paper. Edema of the duodenal walls was also conspicuous. The ulcers were multiple and distributed on every part of the duodenum. The largest ulcer was usually located on the first portion of the duodenum. The number of ulcers, their distance from the pylorus, and their intensity were related to the doses of histamine infused (Figure 2). In the group of *Mastomys* infused with the largest doses of histamine, simultaneous perforation of two duodenal ulcers was frequent and digestive juices in the duodenum escaped into the peritoneal cavity. There was no sex difference as to susceptibility in the development of duodenal ulcers in *Mastomys*. The production of chronic duodenal ulcers was also possible by constant infusion of histamine (5 mg/kg/24 hr) for a month. One or two deep ulcers on the first portion of the duodenum firmly adhered to the liver and penetrated it, followed by the formation of a liver abscess communicating with the base of the ulcer (Figure 3). The distention of the duodenum, the edematous swelling of its entire wall, and the granularity of its mucosa were more marked than those found in the acute experiment.

On the other hand, mice and rats were completely resistant to histamine-induced duodenal ulcers, though they were infused with 20 times more histamine than the group of *Mastomys* administered the smallest doses (5 mg/kg/24 hr). In the guinea pig group, the duodena were moderately distended and superficial mucosal erosion was found in four of ten animals.

Later, Mongolian gerbils were also tested with our histamine duodenal ulcer model. This animal can now be listed as a rodent species resistant to histamine, since five females that were infused with 30 mg of histamine per kilogram for 24 hr were completely free from the duodenal lesions. Table 1 also shows that the endogenous levels of urinary histamine of *Mastomys* were far lower than those of other rodent species.

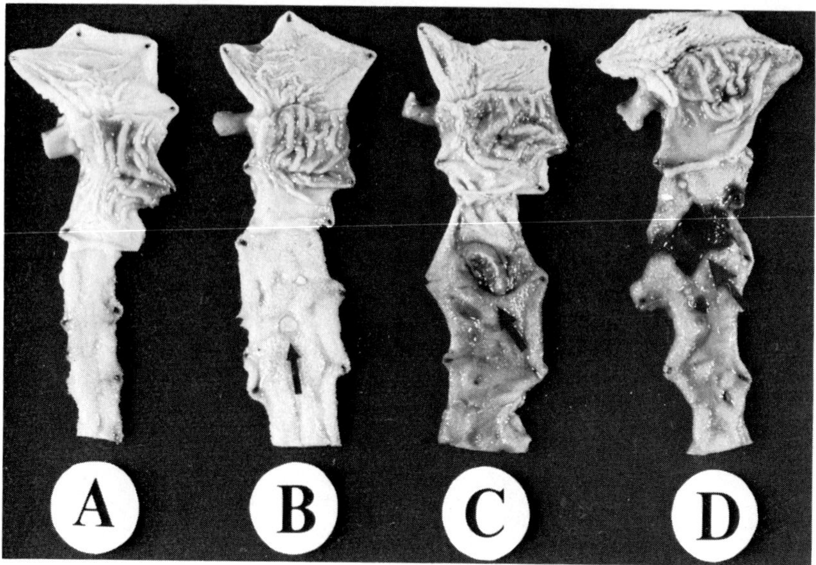

FIGURE 2.   Stomachs and duodena of *Mastomys* after opening along the lesser curvature (stomach) and anterior wall (duodenum). (A) Normal organs from animal infused with water. (B, C, and D) Infusion with 5, 10, and 15 mg/kg/24 hr of histamine, respectively. The severity of duodenal ulcers paralleled the amount of histamine infused: the stomachs are noted to be almost intact. The arrow indicates the largest of the multiple ulcers developed in each duodenum.

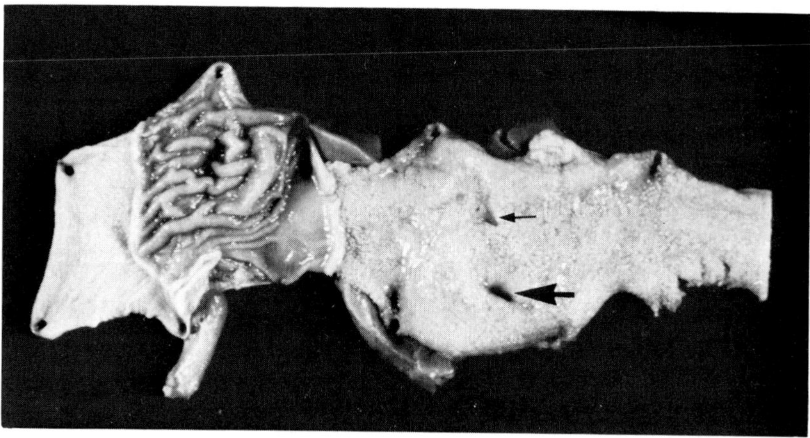

FIGURE 3.   Two deep ulcers developed in the proximal portion of the duodenum. The large one (large arrow) penetrated the liver, forming a liver abscess. Note marked distention of the duodenum, edema of its wall, and granular appearance of its mucosa.

The recovery of histamine, given exogenously through osmotic minipump(s), from urine was <20% in all rodent species (Table 1).

B. Gastric Lesions Associated with Duodenal Ulcers

One or two small, slightly elevated whitish lesions were occasionally observed in the antral mucosa near the pyloric ring of *Mastomys* which had been infused with the largest doses of histamine and which had developed large perforating duodenal ulcers (Figure 4). Histologically, the lesions showed full-thickness hemorrhagic necrosis of

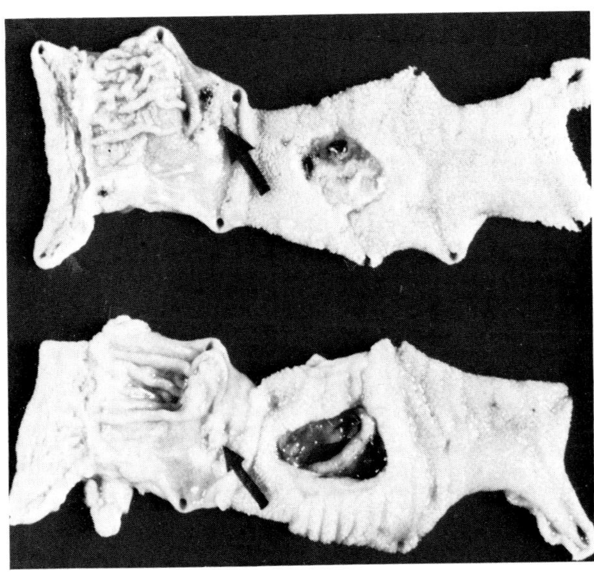

FIGURE 4.   There were slightly elevated focal lesions (arrows) in the antral mucosa associated with a large perforated ulcer in the proximal portion of duodena of *Mastomys* which were infused with 15 mg/kg/24 hr of histamine.

the mucosa or necrosis limited to the superficial part of the submucosa with acute inflammatory cell infiltration. No definite ulcer, either involving the muscularis or perforating the entire gastric wall, was demonstrable.

C. Induction of Duodenal Ulcers By Gastrin Peptides and Enhancement by Fasting on Development of Histamine-Induced Duodenal Ulcers

The effect of various gastrin peptides infused through the same minipump(s) on the development of duodenal ulcers in *Mastomys* was investigated. This time, however, small younger males were chosen because of the low solubility of tetra- and pentagastrins in water and the high cost of human synthetic gastrin I. Ten animals in each group were implanted with two osmotic minipumps filled with tetragastrin or pentagastrin. Under the conditions employed, the amounts of tetragastrin and pentagastrin infused through two minipumps were 0.8 and 0.4 mg/kg/24 hr, respectively. No definite ulcer was induced in the duodenum of *Mastomys* of either group, although two animals in the tetragastrin group and four in the pentagastrin group had superficial mucosal erosions on the proximal portion of the duodenum, which was moderately distended.

Recently, the Alza Corporation produced a new model, the 2 ML1 osmotic pump, which has a tenfold greater reservoir and pumping rate than the earlier osmotic minipump. We have tested this apparatus for the induction of duodenal ulcers by pentagastrin using several adult male *Mastomys* weighing around 70 g. The amounts of pentagastrin infused through the pumps were 0.86 mg/kg/24 hr. However, even under these conditions no definite ulcers were induced in the duodena of *Mastomys*. On the other hand, when two *Mastomys* in each group were infused with 0.4, 0.8, and 1.6 mg/kg/24 hr, of human synthetic gastrin I, respectively, all developed pathologic lesions in the duodenum. There were superficial mucosal erosions in the 0.4-mg group, one or two ulcers in the 0.8-mg group, and multiple perforated ulcers in the 1.6-mg group. The macroscopic and histologic appearances of these lesions were essentially similar to those found in histamine-induced duodenal ulcers (Figure 5). Under similar

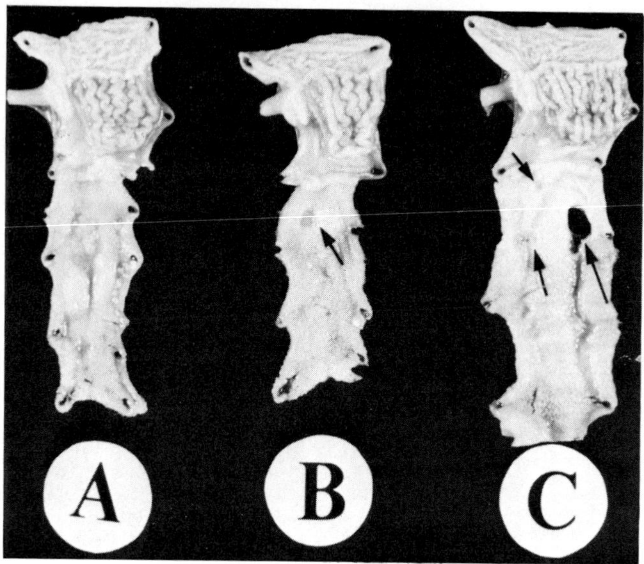

FIGURE 5.   Pathologic changes induced in duodena of *Mastomys* by constant subcutaneous infusion of 0.4 mg (A), 0.8 mg (B), and 1.6 mg (C) per kilogram per 24 hr of human synthetic gastrin I. Arrows indicate induced duodenal ulcers, one of which is perforated (C).

experimental conditions, five small young males in each group were implanted with the minipump which released 1, 2, 3, and 4 mg of histamine per kilogram per 24 hr, respectively. The pathologic changes in their duodena found at necropsy after 48 hr were superficial mucosal erosions without ulcers in all animals of the 1- and 2-mg groups, superficial mucosal erosions and ulcers in four of the 3-mg group, and ulcers in all of the 4-mg group (perforating in two). When the doses of infused histamine were increased to more than 5 mg/kg/24 hr, these animals consistently developed one or two large perforated ulcers in their duodena.

D. Enhancement by Carbachol of Histamine-Induced Duodenal Ulceration

In this experiment, female *Mastomys* were used. First, it was confirmed that under normal feeding conditions none developed a duodenal ulcer after constant infusion of carbachol given in the range of 0.05 and 15 mg/kg/24 hr. At doses of carbachol exceeding 25 mg/kg/24 hr, all *Mastomys* died within a week without the formation of duodenal ulcers. On the other hand, when *Mastomys* were fasted as in the infusion experiments of gastrin peptides, as little as 1.5 mg of carbachol per kilogram per 24 hr could induce duodenal ulcers.

Table 2 shows the potentiating effect of carbachol on the development of histamine-induced duodenal ulcers of *Mastomys* under the fed condition. Though the ulcerogenic effect of histamine in the 1-mg group was less pronounced, the duodenal ulcers developing in the 2-mg group were related to the doses of carbachol infused simultaneously.

E. Application of the Cysteamine-Induced Duodenal Ulcer Model of the Rat to *Mastomys*

When ten males in each group were subcutaneously given 20 and 40 mg of cysteamine per 100 g, respectively, after 48 hr all *Mastomys* in the latter group developed a single deep ulcer with transmural necrosis just distal from the pylorus, and those in the former group exhibited only slight edema of the duodenal mucosa (Figure 6). All *Mas-*

Table 2
DUODENAL ULCERS AFTER SIMULTANEOUS
INFUSION OF A COMBINATION OF HISTAMINE
AND CARBACHOL

Mastomys group	Amount infused (mg/kg/24 hr)		Duodenal ulcer	
	Histamine	Carbachol	Incidence (positive/total)	Severity
1	1	0	0/5	0 [a]
2	1	0.48	0/5	0
3	1	0.96	1/5	0.4
4	1	1.44	1/5	0.8
5	2	0	0/5	0
6	2	0.48	1/5	0.8
7	2	0.96	2/5	1.4
8	2	1.44	4/5	2.2

[a] All values are the mean.

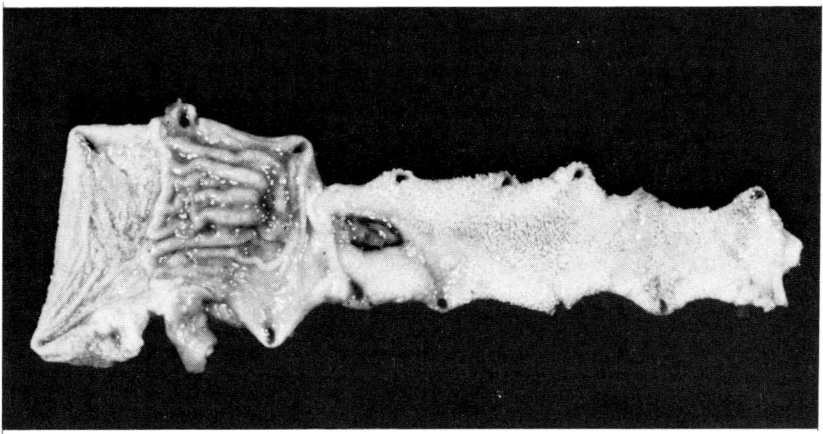

FIGURE 6. A single deep ulcer with transmural necrosis has developed just distal to the pyloric ring of a *Mastomys* which received two subcutaneous injections of 40 mg/kg cysteamine monohydrochloride on a single day.

tomys in each group survived without any serious signs during the period of observation.

F. Suppression of Histamine-Induced Duodenal Ulcers by Various Agents or Vagotomy

Cimetidine — With regard to the effect of cimetidine on histamine-induced duodenal ulcers of *Mastomys,* two of ten males given cimetidine via *ad libitum* drinking showed no ulcer development. When the experiment was repeated and the daily consumption of cimetidine solution was measured, we found that only the *Mastomys* without the ulcers had consumed 15 mℓ of cimetidine per day throughout the experiment. Another ten male *Mastomys* implanted with the same minipumps were given 0.4 g of cimetidine per kilogram per day subcutaneously for a week. None manifested toxic symptoms specific for this drug during the period of observation and no ulcers were induced in their duodena.

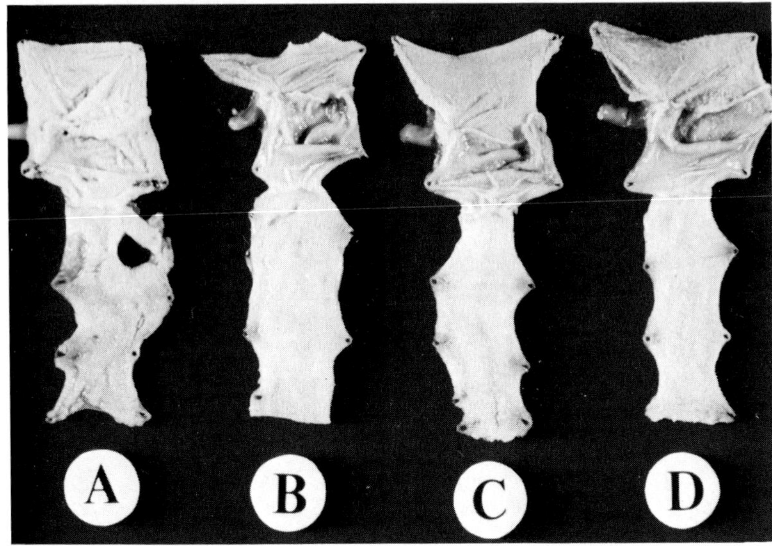

Top

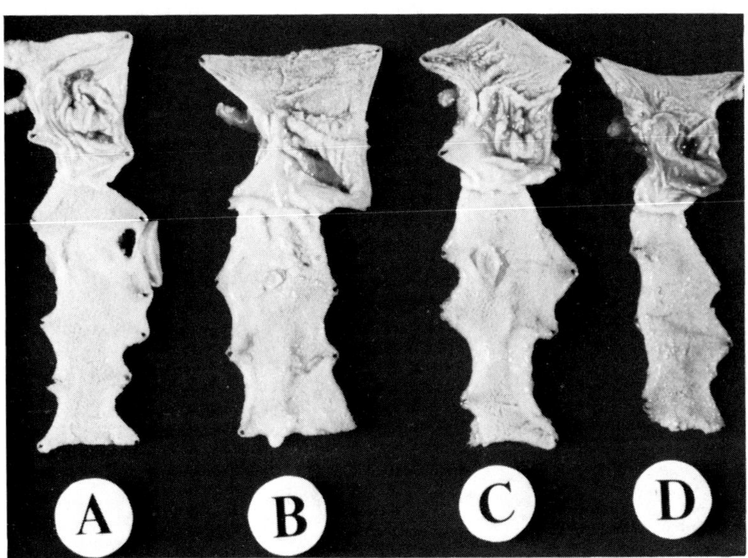

Bottom

FIGURE 7.   Protective effect of various doses of atropine (top) or probanthine (bottom) on duodenal ulcers induced by histamine (15 mg/kg/24 hr). (A) Infusion with histamine alone. (B, C, and D) Infusion with 2.5, 5, and 15 mg/kg/24 hr of atropine, respectively; or 0.07, 0.14, and 0.28 mg/kg/24 hr of probanthine, respectively.

Atropine and probanthine — Atropine and probanthine were selected as representative anticholinergic agents to prevent the development of histamine-induced duodenal ulcers of *Mastomys*. Both agents exerted a dose-related antiulcer effect (Figure 7). Since the doses of atropine and probanthine required for complete suppression of histamine-induced duodenal ulcers of *Mastomys* were 15.0 and 0.28 mg/kg/24 hr, respectively, it was calculated that probanthine was 53.6 times as potent as atropine for inhibiting duodenal ulcers.

Vagotomy — Ten vagotomized *Mastomys* were implanted with minipumps which released 15 mg of histamine per kilogram per 24 hr. After a week all animals still survived. At necropsy their stomachs were distended and distorted with adhesions to the liver and diaphragm. The pathologic changes in their duodena were no ulcers in three animals, superficial mucosal erosions in four, and ulcers in three animals. When these duodenal lesions were scored for severity, using a scale of 0 to 3, the ulcer severity was calculated to be 1.0 ± 0.78 (mean $\pm$ SD). When the authors compared these values with those of nonvagotomized *Mastomys* (2.8 ± 0.4 in Table 1) by a two-sided Student t-test, the probability level was found to be statistically significant ($p < 0.001$).

Morphine — Ten *Mastomys* were implanted with two osmotic minipumps which each supplied 15 mg of histamine and morphine per kilogram per 24 hr. All but one *Mastomys* survived for a week. Their duodenal responses were no ulcer in two animals, superficial mucosal erosions in three animals, and ulcers in five (perforating in two). The mean $\pm$ SD of the calculated ulcer severity score was 1.5 ± 1.02. By use of the Student t-test, the difference between the values and those of the control group was found to be statistically significant ($p < 0.01$).

Somatostatin — Ten *Mastomys* were implanted with two osmotic minipumps which separately released 15 mg of histamine and 1.4 mg of somatostatin per kilogram per 24 hr, respectively. Two animals died of perforated duodenal ulcers within a week. The pathologic changes detected in their duodena were no ulcer in one animal, superficial mucosal erosions in four animals, and ulcer in five. The ulcer severity was calculated as 1.6 ± 0.92. These values were also statistically significant ($p < 0.01$), compared with those in the control group.

Other peptide hormones — Investigations to suppress the histamine-induced duodenal ulcers of *Mastomys* were also carried out by simultaneous infusion of secretin (15 U/kg/24 hr), VIP (0.2 mg/kg/24 hr), or GIP (0.17 mg/kg/24 hr) with histamine (15 mg/kg/24 hr). In both the secretin (ten animals) and VIP (five animals) groups, however, all animals developed deep ulcers (perforating in six in the former and in four in the latter) in their duodena. Two *Mastomys* that were each given 100 μg of GIP developed a single large ulcer in the proximal portion of the duodenum which was graded as 2, in terms of the lesion score.

IV. DISCUSSION

Among rodents, the mouse and the rat have usually been resistant to the induction of duodenal ulcers by gastric secretagogues such as histamine and gastrin,[26,27] whereas the guinea pig has generally been more susceptible to duodenal ulceration with histamine stimulation.[28] We confirmed these facts by the technique of constant infusion of histamine and showed that *Mastomys* was more susceptible to the induction of duodenal ulcers with histamine stimulation than the guinea pig (Table 1). Our preliminary experiment of acute toxic effects of histamine on *Mastomys* showed that the animals could tolerate a single subcutaneous injection of 50 mg of histamine per kilogram of body weight, whereas the LD_{50} of guinea pigs with the same treatment indicated a LD_{50} of 0.5 mg of histamine per kilogram of body weight.[23] In this respect, *Mastomys* may be a rodent species relatively refractory to the direct circulatory and bronchoconstrictor actions of histamine, and has the advantage that it obviates unfavorable side effects of histamine during the study of histamine-induced duodenal ulcers.

In the study of urinary levels of endogenous histamine in the rodent species examined, *Mastomys* was found to excrete the smallest amount of histamine in urine (Table 1). When these levels were adjusted for body weight, the mouse, rat, and guinea pig excreted approximately 600, 100, and 10 times more histamine respectively, in the urine than *Mastomys*. Nevertheless, relative urinary levels of endogenous histamine in *Mas-*

tomys appeared to be several times higher than those reported for humans (average 42 and 49 μg/day in normal males and females, respectively).[24] It was of interest that there was an inverse relationship between the urinary levels of endogenous histamine and the severity of duodenal lesions in these rodents (Table 1). We also noted that each rodent group excreted in the urine less than 20% of the histamine released from the mini-pumps suggesting rapid degradation in vivo (Table 1).

In our earlier study using *Mastomys* bearing either primary or transplantable gastric carcinoid, *Mastomys* excreting larger amounts of histamine often developed small hemorrhagic ulcers in the antrum of the stomach associated with a large perforating ulcer of the duodenum. Further, those bearing a slowly growing tumor transplant occasionally developed one or two chronic duodenal ulcers penetrating into the liver and the descending colon.[20] These findings suggest that the gastric mucosa may be involved in a situation where the more histamine that is released from the carcinoid cells, the more gastric acid secreted from the parietal cells. On the other hand, duodenal ulcers may become chronic during the condition where the carcinoid cells produce relatively smaller amounts of histamine, and secrete it at a slow, steady rate over a month. These findings were confirmed in the histamine duodenal ulcer model investigated, since *Mastomys* infused with 15 mg of histamine per kilogram per 24 hr occasionally developed several small hemorrhagic ulcers in the antrum associated with large perforating duodenal ulcers. Those infused with 5 mg of histamine per kilogram per 24 hr for a month consistently developed one or two chronic duodenal ulcers penetrating the liver.

It has been reported that histamine augmented gastric ulceration produced by intravenous aspirin in cats, and topical aspirin plus hydrochloric acid produced acute gastric mucosal lesions in rats.[30,31] These observations support our earlier findings in the gastric mucosa associated with histamine-induced acute duodenal ulcers in *Mastomys*. Therefore, our acute duodenal ulcer model would also be applicable for further study of the chronic duodenal ulcers resembling those seen in humans and which can readily be produced by varying the dose and duration of histamine infused. Also, the experimental gastric ulcer model might be an advanced form of the preceding focal gastric lesions already mentioned and was presumably induced by an aspirin supplement which inhibited the synthesis of prostaglandins, as in the aspirin-induced gastric ulcer model in cats and rats.[30,31]

The experiments to verify possible induction of duodenal ulcer by tetra- and pentagastrins in *Mastomys* were unsuccessful, probably because the maximal subcutaneous doses of these peptides infused through the two minipumps were too small to maintain gastric hyperacidity leading to duodenal ulceration. Previous investigations have shown that the constant infusion of pentagastrin into rats, as in our experiment, in doses of 5.76 mg/kg/24 hr, resulted only in inconsistent and slight duodenal ulceration.[26,27] Unlike tetra- and pentagastrins, however, human synthetic gastrin I, when administered through the same subcutaneous route, induced duodenal lesions in a dose-related manner, though only two animals in each group were tested in the present experiment because of the cost of this commercially available peptide. From this finding, taken together with the severity of histamine-induced duodenal ulcers of *Mastomys* similarly treated, one may conclude that human synthetic gastrin I was approximately three to four times as potent as histamine for inducing duodenal ulcers in *Mastomys*. It is uncertain, however, whether *Mastomys* is more apt to develop duodenal ulcers with this hexadecapeptide than other animal species, since we found no previous reports in which human synthetic gastrin I, when given by constant subcutaneous infusion, induced duodenal ulcers in laboratory animals.

Robert et al.[26] reported that carbachol, as a cholinergic agent, was duodenoulcerogenic when infused continuously at low but not at high doses in fasted female Sprague-Dawley rats ($ED_{50} = 2.88$ mg/kg/24 hr). Under similar conditions, 1.44 mg of carbachol per kilogram per 24 hr (i.e., one half of the ED_{50} in rats) invariably induced ulcers in the duodenum of female *Mastomys*. Under the normally fed condition, however, *Mastomys* never demonstrated significant pathologic changes in the duodenum when carbachol was infused in the range from 0.05 to 15 mg/kg/24 hr. In this respect, the duodenoulcerogenic action of carbachol differed from that of histamine, since histamine produced duodenal ulcers in *Mastomys* in a dose-related fashion when animals were either fed or fasted. It was deemed worthwhile to determine whether adding carbachol to the continuous subcutaneous infusion of nonulcerogenic low doses of histamine to fed *Mastomys* would produce duodenal ulcers. In fact, carbachol greatly augmented the ulcerogenic action of histamine in the duodena of normally fed *Mastomys* in a dose-related manner (Table 2).

Mastomys were also tested as a cysteamine-induced duodenal ulcer model, which is currently considered simple and reliable for the experimental production of duodenal ulcer in rats.[25,32] The results obtained showed that the intensity of duodenal ulcer induced in *Mastomys* appeared to be comparable to that induced in rats, as reported previously.[25] This fact is somewhat puzzling, since in the present experiment the rats used, which were the same strain employed by previous workers, were completely resistant to histamine-induced duodenal ulcer; and the duodenal ulcerations of rats by cysteamine is also associated with increased gastric acid output.[25,32] According to a recent study by Szabo,[33] cysteamine-induced duodenal ulcers were prevented by dopamine agonists, whereas the severity of duodenal ulcers was enhanced by a dopamine receptor antagonist. He suggested that changes in peripheral and/or central dopamine concentration and/or receptor activity may have a role in the secretion of gastric acid and the pathogenesis of duodenal ulceration. From our study of the urinary levels of endogenous histamine, it was evident that the body histamine pools in the rat were considerably larger than those of *Mastomys*. It is possible, therefore, that the great difference in body histamine content between these two rodent species may result in their different susceptibility to the formation of duodenal ulcers after histamine stimulation, probably through some modulation of the dopamine concentration and/or the activities of dopamine receptors in the peripheral and/or central systems. Further study along this line is underway. Apart from the susceptibility of *Mastomys* to the induction of duodenal ulcer by cysteamine that was comparable to that of rat, it should be mentioned that histamine-induced duodenal ulcers of *Mastomys* were multiple and distributed on every part of the duodenum. This was similar to those induced in rats by two secretagogues in combination (e.g., pentagastrin plus histamine or carbachol), which were also multiple and limited to the proximal duodenum, whereas the cysteamine-induced duodenal ulcers of *Mastomys* or rats were virtually always solitary or double on the anterior and posterior wall of the proximal duodenum. Hence, histamine ulcers in *Mastomys* or rats could serve as an animal model for duodenal ulcers in the Zollinger-Ellison syndrome or similar conditions, while the cysteamine ulcers may be a good example of "peptic" (solitary or kissing) ulcers.

With respect to the use of cimetidine, a H_2-receptor antagonist,[34] we initially gave this drug by free drinking of a 0.3% aqueous solution (solubility in water: 0.45 g/dℓ at 19°C) in place of water to *Mastomys* infused with histamine. Under the conditions employed, the action of cimetidine was less consistently effective in *Mastomys* in suppressing their duodenal ulceration. More recently, we have found that only those *Mastomys* that were able to consume 15 mℓ of the cimetidine solution daily were free of duodenal ulcers. After we changed the administration route of cimetidine from free drinking to subcutaneous injection, the complete suppression of histamine-induced duodenal ulcers in *Mastomys* was a consistent finding.

The antiulcer properties of the anticholinergic agents, atropine and probanthine, were more potent than expected, since the histamine-induced duodenal ulcers of *Mastomys* were completely inhibited by infusion with the same concentration of atropine (15 mg/kg/24 hr) and with a far lower concentration of probanthine (0.28 mg/kg/24 hr). The reduction in ulcer severity by vagotomy was also marked ($p < 0.001$). These findings support the previous view that anticholinergic agents in vivo and vagotomy decrease basal acid secretion and the response to histamine,[35-37] thus providing further evidence of the important role of gastric acid hypersecretion in the etiology of the present histamine duodenal ulcer model. This supports the conventional medical therapy for patients suffering from a duodenal ulcer disease associated with gastric hyperacidity: either anticholinergic drugs or vagotomy.

Earlier studies have shown that somatostatin markedly prevented the formation of duodenal ulcers induced by cysteamine in rats and by histamine or pentagastrin in cats.[38,39] The inhibition by somatostatin of histamine-induced duodenal ulcers in *Mastomys* was not marked, but was significant ($p < 0.01$). Since the dose, route, and mode of administration of somatostatin has varied greatly among previous investigators, a direct comparison of our results with those of others is impossible. In this respect, more studies are needed for the potentiation of the antiulcer effect of somatostatin in our histamine duodenal ulcer model of *Mastomys.*

In contrast to the antiulcer effect of somatostatin, the antiulcer potency of secretin and VIP on histamine-induced duodenal ulcers of *Mastomys* was insignificant, possibly because of the use of smaller doses of these latter two peptides. Each large ulcer which developed in the two *Mastomys* infused with GIP (which was available for use only in limited quantities, i.e., 200 μg) was situated singly in the first portion of the duodenum and did not perforate. Its appearance resembled that of a cysteamine-induced solitary or kissing ulcer. Because only two *Mastomys* were employed in this experiment, however, the question of whether GIP plays some modulating role in the duodenal ulcerogenesis of this sort is still open.

Morphine and related drugs have long been known as inhibitors of gastric secretion in spite of several dissenting reports.[40] Since we considered that the opiate-mediated action on gastric secretion, regardless of its inhibitory or stimulatory nature, may partially represent the cephalic phase, the effect of morphine on histamine-induced duodenal ulcers of *Mastomys* was examined during constant and simultaneous infusion of equimolar concentrations of histamine and morphine. Under the experimental conditions employed, the results imply that morphine may exert an inhibitory effect on the secretion of gastric acid, since the formation of duodenal ulcers in *Mastomys* due to hypersecretion of gastric acid was significantly prevented.

In recent years increasing evidence for the existence of three receptors for gastrin, acetylcholine, as well as histamine, on the parietal cells in the gastric fundus has been supported from isolated cell studies.[41] The available studies with isolated parietal cells have indicated that activation of parietal cell function (i.e., secretion of acid) by histamine but not by carbachol or gastrin is closely linked to stimulation of cyclic AMP generation, whereas cholinergic but not histaminic stimulation of parietal cell function is closely related to enhanced influx of extracellular calcium.[42,43] The nonspecific inhibition of augmented acid secretion in response to many stimulants by atropine and cimetidine in vivo has also been demonstrated in isolated parietal cells in vitro.[35-37,44] These data in vivo and in vitro suggest the existence of either potentiating or inhibitory interactions between specific receptors for histamine, acetylcholine, and gastrin on the parietal cell, though the mechanisms underlying these interactions have not been clarified.

With both the current view of parietal cell function and the present findings in mind, the following scheme is postulated for development of histamine-induced duodenal ulcers in *Mastomys,* and its suppression by various agents and vagotomy (Figure 8). The scheme is a tentative one, and does not precisely express the relative numbers and spatial organization of each receptor on the parietal cell membrane. In this scheme the activity of histamine receptor(s) is presumably variable and the sites are not limited to

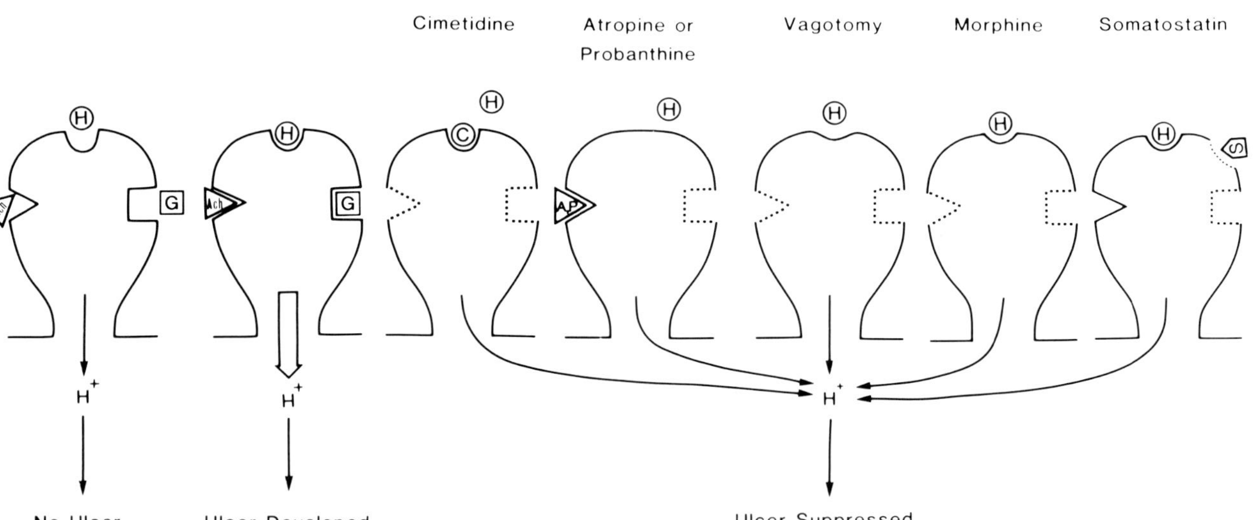

FIGURE 8.   Schematic illustration of inhibitory influences of various agents and vagotomy through gastric parietal cell function, on the development of histamine-induced duodenal ulcers in *Mastomys*. The binding sites of acetylcholine, gastrin, and somatostatin on the parietal cell in modified states are indicated with dotted lines. The present study has not provided data about relative activity of each receptor in these three binding sites under experimental conditions where activity of the histamine receptor site varied. Abbreviations used: A = atropine; Ach = acetylcholine; C = cimetidine; G = gastrin; H = histamine; P = probanthine; S = somatostatin.

a specific region of the cell membrane, depending on either enhanced or suppressed states of other receptors on the parietal cell.

Recent advances in receptor site theory have helped clarify the nature of the production, reduction, and mobility of the receptors. Evidence has already been provided that the receptor, both in vivo and in vitro, represents a dynamic rather than a static population in which the concentration of a receptor may be influenced by a variety of physiological and pharmacological factors. For example, thyroid hormones in vivo increase the number of β-adrenergic receptors in cardiac membranes of the rat[45] and, conversely, the hormones in vitro decrease intranuclear chromatin-associated receptor levels in cultured GH_1 cells secreting growth hormone.[46]

From the results discussed here, we believe that *Mastomys* may well serve as an animal model for the study of not only the etiology and treatment of duodenal ulcer disease, but also the secretory mechanism of gastric acid in humans.

V. SUMMARY

Praomys (Mastomys) natalensis, an African rodent ranging in size between a mouse and rat, is more susceptible to the induction of duodenal ulcers by constant infusion of exogenous histamine through an osmotic minipump implanted subcutaneously than other rodent species tested such as the mouse, rat, guinea pig, or Mongolian gerbil. By increasing the dose of infused histamine, there were increases in the incidence, severity, and perforation rate of duodenal ulcers in *Mastomys*. When animals were fasted during an infusion experiment, the ulcerogenic effect of histamine was highly augmented. Carbachol alone did not cause duodenal ulcers in fed animals, but when given simultaneously with histamine the dose of histamine required for induction of duodenal ulcers could be greatly reduced. The production of chronic duodenal ulcer was also possible by infusion of smaller doses of histamine for 1 month. The induction of duodenal ulcers in *Mastomys* by tetra- and pentagastrins was unsuccessful, probably because of the limited releasing capacity of the present minipumps for use of these two peptides, which are sparingly soluble in water. Human synthetic gastrin I, which is more soluble, was approximately three to four times as potent as histamine in the induction of duodenal ulcers in *Mastomys*. The susceptibility of *Mastomys* to the induction of duodenal ulcer by cysteamine appears to be comparable to that of the rat. The complete suppression of histamine-induced duodenal ulcers of *Mastomys* was possible by repeated subcutaneous injections of cimetidine. Atropine and probanthine also exerted a dose-related antiulcer effect. Vagotomy, morphine, and somatostatin, in this order, decreased the severity of histamine-induced duodenal ulcers at a statistically significant level.

REFERENCES

1. Davis, S. H. C. and Oettlé, A. G., The multimammate mouse *Rattus (Mastomys) natalensis, Proc. Zool. Soc. London,* 131, 293, 1958.
2. Coetzee, C. G., The biology, behavior and ecology of *Mastomys natalensis* in southern Africa, *Bull. WHO,* 52, 3394, 1975.
3. Amies, C. R., The envelope substance of *Pasteurella pestis, Br. J. Exp. Pathol.,* 32, 257, 1951.
4. Lurie, H. I. and DeMeillon, B., Experimental bilharziasis in laboratory animals. III. A comparison of the pathogenicity of *S. bovis,* South African Egyptian strain of *S. mansoni* and *S. haematobium, S. Afr. Med. J.,* 30, 79, 1956.

5. Oettlé, A. G., Spontaneous carcinoma of the glandular stomach in *Rattus (Mastomys) natalensis.* An African rodent, *Br. J. Cancer,* 11, 415, 1957.
6. Soga, J. and Sato, H., Eds., *Praomys (Mastomys) Natalensis: The Significance of Their Tumors and Diseases For Cancer Research,* Daiichi Printing Co., Niigata, Japan, 1977.
7. Solleveld, H. A., *Praomys (Mastomys) Natalensis in Aging Research,* The Institute for Experimental Gerontology TNO, Rijswijk, The Netherlands, 1981.
8. Snell, K. C. and Stewart, H. L., Malignant argyrophilic gastric carcinoids of *Praomys (Mastomys) natalensis, Science,* 163, 470, 1969.
9. Soga, J., Tazawa, K., and Ito, H., Ultrastructural demonstration of specific secretory granules of *Mastomys* gastric carcinoids. Preliminary report, *Acta Med. Biol.,* 17, 119, 1969.
10. Snell, K. C. and Stewart, H. L., Histology of primary and transplanted argyrophilic carcinoids of the glandular stomach of *Praomys (Mastomys) natalensis* and their physiologic effects on the host, in *Gann Monograph,* No. 8, Morris, H. P. and Yoshida, T., Eds., Maruzen Co., Tokyo, 1969, 39.
11. Feldberg, W. and Harris, G. W., Distribution of histamine in mucosa of gastrointestinal tract of dog, *J. Physiol. (London),* 120, 352, 1953.
12. Smith, A. N., The distribution and release of histamine in human gastric tissues, *Clin. Sci.,* 18, 533, 1959.
13. Kim, Y. S. and Glick, D., Determination of histidine decarboxylase in microgram samples of tissue, properties and quantitative histochemistry of the enzyme and histamine in the rat stomach, *J. Histochem. Cytochem.,* 15, 347, 1967.
14. Gregory, R. A. and Tracy, H. J., The constitution and properties of two gastrins extracted from hog antral mucosa, *Gut,* 5, 103, 1964.
15. Waldenström, J., Pernow, B., and Silwer, H., Case of metastasizing carcinoma (argentaffinoma?) of unknown origin showing peculiar red flushing and increased amounts of histamine and 5-hydroxytryptamine in blood and urine, *Acta Med. Scand.,* 156, 73, 1956.
16. Oates, J. A. and Sjoerdsma, A., A unique syndrome associated with secretion of 5-hydroxytryptophan by metastatic gastric carcinoids, *Am. J. Med.,* 32, 333, 1962.
17. Hosoda, S., Nakamura, W., Snell, K. C., and Stewart, H. L., Histamine production by transplantable argyrophilic gastric carcinoid of *Praomys (Mastomys) natalensis, Science,* 170, 454, 1970.
18. Hosoda, S., Nakamura, W., Snell, K. C., and Stewart, H. L., Histidine decarboxylase in the transplantable argyrophilic gastric carcinoid of *Praomys (Mastomys) natalensis, Biochem. Pharmacol.,* 20, 2671, 1971.
19. Hosoda, S., Suzuki, K., Sudo, K., Yoshida, N., and Tanaka, C., Transplantable argyrophilic gastric carcinoids of *Mastomys natalensis* secreting both histamine and serotonin, *J. Natl. Cancer Inst.,* 63, 1447, 1979.
20. Hosoda, S., Saito, T., Suzuki, H., and Hara, K., *Praomys (Mastomys) natalensis* with transplantable gastric carcinoid secreting histamine and 5-hydroxytryptamine and primary gastric carcinoid secreting histamine, *S. Afr. Cancer Bull.,* 24, 394, 1980.
21. Hosoda, S., Ikedo, H., and Saito, T., *Praomys (Mastomys) natalensis:* animal model for study of histamine-induced duodenal ulcers, *Gastroenterology,* 80, 16, 1981.
22. Snell, K. C. and Stewart, H. L., Neoplastic and nonneoplastic renal disease in *Praomys (Mastomys) natalensis, J. Natl. Cancer Inst.,* 39, 95, 1967.
23. Nakamura, W., Kankura, T., and Eto, H., Occult blood appearance in feces and tissue hemorrhage in mice after whole body X-irradiation, *Radiat. Res.,* 48, 169, 1971.
24. Oates, J. A., Marsh, E., and Sjoerdsma, A., Studies on histamine in human urine using a fluorometric method of assay, *Clin. Chem. Acta,* 7, 488, 1962.
25. Szabo, S., Animal model: cysteamine-induced acute and chronic duodenal ulcer in the rat, *Am. J. Pathol.,* 93, 273, 1978.
26. Robert, A., Stout, T. J., and Dale, J. E., Production by secretagogues of duodenal ulcers in the rat, *Gastroenterology,* 59, 95, 1970.
27. Joffe, S. N., Gaskin, R. J., Barros D'Sa, A. A. J., and Barron, J. H., Secretagogue-produced duodenal ulcers in the rat, *Br. J. Surg.,* 64, 218, 1977.
28. Hay, L. J., Varco, R. L., Code, C. F., and Wangensteen, O. H., The experimental production of gastric acid duodenal ulcers in laboratory animals by the intramuscular injection of histamine in beeswax, *Surg. Gynecol.,* 75, 170, 1942.
29. National Defence Research Committee, *Office of Scientific Research and Development,* Washington, D.C., 1943, 115.
30. Hansen, D. G., Aures, D., and Grossman, M. I., Histamine auguments gastric ulceration produced by intravenous aspirin in cats, *Gastroenterology,* 74, 540, 1978.
31. Guth, P. H., Aures, D., and Paulsen, G., Topical aspirin plus HCl gastric lesions in the rat, *Gastroenterology,* 76, 88, 1979.
32. Selye, H. and Szabo, S., Experimental model for production of perforating duodenal ulcers by cysteamine in the rat, *Nature (London),* 244, 458, 1973.

33. Szabo, S., Dopamine disorder in duodenal ulceration, *Lancet,* 2, 880, 1979.
34. Wood, C. J. and Simkins, M. A., Eds., *Int. Symp. Histamine H₂-Receptor Antagonist,* Smith, Kline & French Laboratories, London, 1973.
35. Code, C. F., Hightower, N. C., and Hallenbeck, G. S., Comparison of the effects of methantheline bromide (Banthine) and atropine on the secretory responses of vagally innervated and vagally denervated gastric pouches, *Gastroenterology,* 19, 254, 1951.
36. Dotevall, G., Schroder, G., and Walan, A., The effect of poldine, glycopyrrolate and 1-hyoscyamine on gastric acid secretion in man, *Acta Med. Scand.,* 177, 169, 1955.
37. Hirschowitz, B. I. and Sachs, G., Atropine inhibition of insulin, histamine, and pentagastrin stimulated gastric electrolyte and pepsin secretion in the dog, *Gastroenterology,* 56, 693, 1969.
38. Schwedes, U., Usadel, K., and Szabo, S., Somatostatin prevents cysteamine-induced duodenal ulcer, *Eur. J. Pharmacol.,* 44, 195, 1977.
39. Konturek, S. J., Radecki, T., Pucher, A., Coy, D. H., and Schally, A. V., Effect of somatostatin on gastrointestinal secretions and peptic ulcer production in cats, *Scand. J. Gastroenterol.,* 12, 379, 1977.
40. Konturek, S. J., Somatostatin and opiate peptides: their action on gastrointestinal secretions, in *Gastrointestinal Hormones,* Glass, G. B. J., Ed., Raven Press, New York, 1980, 693.
41. Soll, A. H., Physiology of isolated canine parietal cells: receptors and effectors regulating function, in *Physiology of the Gastrointestinal Tract,* Vol. 1, Johnson, L. R., Christensen, J., Grossman, M. I., Jacobson, E. D., and Schultz, S. G., Eds., Raven Press, New York, 1981, 673.
42. Soll, A. H. and Wollin, A., Histamine and cyclic AMP in isolated canine parietal cells, *Am. J. Physiol.,* 237, E444, 1979.
43. Soll, A. H., Extracellular calcium and cholinergic stimulation of isolated canine parietal cells, *J. Clin. Invest.,* 68, 270, 1981.
44. Soll, A. H., Potentiating interactions of gastric stimulants on ¹⁴C-aminopyrine accumulation by isolated canine parietal cells, *Gastroenterology,* 83, 216, 1982.
45. Williams, L. T., Lefkowitz, R. J., Watanabe, A. M., Hathaway, D. R., and Besch, H. R., Jr., Thyroid hormone regulation of β-adrenergic receptor number, *J. Biol. Chem.,* 252, 2787, 1977.
46. Samuels, H. H., Perlman, A. J., Raaka, B. M., and Stanley, F., Organization of the thyroid hormone receptor in chromatin, in *Recent Progress in Hormone Research,* Vol. 38, Greep, R. O., Ed., Academic Press, New York, 1982, 557.

Chapter 19

THE RELEVANCE OF THE DIAMINE OXIDASE-HISTAMINE SYSTEM FOR SHOCK DEVELOPMENT FOLLOWING INTESTINAL ISCHEMIA

Jürgen Kusche, Wilfried Lorenz, and Rudolph Hesterberg

TABLE OF CONTENTS

I. INTRODUCTION

Intestinal ischemia generally refers to the acute occlusion of the superior mesenteric artery following thrombosis and embolism. However, the acute mesenteric infarction is only the "tip of the iceberg" in intestinal ischemia. Bounous,[1] in his review of acute necrosis of intestinal mucosa reported, from autopsy studies, occurrence up to 90% of ischemic lesions of the intestine following postoperative hypotension, heart failure, or sepsis.[1,2] Clinically, these lesions appeared as a pseudomembranous enterocolitis, which disease must not be confused with the quite different staphylococcal diarrhea or pseudomembranous colitis related to modern antibiotic therapy. The most common cause of pseudomembranous enterocolitis is postoperative hypotension in debilated patients. The prevalence of this disease is increasing.

Even if acute mesenteric infarction is rarely observed in the clinic, the review of Bounous[1] emphasizes that dealing with acute intestinal failure means dealing with an important pathophysiological event. The superior mesenteric artery occlusion (SMAO), however, is the most suitable experimental model for this disease.

Although there is convincing evidence from many publications (for review, see Reference 3) that the development of shock following SMAO is related to ischemic damage of the intestinal mucosa, the exact pathogenic mechanism is still under discussion. We have the problem that many vasoactive substances and related factors have been described which are released into the blood circulation and may be considered responsible for blood pressure and cardiac depression.[4] One way to escape the dilemma of the excessive effect of intestinal shock factors was proposed by Lefer,[5] who postulated certain conditions which a vasoactive agent has to fulfill before its pathophysiological significance can be accepted. Unfortunately, the myocardial depressant factor, detected by Lefer himself, seems to be a victim of point two of these postulations.[6] In Table 1, these criteria are outlined for the diamine oxidase-histamine system. Regarding the well-known facts that (1) histamine and the histamine destroying enzyme, diamine oxidase (EC 1.4.3.6) (DAO), are present in the intestinal mucosa of human subjects and animals, and (2) histamine is a powerful vasoactive agent, it was the aim of a series of experiments to test the postulations of Table 1 and thereby to establish the relevance of the DAO-histamine system for shock development following intestinal ischemia.

II. MATERIALS AND METHODS

A. Materials

1. Animals

The animals used in this series were (1) dogs: male mongrels, 14 to 30 kg body weight; (2) miniature pigs: female, strain Hannover-Göttingen, 31 to 55 kg body weight; and (3) rabbits: male and female purebreds, race: Big-Silver, 2.4 to 5.5 kg body weight. All animals were adapted to their environment. They were fed with commercially available standard diet until 12 hr before the start of the experiment and with tap water *ad libitum.*

The animals were anesthetized with sodium pentobarbital, using 20 to 30 mg/kg body weight for dogs and miniature pigs and 15 to 25 mg/kg for rabbits. All animals were maintained and tested during spontaneous breathing.

2. Tissue and Plasma Samples

Tissue samples for the assay of DAO activity and histamine content, weighing about 1 g, were either frozen in CO_2 snow (for assaying enzymic activity) or homogenized with 9 volumes of 0.4 mol/l $HClO_4$ (for histamine determination) within 10 min after

Table 1

CRITERIA FOR DEMONSTRATION OF THE
RELEVANCE OF THE DIAMINE OXIDASE-
HISTAMINE SYSTEM IN SHOCK
DEVELOPMENT FOLLOWING INTESTINAL
ISCHEMIA[5]

1. Alterations of tissue histamine concentration and metabolism during and following intestinal ischemia
2. Quantitative determination and identification of histamine in blood plasma during shock development
3. Increase of plasma histamine level and aggravation of shock development by an inhibition of histamine catabolism
4. Mitigation of shock development by elimination or antagonism of histamine
5. Relation of the clinical symptoms to histamine release
6. Conclusions drawn from more than one species

withdrawal and stored at −20°C. Tissue samples from *human subjects* were obtained during abdominal operations. Care was taken to keep the time between the disconnection of the organ from the blood circulation and the sample treatment as constant and as short as possible.[7]

For the histological study in miniature pigs, tissue samples of the whole intestinal wall, weighing about 1 g, were taken from the terminal ileum and fixed in a 4% formaldehyde solution. Staining was processed with hematoxylin-eosin, according to Romeis.[8] Plasma for the determination of the histamine concentration in dogs and miniature pigs was prepared according to Lorenz et al.[9]: 19.5 mℓ of blood were withdrawn slowly and with care to avoid producing bubble formation via a polyethylene syringe containing 2 mg of heparin dissolved in 0.5 mℓ of 0.9% NaCl solution. After gently mixing, the sample in the syringe was transferred slowly and with only slight pressure into a 30-mℓ polyethylene centrifuge tube, precooled thoroughly in an ice-cold water bath, and centrifuged immediately for 30 min at 1000 × g and 1 to 2°C. Then 6 mℓ of plasma was withdrawn, mixed immediately with 3 mℓ of 2 mol/ℓ HClO$_4$, and centrifuged for 10 min at 1800 × g. The whole supernatant was passed through a paper filter and either used immediately for histamine assay or stored in a freezer at −20°C, after which histamine was determined several days later.

Plasma for the determination of the histamine concentration in rabbits was prepared by a modification of the technique developed by Da Prada and Pletscher.[10] The histamine-rich platelets in rabbits interfere considerably with the ordinary assay of histamine in plasma. Degradation of histamine by DAO was prevented by injection of 100 mg/kg aminoguanidine into an ear vein. Thereafter, to prevent platelet aggregation, dextran-60 was infused into the right atrium of the anesthetized animal through a short, wide polypropylene catheter inserted via the left jugular vein. Blood samples were taken from the same catheter. For each measurement, 5.4 mℓ was collected in a polypropylene syringe containing 0.6 mℓ of 5% (wt/vol) sodium ethylenediaminetetraacetic acid solution instead of heparin, gently mixed, and immediately cooled in a water bath at 10°C. A few minutes later the first centrifugation step was performed in a Sorvall RC2B centrifuge at 7800 × g and 10°C for 5 min (no visible hemolysis). From the supernatant, the upper 4 mℓ was transferred to a second polypropylene tube and centrifuged at 48,000 × g and 10°C for another 20 min. The upper 3 mℓ of the supernatant was finally taken, mixed with 1.0 mℓ of 2 mol/ℓ HClO$_4$ in glass tubes, and stored at −20°C.

3. Reagents

For the isotope assay of diamine oxidase activity, and the histamine determination in tissues and plasma, the reagents previously described were used.[10-13] Pentobarbitone (Abbott Laboratories, St.-Remy-sur-Auve, France), dextran-60 (Macrodex®, Knoll Chemische Fabriken AG, Ludwigshafen, Germany) were also administered. Amino-guanidine sulfate monohydrate (Schuchardt AG, Munich), dimethpyrindene (Forhistal®, Fenistil®, Zyma, Munich), cimetidine (Smith Kline & French, Welwyn Garden City, England), and sodium EDTA (E. Merck AG, Darmstadt, Germany) were freshly prepared before each experiment according to the manufacturer's recommendations.

B. Methods

1. Models of Intestinal Ischemia

a. Superior Mesenteric Artery Occlusion in Dogs

The aims of this experimental model have been to study: (1) alterations of the histamine concentration of the peripheral blood plasma during and following SMAO, and (2) the influence of an inhibition of the DAO-catalyzed oxidative histamine degradation as induced by aminoguanidine. Following anesthesia, polypropylene catheters were inserted into the abdominal aorta via the femoral artery (for blood pressure measurement) and into the suprahepatic part of the inferior vena cava via the femoral vein (for blood sampling). The abdominal wall of the dog was prepared by shaving and disinfection with phenyl hydrargyrum. After a medial laparotomy the superior mesenteric artery was exposed about 1 to 2 cm after branching from the abdominal aorta, and clamped with hemostats (beginning of the intestinal ischemia). The laparotomy wound was quickly closed with towel clips and covered with sterile cloths.

The duration of the arterial occlusion had been determined in a previous pilot study and 4 hr was taken as the optimal time, since all other animals had died within a few minutes of each other when the occlusion lasted longer (for example, 5 hr), whereas when the occlusion lasted a shorter time (e.g., 2 and 3 hr) the survival time was prolonged to such an extent that nonspecific factors caused solely by surgery, anesthetics, and postoperative treatment had a great influence on the survival time.

The end of arterial occlusion and the start of the reperfusion of the mesenteric vessels were determined by the removal of the hemostats. Circulatory arrest was noticed when the pulse wave, as registered on an oscilloscope, stayed on the base line. Survival time was measured from the removal of the hemostats until appearance of the base line by a stopwatch. Generally, we waited for the spontaneous death of the animal to determine the survival time. However, when the animal lived longer than 10 hr following the reperfusion of the superior mesenteric artery, it was sacrificed by injection of an overdose of pentobarbital.

The experiment included 20 dogs in a randomized, blind trial. Aminoguanidine sulfate, the specific DAO inhibitor, was administered i.v. to ten animals at a dose of 100 mg/kg, 5 min before SMAO and 5 min before the release of the SMAO. The other ten dogs received saline at the same time. The operator was not aware whether he applied the drug or the NaCl solution. Furthermore, investigators determining the plasma histamine concentration did not know to which test group the sample related.

b. Superior Mesenteric Artery Occlusion in Miniature Pigs

The aims of the experimental model in miniature pigs were to study: (1) alterations of histamine concentration and DAO activity in the portal vein blood, (2) alterations of the histamine content and DAO activity of the intestinal mucosa, and (3) the influence of inhibition of the DAO, by aminoguanidine, on the development of shock.

Following anesthesia and disinfection of the abdominal wall, polyethylene catheters were inserted into the femoral artery and vein. The arterial catheter was used for blood pressure measurement, the venous catheter for the application of drugs. After a medial laparotomy, the superior mesenteric artery was prepared for occlusion. Subsequently, a polyethylene catheter was inserted into the vena lienalis and manually positioned in the portal vein. Having finished these preparations in the upper abdominal cavity, a blind loop was prepared 40 to 50 cm proximal of the ileocecal valve by a side-to-side anastomosis of the ileum. From this blind loop, tissue samples could be withdrawn during the experiment without interruption of the continuity of the alimentary channel. The start and finish of the ischemic period were determined as described in dogs by clamping the superior mesenteric artery and removing the clamps. For experimental purposes, a 3-hr period of intestinal ischemia was evaluated as most suitable in a pilot study. The definition of the survival time was the same as described in dogs.

The experiment involved 20 animals, which were treated with aminoguanidine or saline in an alternating series. This design had to be chosen because of the facilities available in our animal stable. Dose and mode of aminoguanidine or saline application were the same as described in dogs.

c. Superior Mesenteric Artery Occlusion and Perfusion in Rabbits

The aims of the model of intestinal ischemia in rabbits were to study: (1) alterations of the peripheral plasma histamine concentrations, (2) alterations of the histamine content and the DAO activity of the intestinal wall, and (3) the influence of DAO inhibition, removal of histamine, and pharmacological blockade of histamine action on shock development.

Male rabbits were anesthetized with pentobarbital as described above, placed on a warmed operating table in order to maintain body temperature, and allowed to breathe spontaneously. In order to check the body temperature, which proved to be a critical point in the whole experiment, the esophageal and, in some cases, the rectal temperature was measured. A polyethylene catheter was inserted into the right femoral artery up to the abdominal aorta in order to determine arterial blood pressure. Pulse and arterial blood pressure were controlled continuously during the whole experiment. Before laparotomy, various doses of aminoguanidine (see below) were injected into an ear vein.

Disinfection of the abdominal wall and preparation of the superior mesenteric artery were performed as described for dogs. An arterial occlusion of 90 min duration was found to be suitable for the experiment, according to a pilot study. The duration of intestinal ischemia and the survival time were defined as described above.

Altogether, four series of experiments were performed. In the first study, 20 animals were randomly allocated to groups treated with aminoguanidine (25 mg/kg) or saline. A parallel group of five sham-operated animals was used, in which the superior mesenteric artery was not ligated, but was exposed and was softly held by a sling.

In a second study the dose-response curve for aminoguanidine and survival time was determined. Six groups of five rabbits were used. In this study, 2 mℓ of saline or 10, 25, 30, 50, or 100 mg/kg aminoguanidine in the same volume of saline was injected into an ear vein. Laparotomy, as described above, was started 1 hr later. The various drug treatments were administered to the animals by using a balanced random allocation of experimental units by forming a random permutation.[15]

In a third study the mesenteric vessels were perfused with Ringer-lactate solution before the restoration of the mesenteric circulation. The perfusate was removed from the circulation. With this experimental model the release of histamine from the mesenteric system was studied as well as the possible benefit of the withdrawal of vasoactive substances (probably of histamine) from the circulatory system. The operative technique was essentially the same as described above up to the preparation of the superior mesenteric artery.

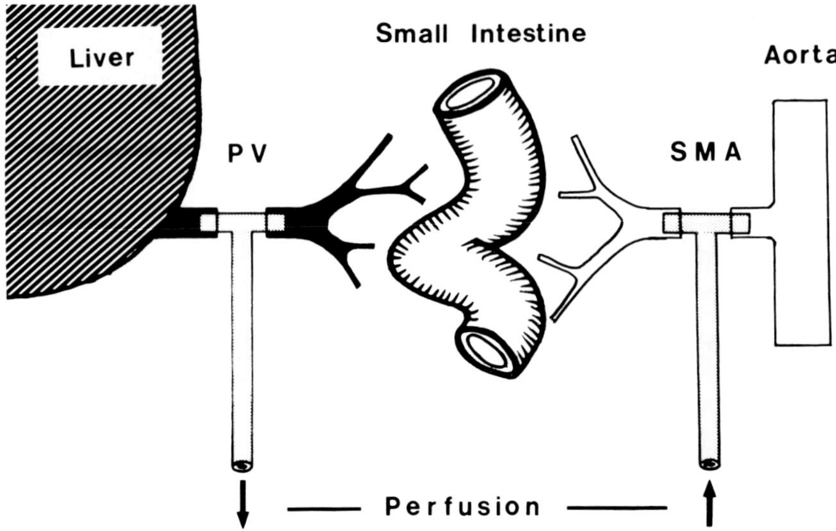

FIGURE 1.   Model of perfusion of the mesenteric vascular system. PV = portal vein; SMA = superior mesenteric artery. During the time of intestinal ischemia, the SMA was occluded between the T-drain and the aorta, and the long sides of the T-drains were also closed. During the perfusion of the mesenteric vessels with Ringer-lactate solution, the portal vein between the T-drain and liver was also occluded. The long sides of the T-drains were open. The arrows mark the infusion and elimination of the Ringer-lactate solution. Restitution of blood supply was achieved by occluding the long parts of the T-drains and opening the SMA and PV.

Following the occlusion of the superior mesenteric artery by an hemostat (start of intestinal ischemia) a T-drain was inserted into the superior mesenteric artery with the long side turned out from the peritoneal cavity (Figure 1). The same procedure was performed at the portal vein. The vena lienalis was ligated because of the high risk of bleeding. The long side of this second T-drain was again turned out from the abdomen. During the period of intestinal ischemia, the superior mesenteric artery and the long sides of the T-drains were kept closed. Following the 90-min SMAO, 16 animals were randomly allocated into two groups — one with immediate restoration of the blood supply and the other with perfusion of the mesenteric vessels. During the time of perfusion the superior mesenteric artery was kept closed for an additional 15 min (median) and 500 mℓ of Ringer-lactate (37°C) was infused into the long side of the T-drain of the superior mesenteric artery which was now opened. During the time of perfusion the portal vein was closed with an hemostat distal to the T-drain, but the long part of this drain was also opened. About 450 mℓ of the infusion fluid was removed in five fractions via the drain in the portal vein. After this procedure the portal vein and the superior mesenteric artery were opened for free blood flow and the long parts of the T-drains closed again (start of the survival time). The perfusate was tested for its content of histamine. Five sham-operated animals, which were treated by T-drain insertion but not with SMAO, were run in parallel.

The fourth study tested the influence of H_1- plus H_2-receptor antagonists on the survival time. Both H_1- and H_2-receptors are present in the rabbit cardiovascular system and therefore the effects of histamine release from ischemic gut are only likely to be prevented by the combined administration of H_1- plus H_2-receptor antagonists.[16] This has previously been verified in the dog.[17,18]

In the fourth study, two randomized controlled trials were performed consecutively to show the effects of the antagonists on saline- or aminoguanidine-pretreated rabbits. In contrast to our previous findings in dogs, the dose of the H_1-antagonist (0.1 mg/kg) was not high enough to exert a statistically significant effect ($2\alpha = 0.05$) although a clear trend was observed in the aminoguanidine-pretreated animals.[18] Thus, in the second trial 0.5 mg/kg dimethpyrindene was used.

In the first trial four groups of ten rabbits were used. Each animal received either saline (2 mℓ) plus saline (0.6 mℓ), saline (2 mℓ) plus H_1- plus H_2-receptor antagonists (dimethpyrindene 0.1 mg/kg dissolved as 1 mg/mℓ saline plus cimetidine 5 mg/kg dissolved finally as 10 mg/mℓ saline), plus saline (0.6 mg), or aminoguanidine plus H_1- plus H_2-receptor antagonists. The four treatments were applied to animals in random order by using a continuous series of random digits.

In the second trial two groups of ten rabbits each were used. Each animal received either 100 mg/kg aminoguanidine plus 2.0 mℓ saline, or 100 mg/kg aminoguanidine plus H_1- plus H_2-receptor antagonists (dimethpyrindene 0.5 mg/kg plus cimetidine 5 mg/kg). The order of the two treatments was randomized. In both trials the experiments started with the injection of saline or aminoguanidine into an ear vein. This was followed by anesthesia with pentobarbital. Polyethylene catheters were inserted into the femoral artery (for blood pressure recording) and femoral vein (for infusion of the H_1- plus H_2-receptor antagonists). After exactly 1 hr the laparotomy was started, and H_1- plus H_2-receptor antagonists or saline was infused slowly for 2 min immediately before clamping of the superior mesenteric artery. After exactly 90 min of ischemia, the clamp was removed. The survival time was recorded from the monitor as described above.

2. Determination of Diamine Oxidase Activity and Histamine Concentration in Tissue and Plasma

For the determination of diamine oxidase activity frozen tissues were homogenized with an Ultraturrax homogenizer with 9 parts by volume of ice-cold phosphate buffer (KH_2PO_4/Na_2HPO_4, 0.2 mol/ℓ) at pH 6.9 for rabbits and pH 7.6 for dogs and pigs. The homogenate was centrifuged in a Sorvall RC2B centrifuge for 30 min at 48,000 × g and 4°C. The enzymic activity was measured in the supernatant.

The DAO activity was measured by our modification of the isotope assay of Okuyama and Kobayashi,[19] which was revised recently.[11,12] A mixture of [1,4-^{14}C] putrescine and unlabeled putrescine was used as substrate at a final concentration of 10^{-3} mol/ℓ.[20] The reaction was stopped with perchloric acid. One of the reaction products, Δ_1-pyrroline, together with its polymers, was extracted into toluene and measured by liquid scintillation counting. In addition to cpm-values/unit of time, as reported by Okuyama and Kobayashi,[19] we also determined the nanomoles of product formed per minute by calibrating the isotope assay with the glutamate-dehydrogenase method.[11,12,21] In this way the enzymic activity was expressed as nanomoles per minute × grams of fresh weight.

Histamine was measured fluorometrically in tissue specimens and in plasma, as described by Lorenz et al.[9,22] The histamine concentrations were expressed as micrograms of histamine dihydrochloride per gram of fresh weight, or as nanograms of histamine base per milliliter of plasma. Specificity of the assay for tissues and plasma was shown by fluorescence spectra, the heating test, and fluorescence spectra after heating for 2 hr.[14]

3. Parameters For the Control of Intestinal Ischemia and Reperfusion

The purpose of our animal model was to demonstrate the relevance of the DAO-histamine system for the shock development following SMAO. Therefore, the most important parameters were plasma and tissue histamine concentrations, DAO activity, and the survival time as an indicator of the severity of shock. However, additional parameters were necessary to obtain more information about effectiveness of the occlusion of the superior mesenteric artery and especially of a true onset of the mesenteric reperfusion. These parameters follow:

1. Body temperature, which was especially important in small animals like rabbits. It was tested by a flexible probe in the rectum or esophagus and was recorded continuously.
2. Tissue oxygen tension was determined polarographically using a platinum surface electrode, according to Kessler.[23] This electrode contained 16 wires of 15-μm diameter each; the signals were integrated to give a single value of oxygen tension. The area of measurement for each wire was about 60 μm. The electrode was calibrated by nitrogen and room air (20.4% oxygen) with regard to actual temperature of the gut and the actual barometric pressure. The average tissue oxygen tension was determined by calculating the arithmetic mean of the values from 8 to 15 areas, each of them separated by about 0.5 cm, and was expressed in torr.
3. Blood pressure and pulse rate were assayed directly by a Statham pressure transducer, P 23 Db, and recorded on a Hellige compensograph. The mean arterial pressure was calculated according to Burton.[24]
4. The hematocrit, which was determined according to Richterich.[25]

4. Statistics

In the majority of cases the median-percentile system was used for parameters of locations and variance. The $\bar{x} \pm$ SD system was used only if the distribution of the data was approximately normal. For regression analysis (Figure 7), hyperbolic and exponential models were chosen by the method of least squares. The different parts of the study were performed over a period of 5 years, thus various inductive statistical techniques were used to test H_o and alternative hypotheses: if normal distribution was suggested (e.g., Figure 2), the t-test for paired data was used ($\alpha = 0.05$) in spite of the problem of time-dependent measurement. The statistical treatment of such a series remains a matter of dispute.[26] In the trial shown in Figure 9a, the problem of comparing all possible pairs could be overcome only by an asymptotic test described by Steel[27] (K $\leqslant$ 4), and H_o was repeatedly tested being rejected at a nominal significance level of $2\alpha = 0.05$.[27,28] In the trial of Figure 9b, however, the Mann-Whitney test could be chosen without restriction.

III. RESULTS

A. Intestinal Ischemia and the Diamine Oxidase-Histamine System
1. Normal Values of Diamine Oxidase Activity and Histamine Concentration in the Intestinal Tract of Human Subjects, Dogs, Miniature Pigs, and Rabbits

Before alterations of DAO and histamine by intestinal ischemia could be observed, it was necessary to study the system under normal conditions. Table 2 shows that the amine, as well as the enzyme responsible for its oxidative catabolism, is present in the intestinal mucosa of mammals and human subjects. This means that the three species in this study, from a biochemical point of view, had comparable preconditions. Furthermore, it can be suggested that in human subjects the DAO-histamine system will be similarly influenced by intestinal ischemia. Among the species investigated, the rabbit is to some extent unique because the DAO activity was found solely in the intestinal mucosa, whereas in pigs, dogs and human subjects the enzyme was also detected at high activity in the kidney.

2. Tissue Diamine Oxidase, Histamine, and Intestinal Ischemia

The alterations of the DAO-histamine system were studied in rabbits and miniature

Table 2
DAO ACTIVITY AND HISTAMINE CONTENT OF THE INTESTINAL TRACT

	Human subjects	Dogs	Miniature pigs	Rabbits
DAO activity (nmol/min/g)				
Jejunum	132.0	12.3 (5)	14.6 (3)	7.3 (6)
Ileum	102.0	19.2 (5)	13.9 (3)	3.4 (6)
Colon	57	19.7 (9)	2.9 (3)	—
Histamine content (μg/g)				
Jejunum	29.8	26.2 (10)	—	3.0 (10)
Ileum	31.1	7.0 (10)	200 (10)	—
Colon	14.4	—	—	—

Note: The values represent the median ($\tilde{x}$) from 64 human subjects[7] and the mean ($\bar{x}$) from animals. The number of individuals is given in parentheses. Data for dogs, miniature pigs, and rabbits are from References 39, 55, 63, and 65.

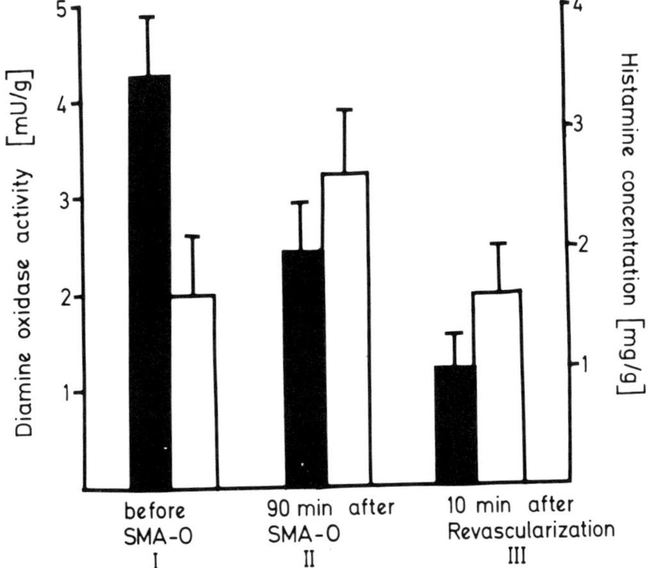

FIGURE 2. Influence of intestinal ischemia and reperfusion on the diamine oxidase activity and the histamine concentration of rabbit small intestine. Each column represents the mean ± SD of five animals. Filled bars represent diamine oxidase activity; open bars represent histamine concentration. Tissue samples were taken from the proximal jejunum. As calculated by the *t*-test for paired data, the alteration of diamine oxidase activity was statistically significant (I/II, $p < 0.005$; I/III, $p < 0.005$; II/III, $p < 0.02$) as well as the increase in the histamine concentration during the ischemic period (I/II, $p < 0.05$). SMAO = superior mesenteric artery occlusion. With kind permission of the American Gastroenterological Association.

pigs (Figures 2 and 3). The DAO activity decreased during the period of intestinal ischemia and again following mesenteric reperfusion. This loss of activity was statistically significant in rabbits and pigs.

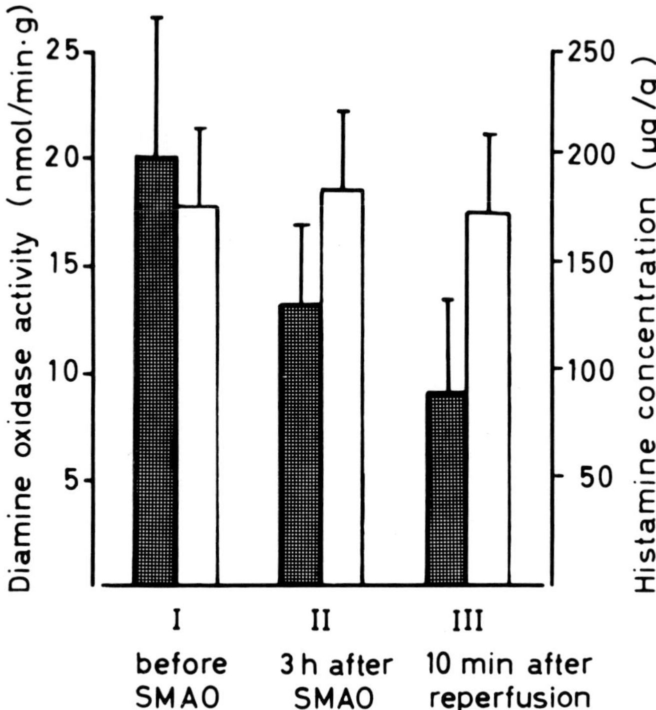

FIGURE 3.   Influence of superior mesenteric artery occlusion and reperfusion on diamine oxidase activity and histamine concentration of the terminal ileum of miniature pigs. Each column represents the mean ± SD of ten animals. Filled bars: diamine oxidase activity; open bars: histamine concentration. As calculated by the Student's *t*-test, the alteration of diamine oxidase activity was statistically significant (I/II, $p < 0.01$; II/III, $p < 0.001$; II/III, $p < 0.01$). SMAO = superior mesenteric artery occlusion.

The content of histamine of the intestinal wall increased during the ischemic period, and this was statistically significant in rabbits but not in miniature pigs. This quantitative difference between the two species may be due to the different initial values of histamine concentration in the gut. In rabbits the initial histamine concentration was in the range of 2 to 3 µg/g, and in miniature pigs in the range of 160 to 180 µg/g. This means that an increase of about 2 µg/g produced a doubling of the intestinal histamine concentration in rabbits, but had no such remarkable effect in pigs.

After reperfusion of the superior mesenteric artery, the intestinal histamine concentration fell back almost to initial values in rabbits and in miniature pigs. This observation suggested a release of the amine from the gut. Indeed, this was confirmed by the study of plasma histamine.

3. Plasma Histamine and Intestinal Ischemia

It should be mentioned here that it was not the primary aim of our study to detect a release of histamine from the ischemic gut, but to investigate the role of the oxidative histamine catabolism. Therefore, the administration of the highly specific DAO inhibitor, aminoguanidine, was inseparably connected with the experiments of SMAO. The results will be interpreted first from a pathobiochemical point of view and then from the perspective of shock development.

In dogs, pigs, and rabbits, a uniform reaction of the plasma histamine levels after mesenteric artery occlusion and reperfusion was observed. During the period of is-

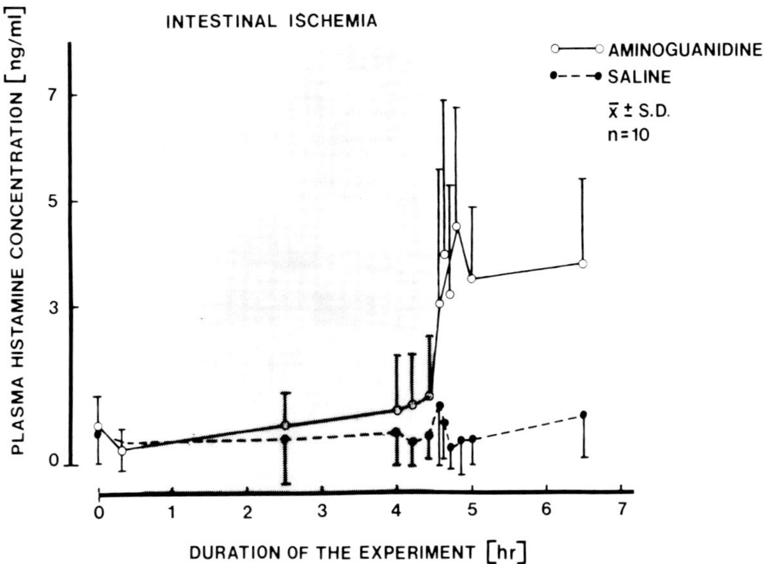

FIGURE 4. Plasma histamine concentration during intestinal ischemia experiments in dogs. Mean values ± SD from ten animals in each group. Statistical significance by the Student's *t*-test between the two groups 30 min after mesenteric reperfusion, $p < 0.001$. (From Kusche, J., Stalknecht, C.-D., Lorenz, W., Reichert, G., and Richter, H., *Agents Actions*, 7, 81, 1977. With permission.)

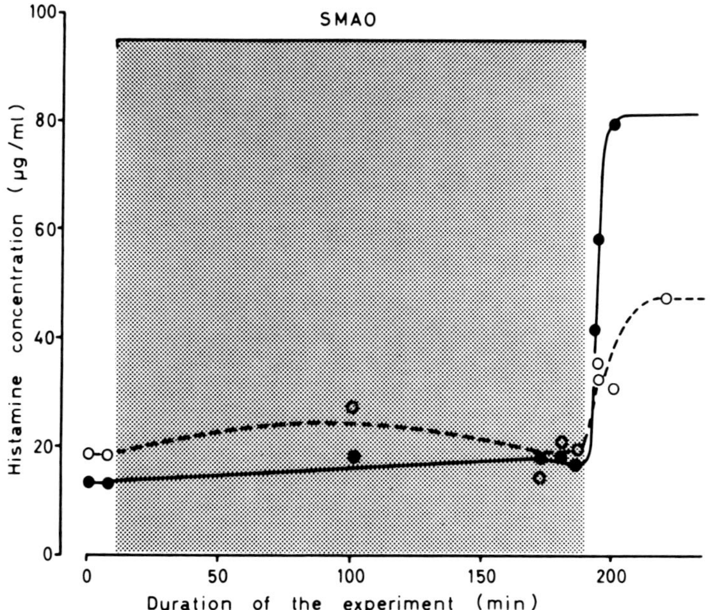

FIGURE 5. Plasma histamine concentrations in the portal vein during intestinal ischemia and after reperfusion of the mesenteric artery in miniature pigs. Median from ten animals in each group; ●—● and aminoguanidine-treated animals; O —— O saline-treated pigs. Statistical significance in the Mann-Whitney test between the two groups 30 min after reperfusion, $p < 0.002$.

chemia the plasma histamine concentration was only slightly elevated in the peripheral and in the portal venous blood (Figures 4 to 6). No statistical difference was produced by the inhibition of DAO.

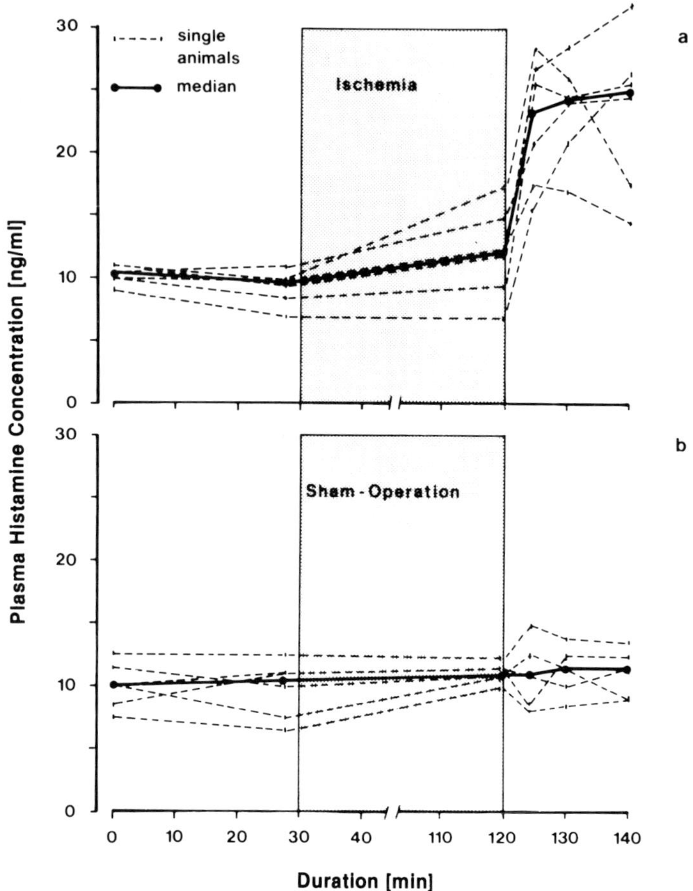

FIGURE 6.   Plasma histamine concentration in experiments with superior mesenteric artery occlusion and reperfusion in rabbits. Single values and median; n = 6 in groups a and b. In the sham-operated group b, the same procedure was performed as in group a, including preparation of the mesenteric artery, except for occlusion of the vessel. With kind permission of the American Gastroenterological Association.

Immediately after the suspension of the mesenteric blockade, however, histamine appeared in the blood circulation of all three species at considerable levels. The elevation of the plasma histamine levels in the blood taken from a peripheral vein was less pronounced when no aminoguanidine was administered, but was highly significant in aminoguanidine-treated dogs and rabbits. In the plasma of the portal vein of miniature pigs, even without aminoguanidine, the histamine levels increased considerably during the reperfusion period. However, in this species the plasma histamine levels were significantly enhanced by aminoguanidine treatment.

These results indicated that in all three species studied a considerable amount of histamine was released into the blood circulation, which must be regarded to be also highly likely in clinical conditions.[29]

4. Diamine Oxidase Inhibition and Reduction of the Survival Time

The survival time was regarded as an important parameter which indicated the severity of shock development. Therefore, it was expected that the survival time would be influenced by the release of histamine if any relevance for shock development could

Table 3

INFLUENCE OF AMINOGUANIDINE ON THE SURVIVAL
TIME FOLLOWING INTESTINAL ISCHEMIA AND
REPERFUSION IN THREE SPECIES

Species	Duration of intestinal ischemia (min)	Minutes of survival time (median range)		Significance
		Aminoguanidine	Saline	
Miniature pigs	180	64 (17—119)	482 (120—620)	$p < 0.001$
Dogs	240	154 (7—339)	490 (137—666)	$p < 0.002$
Rabbits	90	52 (12—113)	147 (97—410)	$p < 0.001$

Note: In all the groups, n = 10. For experimental conditions see Section II in the text.
For statistical evaluation of the survival time, a modification of the Wilcoxon
test was applied in which censored data were used.[64] Data obtained from Reference 65.

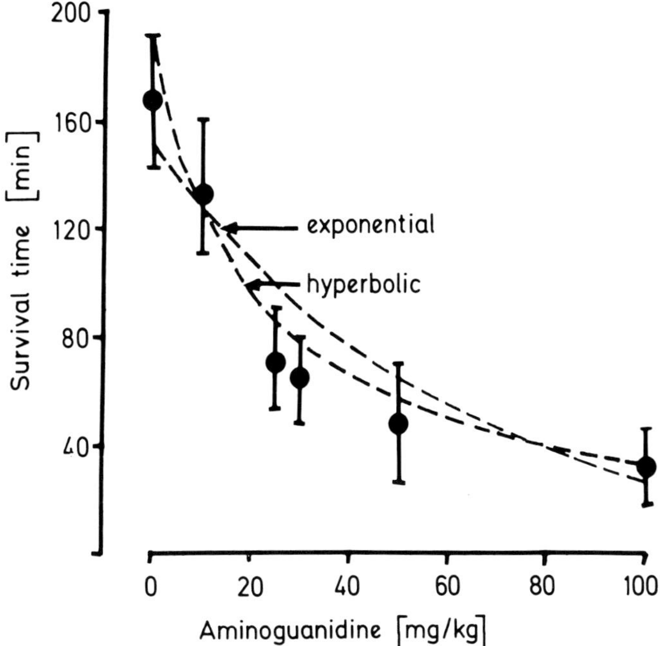

FIGURE 7. Influence of aminoguanidine on the survival time of rabbits
after superior mesenteric artery occlusion and reperfusion. Each value
represents the mean ± SD of five animals. Best correlation ($r^2 = 0.91$) was
obtained by the hyperbolic model according to the equation $1/y =
0.00534 + 0.00025 \cdot x$. However, the exponential model showed the significant coefficient of correlation ($r^2 = 0.81$; equation: $y = 152.108 \cdot
e^{-0.017x}$) which was important for the hypothesis of a one drug-one receptor interrelationship of the aminoguanidine action. With kind permission
of the American Gastroenterological Association.

be ascribed to this amine. As shown before, the plasma histamine concentration was
altered by the inhibition of the enzyme which oxidatively deaminated the amine. Thus,
the DAO inhibitor, aminoguanidine, should also influence the survival time.

In dogs, pigs, and rabbits, aminoguanidine reduced with statistical significance the
survival time after SMAO and reperfusion (Table 3). To clarify the specificity of this
effect, a dose-response curve for aminoguanidine was constructed (Figure 7). The

Table 4

THE INFLUENCE OF PERFUSION OF THE
MESENTERIC VESSELS ON THE
SURVIVAL TIME IN INTESTINAL
ISCHEMIA EXPERIMENTS

Test number	Survival time		
	Perfused (min)	Nonperfused (min)	Sham-operated (hr)
1	95	4	13
2	90	15	11
3	74	28	22
4	135	16	18
5	180	40	15
6	281	1	—
7	81	3	—
8	118	10	—
$\bar{x} \pm SD$	132 ± 69	14 ± 13	14 ± 4

Note: The statistical significance between the group with and without perfusion was $p < 0.005$ (Student's t-test).

shape of the dose-response curve was very similar to that of a monoexponential function, indicating a one drug-one receptor relationship. This would be expected if aminoguanidine exerted its action in a specific way by competitively inhibiting the enzyme responsible for histamine catabolism.

5. Elimination and Receptor Blockade of Histamine and Prolongation of the Survival Time

An attempt was made to aggravate shock development by the inhibition of DAO, as a result enhancing the plasma histamine level. Also, another attempt was made to prolong survival time by the elimination of histamine released into the mesenteric circulation, or by blocking its effects by histamine receptor antagonists.

The elimination of histamine was achieved by an infusion of 500 mℓ Ringer-lactate solution into the mesenteric artery before restitution of the blood supply and removal of the perfusate from the portal vein (see Figure 1). The total amount of histamine which was found in the five fractions of the perfusate reached about 80 μg. With respect to a histamine concentration of 3 μg/g (Table 2), the histamine in the perfusate represented a considerable part of that initially found in the circulatory field of the superior mesenteric artery.

The survival time of perfused rabbits was compared with the survival time of nonperfused or sham-operated animals (Table 4). The perfusion significantly prolonged the survival time despite the fact that it extended the period of intestinal ischemia by about 15 min.

A similar experiment to our rabbit study was performed by Köbler, with dogs,[30] and the result — prolongation of the survival time — was essentially the same as with rabbits.

To demonstrate the effect of histamine H_1- plus H_2-receptor antagonists on the survival time, two trials were needed. In the first trial, the model of experimental intestinal ischemia proved to be fully reproducible (Table 3). Aminoguanidine again shortened the survival time, but in contrast to our findings with dogs and human subjects, the

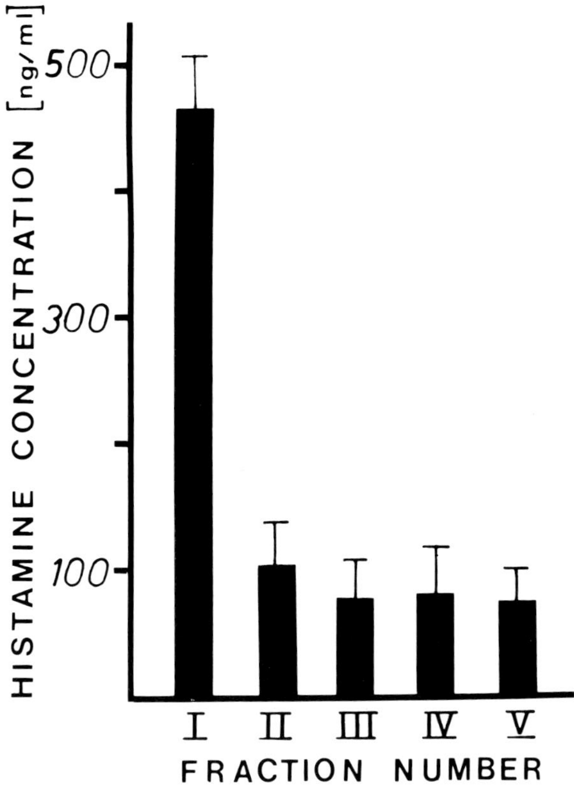

FIGURE 8. Histamine concentration in the perfusate after perfusion of the superior mesenteric vascular system. Fractions I to IV represent 100 m*l* each, fraction V: 50 m*l*. Mean values ± SD; from eight rabbits.

dose of the H_1-receptor antagonist did not significantly prolong survival when administered to the saline plus aminoguanidine-treated animals (Figure 9a).[18,31]

In the second trial, however, a fivefold higher dose of dimethpyrindene completely reversed the aminoguanidine-induced shortening of the survival time (Figure 9b). As dimethpyrindene is a highly specific histamine H_1-receptor antagonist, the protective effect of intestinal diamine oxidase against histamine released during intestinal ischemia seems well established.[32]

B. Histamine-Related Parameters and Intestinal Ischemia

To estimate the relevance to the whole organism, the alterations of the DAO-histamine system were related to "clinical" parameters such as decrease in blood pressure, hematocrit, and histological findings. The arterial blood pressure is highly sensitive to a release of histamine; therefore, its initial decrease immediately after the reperfusion of the mesenteric artery was compared in saline and aminoguanidine-treated animals (Table 5).[33,34] No statistically significant difference, but a tendency toward a more notable decrease in blood pressure, was observed in the aminoguanidine-treated dogs and pigs. Since histamine probably is not the only vasoactive substance released following SMAO, and is not the only factor affecting the blood pressure at this stage of the experiment, this result also supports the hypothesis of shock aggravation by histamine liberation.

Changes in the hematocrit during the experiment were observed in miniature pigs

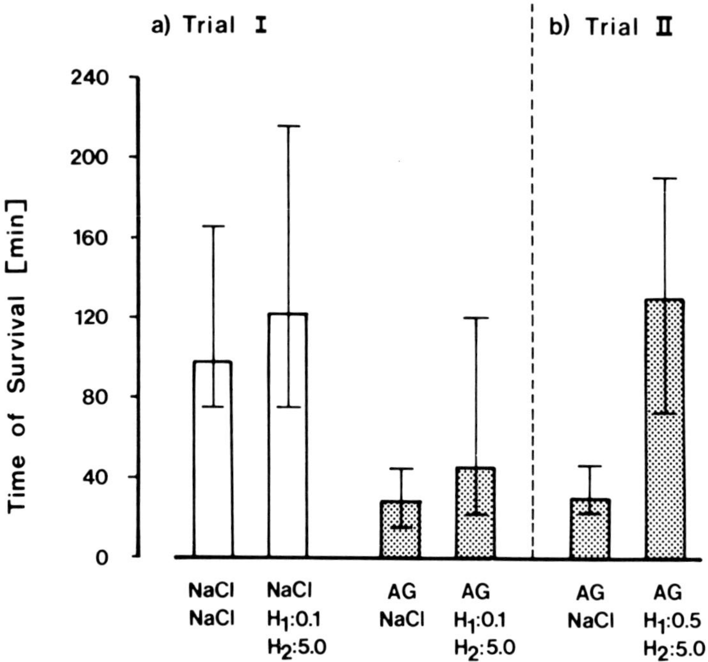

FIGURE 9.   Influence of H_1- and H_2-receptor antagonists on the survival time after mesenteric artery occlusion and reperfusion in rabbits. Interquartile range and median; n = 10 in each group. NaCl = 0.9% sodium chloride solution; AG = aminoguanidine (100 mg/kg); H_1 = dimethpyrindene; H_2 = cimetidine. The doses of the H_1- and H_2-receptor antagonists are given in milligrams per kilogram.

Table 5
THE INFLUENCE OF AMINOGUANIDINE ON THE ACUTE FALL OF ARTERIAL BLOOD PRESSURE IMMEDIATELY AFTER RESTITUTION OF BLOOD SUPPLY

	Saline			Aminoguanidine		
Species	Before restitution	3 min after restitution of mesenteric circulation	Δ mmHg	Before restitution	3 min after restitution of mesenteric circulation	Δ mmHg
Dog	126	95	31	169	120	43
Miniature pig	100	62	38	89	43	47
Rabbit	98	65	33	94	62	32

Note: The values represent the mean ($\bar{x}$) arterial blood pressure calculated according to Burton;[24] n = 10 in each group.

(Figure 10). During the reperfusion period a statistically significant hemoconcentration developed under the influence of aminoguanidine. Hemoconcentration, however, may have been related to histamine concentration since one of the best known effects of histamine is an increase in vascular permeability.[35] The morphological manifestations of an increased vascular permeability are edema and hemorrhagic infiltration of tissue.

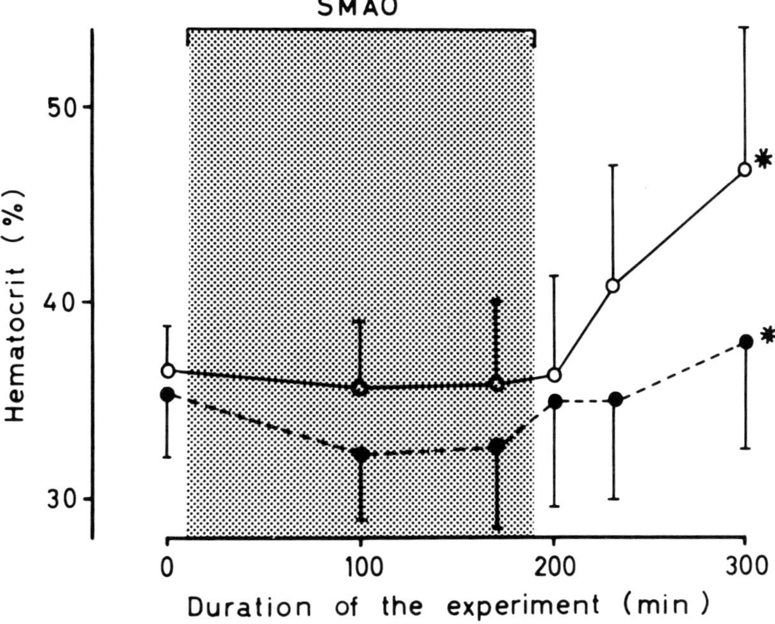

FIGURE 10. Development of hemoconcentration during experimental superior mesenteric artery occlusion (SMAO) and the reperfusion. •- - -• NaCl 0.9%-treated miniature pigs; O——O aminoguanidine-treated pigs; mean values ± SD; n = 10 in each group; * $p < 0.05$ (Student's t-test).

This was also studied in miniature pigs. An independent pathologist, who operated as a statistically "blinded" observer, observed an enhanced dilatation, edema, and hemorrhagic infiltration in the aminoguanidine-treated group. A histological sample of the intestinal mucosa at the end of the survival time demonstrates the acute exfoliation of the villi (Figure 11) in a saline-treated miniature pig and, additionally, the severe hemorrhagic infiltration (Figure 12) under aminoguanidine treatment.

Histamine is regarded as an important factor in the development of acute gastric erosions, which can be prevented by H_2-receptor antagonists.[36] Also, following experimental intestinal ischemia, stress ulcers of the gastric mucosa were observed.[37,38] In our study, this could be confirmed in animals surviving longer than 1 hr after reperfusion of the mesenteric artery. If we consider the observations which coincide with the outcome of the organism following the intestinal ischemia, i.e., shock development, decreased blood pressure, hemoconcentration, and morphological alterations, we obtain the full picture of the severe reaction to histamine release.

C. Control of the Experimental Model

The demands which were made upon the model of experimental ischemia are listed below.

Adaptation to the clinical situation — This was provided by the acute mesenteric artery occlusion which resembles mesenteric infarction due to embolism and thrombosis. Furthermore, the suspension of the mesenteric blockade corresponded to the surgical approach of embolectomy. Our experimental model can therefore be described as an acute and time-limited intestinal ischemia which did produce necrosis of the intestinal villi but not of the crypts, thus preserving the basically regenerative mucosa.

Standardization — The duration of the ischemic period was based upon a reproducible survival time which was not affected by septic complications. Therefore, the ap-

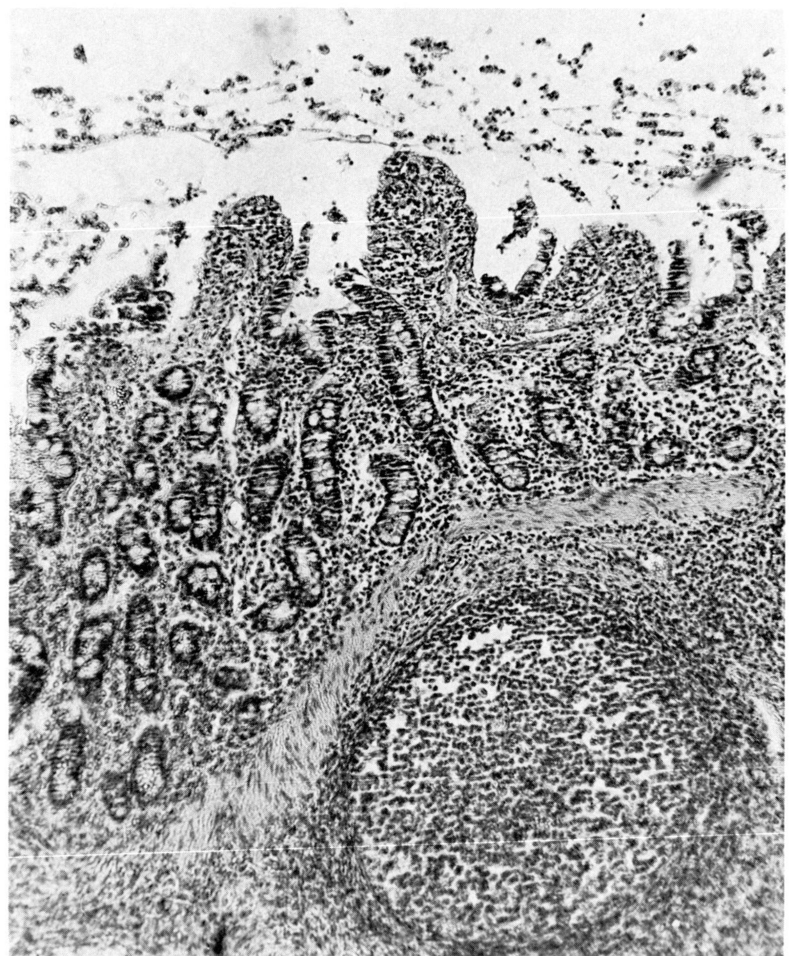

FIGURE 11.   Histology of the mucosa of the ileum. Enlargement about 80-fold; sample from the excluded loop of the terminal ileum of a NaCl-treated miniature pig, 3-hr superior mesenteric artery occlusion, reperfusion and 6 hr survival. There is desquamation of the villi and edema of the rest of the mucosa, but regenerative crypt cells are evident. A lymphatic intestinal follicle in the submucosa is also illustrated.

propriate duration of mesenteric occlusion was established in a pilot study for each species.

Control — Recordings of arterial blood pressure and pulse rate were necessary for the determination of survival time. However, these parameters were also suitable for control of the efficacy of the mesenteric artery occlusion and reperfusion. The arterial blood pressure regularly increased immediately after termination of the mesenteric blood supply. Immediately after reperfusion, however, a rapid fall of blood pressure was observed (Figure 13). If these rapid changes of arterial blood pressure were not recorded, either the artery was not completely occluded or the reperfusion was not established. Another possible method to monitor the blood supply was the determination of oxygen tension at the serosal site of the gut (Figure 14). The oxygen tension was also followed during the course of the experiment.

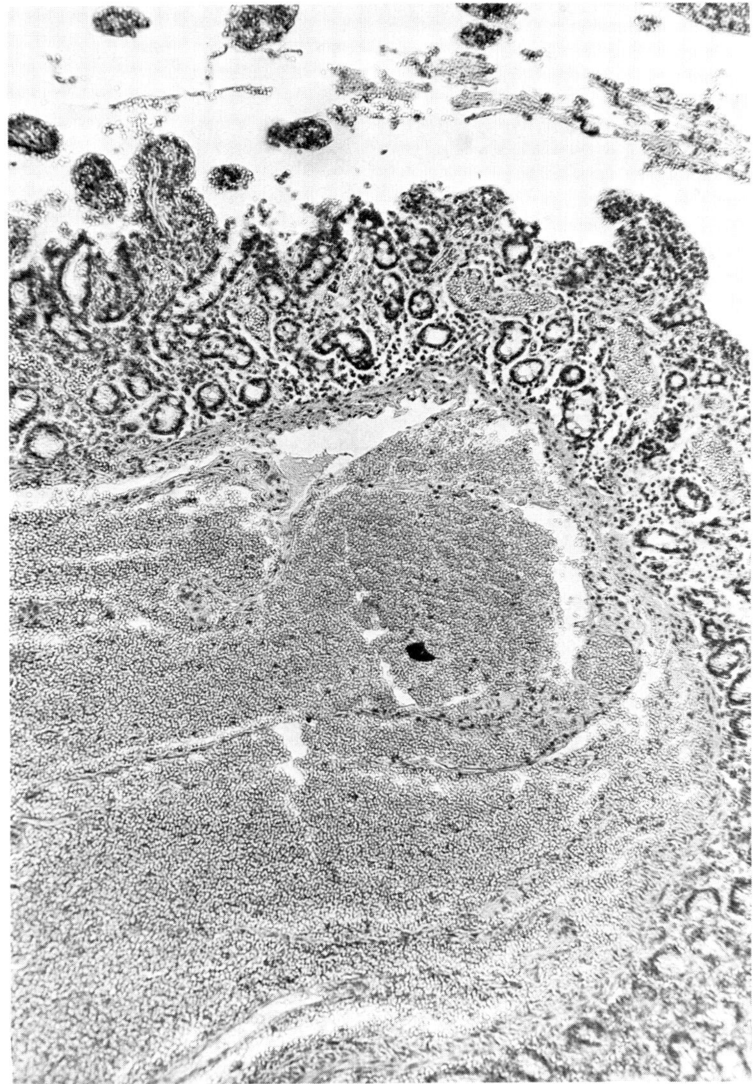

FIGURE 12.   Histology of the mucosa of the ileum. Enlargement about 80-fold; sample from the excluded loop of the terminal ileum of an aminoguanidine-treated miniature pig; 3-hr superior mesenteric artery occlusion; reperfusion and about 1 hr survival. The tissue shows, besides the alterations described for Figure 11, a massive hemorrhagic infiltration of the submucosa and mucosa.

IV. DISCUSSION

A. The Diamine Oxidase-Histamine System

The changes in DAO activity followed a very uniform pattern, i.e., a continuous decrease during the course of the SMAO experiments. However, it was questionable as to where the enzymic activity might have relocated. Attempts to detect the DAO in the peripheral blood following mesenteric artery occlusion were unsuccessful in rabbits and dogs. In the portal venous blood of miniature pigs, the DAO was slightly elevated at the end of the ischemic period and was somewhat more elevated following the reperfusion (Figure 15). Unfortunately, the enzymic activity varied widely and, more

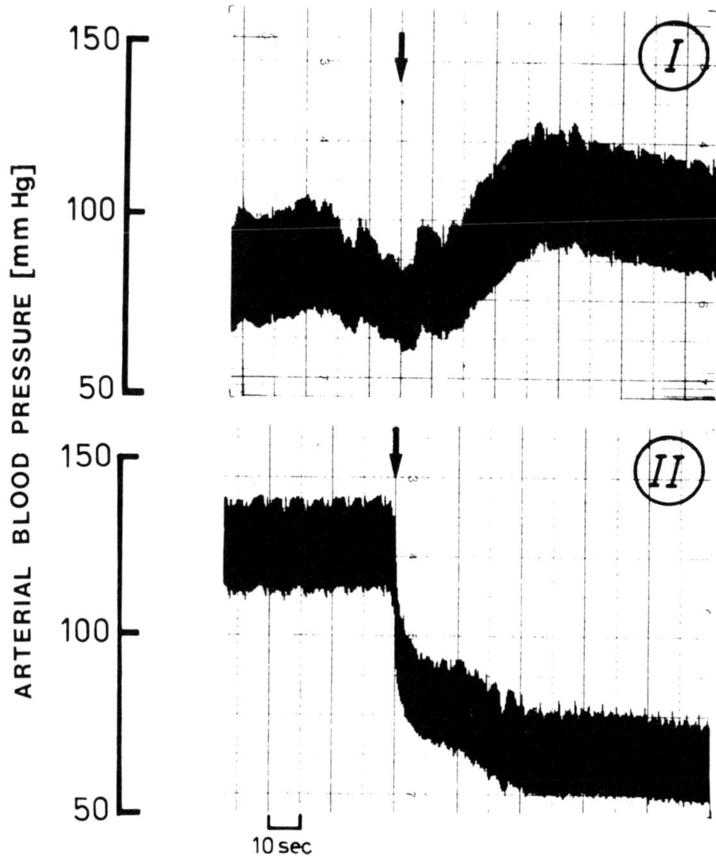

FIGURE 13.   Acute alterations of the arterial blood pressure by mesenteric artery occlusion and reperfusion in miniature pigs. I: the arrow marks the time of occlusion; II: the arrow marks the time of restitution of the blood supply.

importantly, the small activity released into the circulation was not related to the considerable amount of DAO disappearing from the mucosa. Thus, it might be speculated that the enzyme, together with the mucosal cells, was sloughed into the lumen of the gut. This was observed in closed ileal loops of dogs during ischemia and was later confirmed with SMAO in rabbits.[39,40] Tissue and plasma histamine concentrations were to some extent related. The decrease in tissue histamine concentration corresponded to the increase in plasma histamine, as studied in rabbits and miniature pigs.

Following the steep increase in plasma histamine at the beginning of the reperfusion period, however, rapid elimination of the amine was not found, as observed after histamine release induced by various drugs (half life of about 5 min).[34] In contrast, the plasma histamine level remained elevated until the death of the animals. This type of delayed histamine release was similar to that found as a reaction to cremophor EL, the histamine releaser which especially affects the intestinal tract.[31] Furthermore, *de novo* formation of histamine must be discussed. This was indicated during shock by increased activity of histidine decarboxylase.[41] Schauer[42] has provided a morphological demonstration of new formation of histamine. He demonstrated in the rat mesentery, after a 20 min period of ischemia, the appearance of new mast cells which were full of histamine-containing granules.

B. Aminoguanidine

Aminoguanidine is a strong, specific inhibitor of mammalian diamine oxidase.[43] The

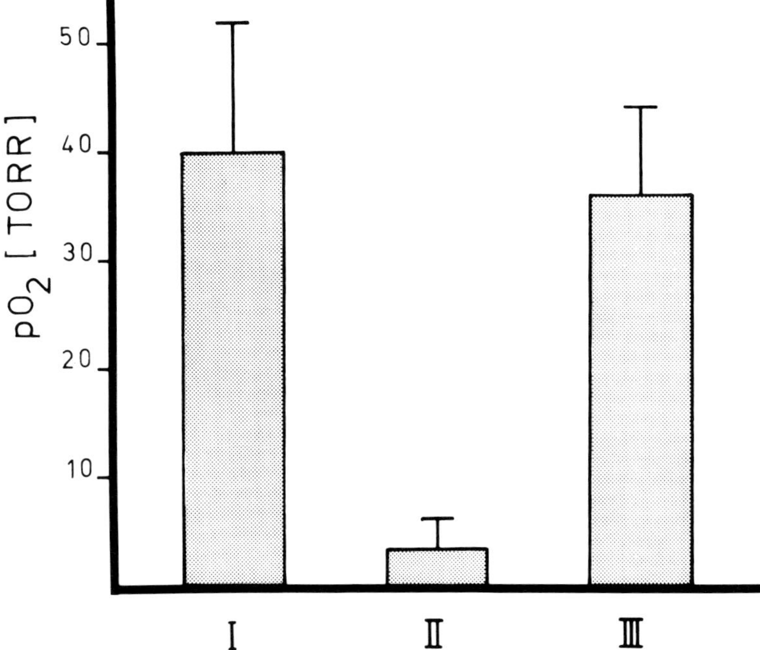

FIGURE 14.   Alterations of the oxygen tension at the serosal side of the jejunum by mesenteric artery occlusion and reperfusion in miniature pigs. I: Initial oxygen tension; II: oxygen tension 10 min after superior mesenteric artery occlusion; and III: oxygen tension 10 min after reperfusion of the mesenteric vessels.

specific and nonspecific effects of this compound, as far as they may influence the SMAO experiments, are compiled in Table 6. The nonspecific inhibition of histidine decarboxylase, if effective, would prolong the survival time as well as cause a transient increase in blood pressure. Aminoguanidine, however, reduced the survival time. It was very important that the DAO inhibitor did not release histamine and had no influence on histamine methyltransferase and monoamine oxidase activities.

The inhibition of diamine oxidase by aminoguanidine has been shown by measuring products of histamine catabolism in tissue and body fluids.[44-46] Aminoguanidine specifically potentiated pharmacological doses of histamine in animals and isolated organs.[47-52] In pathophysiologic situations associated with greatly elevated blood and plasma histamine levels (e.g., during histamine shock in guinea pigs), aminoguanidine considerably enhanced fatality.[53]

The presence of aminoguanidine in the gut was also shown in vivo in a pharmacokinetic study.[54] In our own experiments complete inhibition of diamine oxidase activity was found in tissue samples from rabbits treated with >10 mg aminoguanidine per kilogram. This finding indicated that aminoguanidine was actually present in the tissue where the enzyme was effective. These results, however, do contradict the dose-related reduction of the survival time in vivo over the range of 100 mg/kg. It is reasonable to suggest that, in vivo, not all of the aminoguanidine entered the cytoplasmatic compartment where diamine oxidase is localized.[55] However, these conditions were changed when the tissue samples were disrupted by homogenization and the enzymatic activity was measured in the supernatant.

C. Antihistaminics

Altura and Halevy[56] showed convincingly the H_1-receptor antagonists were benefi-

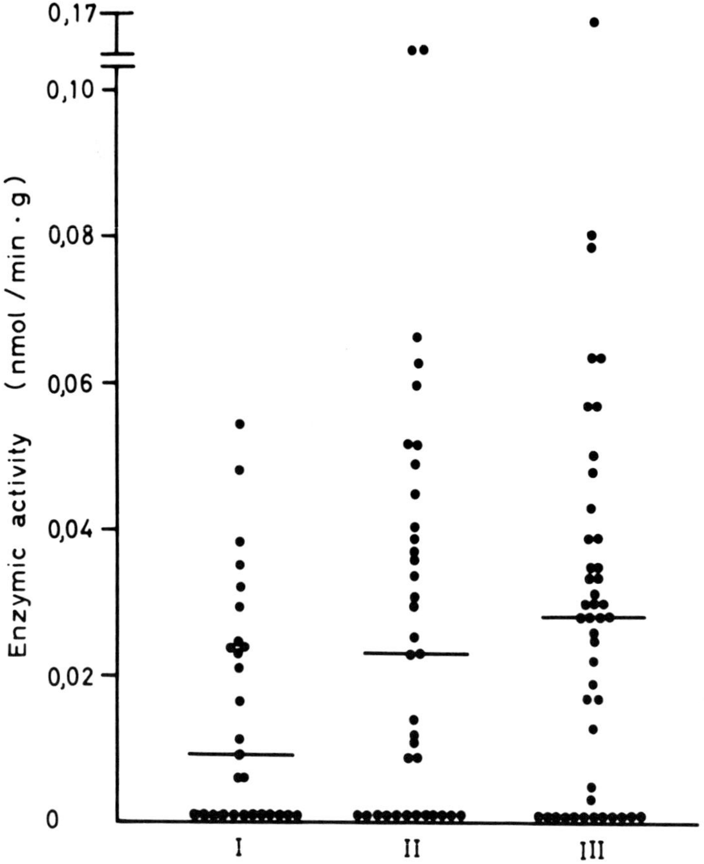

FIGURE 15.   Activity of diamine oxidase in the plasma of the portal vein of miniature pigs. Median and single values for nine animals without aminoguanidine treatment. Three blood samples per animal were taken before intestinal ischemia, four samples during intestinal ischemia, and five samples after reperfusion. Each value of the enzymic activity is shown in the figure. I: Initial values; II: values at the end of the period of mesenteric artery occlusion; and III: values at the end of survival time.

Table 6
EFFECTS OF AMINOGUANIDINE ON THE METABOLISM OF BIOGENIC AMINES

Specific effect:
    Inhibition of diamine oxidases
    $ID_{90} = 8 \times 10^{-6}\ M$ for the intestinal enzyme

Nonspecific effect:
    Inhibition of histidine decarboxylase ($ID_{90}\ 10^{-3}\ M$)

No effect on:
    Histamine liberation
    Histamine methyltransferase
    Monoamine oxidase

Aminoguanidine: $H_2N-C\overset{\displaystyle /\!\!/ NH}{\underset{\displaystyle \backslash NH_2}{}}$

cial in intestinal ischemia, whereas one of the H_2-receptor antagonists, burimamide, was detrimental.[56] However, burimamide is unique among the H_2-receptor antagonists in that it is a strong inhibitor of gastric histamine methyltransferase and intestinal diamine oxidase.[57,58] It seems possible that these effects, rather than H_2-blockade, were responsible for the detrimental effects of burimamide in intestinal ischemia.

D. Postulations

At the end of a series of experiments which can be used as a model to study the relevance of vasoactive substances, it becomes possible to answer the postulations outlined in Table 1.

Alterations in tissue histamine concentration and metabolism which were statistically significant were found in rabbits and in miniature pigs. The mode of histamine determination provided an identification of the amine (Point 1 of Table 1). These changes in tissue histamine concentration were influenced by experimental ischemia, and were related to changes in the plasma histamine concentration. Quantitatively, it could be demonstrated that the plasma histamine reached concentrations which were of clinical significance (Point 2). When the catabolism of histamine was inhibited by administration of the specific DAO inhibitor, aminoguanidine, shock development was aggravated, as shown by a reduction of the survival time. A reverse effect, i.e., prolongation of survival time or abolishment of the aminoguanidine effect, could be obtained by perfusion of the mesenteric vessels — which eliminated histamine from the circulation — or by an application of H_1 plus H_2 histamine receptor antagonists (Points 3 and 4). "Clinical" symptoms such as a decrease in blood pressure, hemoconcentration, and histological findings could be explained by the release of histamine (Point 5). All species which have been studied have reacted in exactly the same manner with our experimental model (Point 6).

Summarizing all results, the aggravation of shock by histamine release and the protective role of intestinal DAO must be regarded as a general pathobiochemical principle in intestinal ischemia. Based on the fact that in human subjects similar pathobiochemical preconditions exist concerning the DAO-histamine system, this principle is probably of clinical importance. Indeed, the administration of H_1- plus H_2-receptor antagonists before mesenteric reperfusion has been successfully applied with some patients in the surgical clinic at Marburg.[59]

The DAO-histamine hypothesis is fully compatible with another convincing hypothesis: the role of proteases during intestinal ischemia.[60] In this hypothesis, Bounous et al.[1,60] ascribes injury to the ischemic mucosa to the action of trypsin and chymotrypsin. Trypsin, however, is a powerful histamine liberator.[61,62] Probably the alteration of the DAO-histamine system and the action of proteases are two important factors of the shock phenomenon following superior mesenteric artery occlusion.

REFERENCES

1. Bounous, G., Acute necrosis of the intestinal mucosa, *Gastroenterology,* 82, 1457, 1982.
2. Wiklund, L., Grevsten, S., Nilsson, F., Norlén, B.-J., and Rimsten, Å., Non-occlusive enteric gangrene associated with severe upper gastrointestinal bleeding, *Acta Chir. Scand.,* 182, 593, 1976.
3. Marston, A., *Intestinal Ischaemia,* Edward Arnold, London, 1977.
4. Gruber, U. F., Intestinale Faktoren im Schock: Darmtoxine, *Langenbecks Arch. Klin. Chir.,* 319, 909, 1967.

5. Lefer, A. M., Blood borne humoral factors in the pathophysiology of circulatory shock, *Circ. Res.,* 32, 129, 1973.
6. Lefer, A. M., Cowgill, R., Marshall, F. E., Hall, L. M., and Brand, E. D., Characterization of a myocardial depressant factor present in hemorrhagic shock, *Am. J. Physiol.,* 213, 492, 1967.
7. Hesterberg, R., Lorenz, W., Sattler, J., Stahlknecht, C.-D., Crombach, M., and Weber, D., Histamine content, diamine oxidase and histamine methyltransferase activities in human tissues: fact or fiction? *Agents Actions,* 14, 325, 1984.
8. Romeis, B., *Mikroskopische Technik,* Oldenburg, Munchen, 1968.
9. Lorenz, W., Reimann, H.-J., Barth, H., Kusche, J., Meyer, R., Doenicke, A., and Hutzel, M., A sensitive and specific method for the determination of histamine in human whole blood and plasma, *Hoppe-Seyler's Z. Physiol. Chem.,* 353, 911, 1972.
10. Da Prada, M. and Pletscher, A., Isolated 5-hydroxytryptamine organelles of rabbit blood platelets: physiological properties and drug induced changes, *Br. J. Pharmacol.,* 34, 591, 1968.
11. Kusche, J., Richter, H., Hesterberg, R., Schmidt, J., and Lorenz, W., Comparison of the ^{14}C-putrescine assay with the NADH test for the determination of diamine oxidase: description of a standard procedure with a high precision and improved accuracy, *Agents Actions,* 3, 148, 1973.
12. Kusche, J. and Lorenz, W., Diamine oxidase, in *Methods of Enzymatic Analysis, Vol. 3,* Bergmeyer, H. U., Ed., Verlag Chemie, Weinheim, 1983, 237.
13. Lorenz, W., Barth, H., Thermann, M., Schmal, A., Dormann, P., and Niemeyer, I., Fluorometric histamine determination in canine plasma under normal conditions, following application of exogenous histamine and during histamine release by Haemaccel® , *Hoppe-Seyler's Z. Physiol. Chem.,* 355, 1097, 1974.
14. Lorenz, W., Barth, H., Karges, H. E., Schmal, A., Dormann, P., and Niemeyer, I., Problems in the assay of histamine release by gelatine: o-phthaldialdehyde-induced fluorescence, inhibition of histamine methyltransferase and H_1-receptor antagonism by Haemaccel® , *Agents Actions,* 4, 324, 1974.
15. Snedecor, G. W. and Cochran, W. G., *Statistical Methods,* 6th ed., Iowa State University Press, Ames, 1967.
16. Parsons, M. E. and Owen, D. A. A., Receptors involved in the cardiovascular responses to histamine, in *Int. Symp. Histamine H_2-Receptor Antagonists,* Wood, J. C. and Simkins, M. A., Eds., Smith Kline & French, Welwyn Garden City, England, 1973, 127.
17. Thermann, M., Lorenz, W., Schmal, A., Shingale, F., Dormann, P., and Hamelmann, H., Influence of H_1- and H_2-receptor antagonists on the circulatory system and on the endogenous plasma histamine concentrations in dogs, *Agents Actions,* 7, 97, 1977.
18. Lorenz, W. and Doenicke, A., Histamine release in clinical conditions, *Mount Sinai J. Med.,* 45, 357, 1978.
19. Okuyama, T. and Kobayashi, Y., Determination of diamine oxidase activity by liquid scintillation counting, *Arch. Biochem. Biophys.,* 95, 242, 1961.
20. Kusche, J., Richter, H., Schmidt, J., Hesterberg, R., Friedrich, A., and Lorenz, W., Diamine oxidase in rabbits small intestine: separation from a soluble monoamine oxidase, properties and pathophysiological significance in intestinal ischemia, *Agents Actions,* 5, 431, 1975.
21. Lorenz, W., Kusche, J., and Werle, E., Über eine neue Methode zur Bestimmung der Diaminoxydase-Aktivität, *Hoppe-Seyler's Z. Physiol. Chem.,* 348, 561, 1967.
22. Lorenz, W., Benesch, L., Barth, H., Matejka, E., Meyer, R., Kusche, J., Hutzel, M., and Werle, E., Fluorometric assay of histamine in tissue and body fluid: choice of the purification procedure and identification in the nanogram range, *Z. Anal. Chem.,* 252, 94, 1970.
23. Kessler, M., Normal and critical O_2 supply of the liver, in *Oxygen Transport in Blood and Tissue,* Lübbers, D. W. and Luft, Ü., Eds., Thieme, Stuttgart, 1967, 242.
24. Burton, A. C., *Physiologie und Biophysik des Kreislaufs,* Schattauer, New York, 1969.
25. Richterich, R., *Klinische Chemie,* 4th ed., S. Karger, Basel, 1978, 435.
26. Bergmeyer, H. U., *Methods of Enzymatic Analysis,* Vol. 1, 2nd ed., Verlag Chemie, Weinheim, 1974, 385.
27. Steel, R. G. D., A rank sum test for comparing all pairs of treatments, *Technometrics,* 2, 197, 1960.
28. Lienert, G. A., *Verteilungsfreie Methoden in der Biostatistik,* 2nd ed., Anton Hein, Meisenheim am Glan, 1973.
29. Lorenz, W., Doenicke, A., and Schöning, B., Anaphylactoid and allergoid reactions related to anesthesia, in *Complications of Anesthesia Operative Risk,* Conseiller, C., Cousin, M. T., Desmonts, J.-M., Duvaldestin, P., Glaser, P., Lienhart, A., Montagne, J., Salamagne, J.-C., Samii, K., Seebacher, J., Scherpereel, Ph., Viars, P., and Vourc'h, G., Eds., Excerpta Medica, Amsterdam, 1982, 173.
30. Köbler, H., Beeinflussung der Überlebenszeit durch regionale Perfusion im AMS Schock, *Bruns Beitr. Klin. Chir.,* 217, 82, 1969.

31. Lorenz, W., Doenicke, A., Dittmann, J., Haug, P., and Schwarz, B., Anaphylaktoide Reaktionen nach Applikation von Blutersatzmitteln beim Menschen: Verhinderung dieser Nebenwirkung von Haemaccel durch Prämedikation mit H_1- und H_2-Rezeptor Antagonisten, *Anaesthesist*, 26, 644, 1977.
32. Werle, E. and Lorenz, W., The antikinin action of some antihistaminic drugs on the isolated guinea-pig ileum, rat uterus and blood pressure of the anaesthetized dog, *Adv. Exp. Med. Biol.*, 8, 447, 1970.
33. Smith, A. N., Release of histamine by histamine liberator 48/80 in cats, *J. Physiol. (London)*, 121, 517, 1953.
34. Lorenz, W., Doenicke, A., Schöning, B., and Neugebauer, E., The role of histamine in adverse reactions to intravenous agents, in *Adverse Reactions of Anaesthetics Drugs*, Thornton, A., Ed., Elsevier-North Holland, Amsterdam, 1981, 169.
35. Goodman, L. S. and Gilman, A., *The Pharmacological Basis of Therapeutics*, 5th ed., Macmillan, New York, 1975.
36. Lorenz, W., Fischer, M., Rohde, H., Troidl, H., Reimann, H.-J., and Ohmann, Ch., Histamine and stress ulcer: new components in organizing a sequential trial on cimetidine prophylaxis in seriously ill patients and definition of a special group at risk, *Klin. Woschr.*, 58, 1, 1980.
37. Funovics, J., Kretschmer, G., Piza, F., Pregez, J., and Zekert, F., Experimentelle Untersuchungen über die pathophysiologischen Folgen der Mesenterialstenose auf den Magen, *Langenbecks Arch. Klin. Chir.*, 332, 92, 1973.
38. Boley, S. J., Cohen, M. J., Winslow, P. R., and Becker, N. H., Treiter, W., McNamara, H., Veith, F. J., and Gliedman, M. L., Mesenteric ischaemia: a cause of increased gastric blood flow, hyperacidity and acute gastric ulceration, *Surgery*, 68, 222, 1970.
39. Richter, H., Kusche, J., Schumann, K.-Th., Schmidt, J., and Lorenz, W., Diaminoxydase, Histamin und Histidin im Dünndarm nach experimenteller Ischämie, *Langenbecks Arch. Chir. Suppl. Chir. Forum*, 295, 1973.
40. Wollin, A., Navert, H., and Bounous, G., Effects of intestinal ischemia on diamine oxidase activity in rat intestinal tissue, *Gastroenterology*, 80, 349, 1981.
41. Schayer, R. W., Relationship of induced histidine decarboxylase activity and histamine synthesis to shock from stress and from endotoxin, *Am. J. Physiol.*, 198, 1187, 1960.
42. Schauer, A., *Die Mastzelle*, Fischer, Stuttgart, 1964.
43. Schuler, W., Zur Hemmung der Diaminoxydase (Histaminase), *Experientia*, 8, 230, 1952.
44. Schayer, R. W., Kennedy, J., and Smiley, R. L., Studies on histamine metabolizing enzymes in intact animals, *J. Biol. Chem.*, 205, 739, 1953.
45. Eliassen, K. A., Metabolism of ^{14}C-histamine in goats and pigs with aminoguanidine, *Acta Physiol. Scand.*, 88, 1, 1973.
46. Granerus, G., Wetterquist, H., and White, T., Histamine metabolism in healthy subjects before and during treatment with aminoguanidine, *Scand. J. Clin. Lab. Invest.*, 104(Suppl. 22), 39, 1968.
47. Westling, H., Potentiation of histamine effects by histaminase inhibitors in the anaesthetized guinea-pig, *Acta Physiol. Scand.*, 38, 91, 1956.
48. Lindell, S. E. and Westling, H., Potentiation by histaminase inhibition of the blood pressure response to histamine in cats, *Acta Physiol. Scand.*, 37, 307, 1956.
49. Amure, B. O. and Ginsburg, M., Inhibitors of histamine catabolism and action of gastrin in the rat, *Br. J. Pharmacol.*, 23, 476, 1964.
50. Hansson, R. and Sundström, G., Diamine oxidase (histaminase) and heparin inhibition of gastric secretion in man, *Scand. J. Clin. Lab. Invest.*, 26, 263, 1970.
51. Severs, W. B., Gordon, J. W., Beaven, M. A., and Jacobson, S., Some observations on aminoguanidine pharmacology, *Pharmacology*, 3, 201, 1970.
52. Arnuslakshana, O., Mongar, I. L., and Schild, H. O., Potentiation of pharmacological effects of histamine by histaminase inhibitors, *J. Physiol.*, 123, 32, 1954.
53. Giertz, H., Hahn, F., Seseke, G., and Schmutzler, W., Über die Wirkung von Heparin und Aminoguanidin auf den anaphylaktischen. Anaphylatoxin- und Histamin-Schock des Meerschweinchens, *Naunyn-Schmiedebergs Arch. Pharmacol.*, 256, 26, 1967.
54. Beaven, M. A., Gordon, J. W., Jacobson, S., and Severs, W. B., A specific and sensitive assay for aminoguanidine, its application to a study of the disposition of aminoguanidine in animal tissue, *J. Pharmacol. Exp. Ther.*, 165, 14, 1969.
55. Kusche, J., Lorenz, W., Stahlknecht, C.-D., Richter, H., Hesterberg, R., Schmal, A., Hinterlang, E., Weber, D., and Ohmann, Ch., Intestinal diamine oxidase and histamine release in rabbit mesenteric ischemia, *Gastroenterology*, 80, 980, 1981.
56. Altura, B. M. and Halevy, S., Beneficial and detrimental actions of histamine H_1- and H_2-receptor antagonists in circulatory shock, *Circ. Res.*, 32, 129, 1973.
57. Barth, H., Niemeyer, J., and Lorenz, W., Studies on the mode of action of histamine H_1- and H_2-receptor antagonists on gastric histamine methyltransferase, *Agents Actions*, 3, 138, 1973.

58. Bieganski, T., Kusche, J., Feussner, K.-D., Hesterberg, R., Richter, H., and Lorenz, W., Human intestinal diamine oxidase: substrate specificity and comparative inhibitor study, *Agents Actions,* 10, 108, 1980.
59. Kusche, J., Data presented at the symposium Histamine and Antihistamines in Anaesthesia and Surgery, Munich, June 3 to 5, 1981.
60. Bounous, G., Proulx, J., Konok, G., and Wollin, A., The role of bile and pancreatic proteases in the pathogenesis of ischemic enteropathy, *Int. J. Clin. Pharmacol. Biopharm.,* 17, 317, 1979.
61. Tauber, R., Maroske, D., Schult, H., Dormann, T., Schmal, A., Häfner, G., and Lorenz, W., Speicherung von Histamin im Blut nach Freisetzung aus Leber und Antrum durch Trypsin: Protektiver Mechanismus oder Faktor in der Genese des pankreogenen Schock? *Langenbecks Arch. Chir. Suppl. Chir. Forum,* 213, 1975.
62. Tauber, R., Lorenz, W., Schmal, A., Uhlig, R., and Maroske, D., Histamine Freisetzung beim Hund durch Trypsin und Kallikrein. Frage einer pathophysiologischen Bedeutung bei der aktiven Pankreatitis, *Langenbecks Arch. Chir. Suppl. Chir. Forum,* 135, 1974.
63. Kusche, J., Stahlknecht, C.-D., Lorenz, W., Reichert, G., and Richter, H., Diamine oxidase activity and histamine release in dogs following acute mesenteric artery occlusion, *Agents Actions,* 7, 81, 1977.
64. Burdette, W. J. and Gehan, E. A., *Planning and Analysis of Clinical Studies,* Charles C Thomas, Springfield, Ill., 1970, 73.
65. Kusche, J., Stahlknecht, C.-D., Lorenz, W., Reichert, G., and Dietz, W., Comparison of alterations in the histamine-diamine oxidase system during acute intestinal ischaemia in pigs, dogs and rabbits: evidence for a uniform pathophysiological mechanism? *Agents Actions,* 9, 49, 1979.

Index

INDEX

A

C

D

H

T